Arteriovenous Malformations of the Brain and Spinal Cord

Arteriovenous Malformations of the Brain and Spinal Cord

Deductive Embryology and Flow Dynamics

VIDYASAGAR CASIKAR

Co-Authors

G.S. RAMASWAMY
D.H. DESHPANDE
M. BHAGWAT

ISBN: 979-8-90094-003-8 (sc)
ISBN: 979-8-90094-004-5 (e)

EXPRESSO
Executive Center 777, Dunsmuir Street Vancouver, BC V71K4
1-888-721-0662 ext 101
info@expressopublishing.com

Arteriovenous Malformations of the Brain and Spinal Cord

This work is dedicated to the memory of my late chief,
Prof. B. H. Dawson, FRCS, who encouraged me into this project.
His analytical approach and the exacting standard he demanded
of me (often painful) have been greatly responsible for this effort.

Contents

Foreword

This is an outstanding and encyclopedic scholarly work that relates arteriovenous malformations of the brain and spinal cord to the vascular anatomy and physiology as well as the embryological development of this anatomy. This work provides an outstanding base for a deeper understanding of arteriovenous malformations for both those making decisions on the treatment of these lesions as well as those involved in their research.

In a world of scientific literature focusing on the comparisons between various treatments and the natural history of AVM, a world that focuses on trials, treatments and variables with statistical associations, the underlying fundamental anatomy and physiology seems to take a back seat. However, the academic approach of this treatise, exploring the basics of anatomy and physiology, is a keystone in making sense of arteriovenous malformations of the brain and spinal cord. Furthermore, keeping the underlying vascular embryology at the forefront of our mind in clinical practice may provide opportunities of enriching our understanding and creating new knowledge in the future.

The current view that arteriovenous malformations may develop following birth may prove not to be so. The arteriovenous shunts themselves may well predate birth but may not result in the physiological responses in the feeding artery and draining vein, upon which the imaging diagnosis depends. The cardiovascular system transforms from low resistance (prior to closure of the ductus arteriosus) to high resistance following birth. This will lead to a greater disparity in resistance between the fistula associated with the arteriovenous malformations and the normal circulation. This, in turn, may result in a post-natal development of the changes in feeding artery and draining vein in response to the low resistance arteriovenous malformations.

Therefore, the embryological understanding of vascular development cannot be ignored even for those cases that appear to develop after birth.

Dr Casikar has been a long-time student of the vascular embryology reporting upon persistent embryonic veins in association with arteriovenous malformations nearly 40 years ago. This book is a culmination of a long study and insightful understanding of one of the pillars of underpinning knowledge, vascular embryology, that we who research arteriovenous malformations, should read and embrace.

Professor Michael K Morgan AO
Professor of Cerebrovascular Neurosurgery

Macquarie University
Sydney
Australia

Preface

It is a common practice to describe the anatomy of the Arterio-venous malformations (AVM) with reference to adult anatomy. The arterial feeders and the venous sinuses into which the arterialised blood drains are easily identifiable. However the arterialised venous channels extending between the arteries and the dural sinuses are just described as “abnormal venous channels”. These AVMs occur due to developmental anomalies in the embryos. It is possible to identify these vessels. These structures normally disappear during the course of development, as they become atritic due to diversion of blood away from them. In the presence of an AVM, these vessels persist because of the abnormal flow created by the fistula. This publication demonstrates the method of identification of these segmental vessels. It is possible to deduct the anatomy if the formations of these malformations are followed through the various stages of the development of the embryo (Simmonds[304], Heine[120]).

Padget[233-235] proposed that accidental defects between the primitive embryonic segmental pial vessels produce these Arterio-venous fistulae. This concept is developed to logically deduce the anatomy. It is not possible to demonstrate all the possible variations. The reader is provided with the methodology that will lead to the identification of the anatomy (Richter[272], Ribbert[271], Roux[278]).

The flow pattern in an AVM is unique. Two fluid systems of different pressures and flow are interconnected. There are numerous reports on the flow characteristics of these malformations based on the assumption that the equations for a flow in a linear tube are applicable. We have demonstrated by experimental evidence and computational fluid dynamic studies that the flow is extremely complex (Steinhein[312], Sugar[317]).

Acknowledgements

I started this research work three years ago at the suggestion of Mr B. H. Dawson, consultant neurological surgeon at The Salford Royal Hospital. He guided the research with much enthusiasm to its conclusion, and I am grateful to him for his continued interest.

My thanks are also due to Mr R. A. C. Jones, consultant neurological surgeon at The Salford Royal Hospital, for permitting me to use his cases and giving me great encouragement at times when I needed it most.

I wish to thank Prof. W. E. Kershaw at the Department of Biology, University of Salford, for his kind permission to allow me to complete this research.

It would be impossible to thank sufficiently Mrs B. Higginson for her secretarial help and assistance. She had the great task of deciphering illegible medical jargon into Standard English.

The efforts and skill of Mr P. J. N. Kilshaw were widely used in producing the illustrations for this work, and I am greatly indebted to him for his cooperation.

I wish to extend my gratitude to The Salford Area Health Authority for permitting me to use the hospital facilities.

We wish to acknowledge the financial assistance granted by the Indian Council for Medical Research. We are grateful to the director of The National Institute Of Mental Health And Neurosciences, the vice chancellor of University of Agricultural Sciences and the Director of St John's Medical College for their support. Figures 5, 6, 7 and 8 were taken from N. C. Prattipati's thesis titled Study of Flow Characteristics of Blood in an Arterio-venous Malformation (University of Sydney).

My special thanks to Dr. Anil GOLKAR, OBE Consultant Neuroradiologist for lending images from his presonal collection.

I wish to thank Wordzworth Limited- for their efforts to convert a PhD thesis with many badly hand drawn diagrams into a book. Multiple rounds of revisions for every chapter, table, image, figure and legend were necessary. Their uncompromising commitment to accuracy and quality has produced this excellent product.

Introduction

An abnormal communication between arteries and veins, diverting the blood from the normally intervening capillary system, results in an arteriovenous fistula (AVF). Such a lesion may occur anywhere in the body. Trauma to the adjacent walls of the vessels is the most frequent aetiological factor in extracranial AVF. The primary objective of the treatment of the condition is to close the fistula and eliminate the short circuit between arteries and veins (Browne[32&33], Callander[36], Corliss[51], Doane[68], Dott[69], Gerbode[90], Gillingham[94], Gurdjian[105], Grinker[103], Jacas[141], Shi YQ[300]).

In contrast to the other regions of the body, most cerebral arteriovenous fistulae occur in intrauterine life. The exact pathogenesis is not known, but in some way, an abnormal communication occurs between the primitive arteries and primitive veins. The most widely accepted concept is that these lesions represent the normal embryonic arteriovenous communications that have failed to undergo the natural process of atresia. I will later contend that a rupture between the primitive artery and the primitive vein occurs and causes the arteriovenous fistula, just as in the cases of extracranial arteriovenous malformation.

Cerebral arteriovenous malformations, like those elsewhere, consist of the following:

1. The arterial feeder
2. The angioma (arterio-capillary tangle)
3. The venous channels draining the blood from the fistula to the dural venous sinuses

The arterial component and the dural venous sinuses are easily identifiable, as they conform to the adult anatomical description.

The venous channels extending from the fistula to the dural venous sinuses do not generally resemble known adult cerebral veins and are, therefore, classified as abnormal veins.

Great attention is usually given to the location and size of the angioma. These vascular tangles are thought to represent the foetal fistula dilated greatly to accommodate an abnormal shunting of the arterial blood into the venous channels. Various modes of treatment are used to eliminate these cerebrovascular tangles, and excision of the entire mass of vessels by surgery is undertaken wherever possible. Lesions not easily accessible to the above procedure are treated by deep X-ray (DXR), in an attempt to reduce the size of the lesion by a process of fibrosis. The risks of damage to the surrounding normal cerebral tissues often limit the scope of the above procedure (Tonnis[326], Boyd[28], Bosher[26], Martin[192], Masherpa[193]).

It will be contended that these angiomas in cerebral arteriovenous malformations are not in any special way different from those found elsewhere in the body. The numerous arteriovenous and capillary collaterals in the region of an arteriovenous fistula are just like those found in arteriovenous malformations in other parts of the body. Excision of these collateral vessels is not regarded as a logical surgical step in extracranial situations because it necessitates quite extensive damage to the surrounding tissues. So it is not more logical to excise such malformations in the nervous system (Mayer[196&197], Meleney[198], Olivercrona[229&230], Osherwitz[232], Perret[244&245], Raimondi[261], Raskin[263], Ray[265]).

An attempt has been made in the present work to determine the pathogenesis of the cerebral arteriovenous malformations by studying the radiological anatomy. Arteriovenous fistula in the brain will be looked upon as abnormal communications between definite embryonic arteries and veins. It is contended in this work that accidental rupture occurs between two definite embryonic segmental pial vessels due to defects in the walls. The pathology of the complex congenital abnormalities occurring in the uro-genital system, the alimentary system and the cardio-vascular system has already yielded to embryological interpretation. It is hoped, therefore, that the study of the congenital abnormalities of the blood vessels of the brain and spinal cord will be similarly beneficial.

The abnormal venous channels, it will be shown, represent the foetal cerebral veins, which, because of abnormal and continuing blood flow as a consequence of the fistula, have failed to undergo their normal process of atresia. These persistent foetal venous channels will be codified by me.

Organisation of the Book

It is suggested that this book could be read in many ways, depending on the needs of the reader.

Knowledge of embryology is not necessary to read this book.

Arteries are in red, adult veins in blue, and the embryonic veins are in green.

1. Identify the arterial feeder in the radiograph. Refer to the chart to locate the embryonic segment of origin. Go to the corresponding chapter. The schematic drawings will help to understand the anatomy of the persistent embryonic vein. The examples indicate the anatomy of these veins.
2. Study any embryonic segment. Each chapter is independent, and the format is the same.
3. Determine the location of the vascular malformation. Refer to the chart to identify the corresponding segment of the developing brain in the embryo. Go to the corresponding chapter to study the various possible varieties of persistent embryonic veins in the area of the brain.
4. You could, of course, start at the very beginning and read through.

1

Review of Classifications of Arteriovenous Malformations

A brief review of various classifications of arteriovenous malformations are made. The inadequacies of these methods of classifications are indicted.

The following classifications are taken from Noran (1945):[215]

Cushing and Bailey (1928)[57]

1. Vascular malformations
   a. Telangiectasis (a group of capillaries)
   b. Angioma venosum (lesions composed principally of veins)
   c. Angioma arteriale (lesions containing vessels resembling arteries as well as veins)
2. Haemangioblastoma (angioblastoma)
   a. Cystic type (associated with cyst formation)
   b. Solid type (not associated with cyst formation)

Each of these two types was again classified into capillary, cellular, and cavernous varieties, according to the microscopic features.

Turner and Kernohan (1941)[328]

1. Vascular malformations
   a. Telangiectasis
   b. Angioma or hamartoma
      i. Angioma venosum
      ii. Angioma arteriovenosum or angioma arteriale
2. Vascular neoplasms
   a. Capillary
      i. Capillary haemangioma
      ii. Haemangio-endothelioma
      iii. Capillary haemangioblastoma
   b. Cavernous
      i. Cavernous haemangioma
      ii. Cavernous haemangioblastoma
   c. Haemangiosarcoma

Rienhoff (1924)[273]

1. Arterial aneurysm (tumour consisting of arteries)
2. Venous aneurysm (tumour consisting of veins)
3. Arteriovenous aneurysm (tumour containing both arteries and veins)

Dandy (1928)[59]

1. Arteriovenous aneurysm
2. Venous abnormality
   a. Venous abnormality or venous anomaly in the brain
   b. Venous abnormality in the dura
   c. Angioma
      i. Cyst with angioma in the wall (actually angioblastoma)
      ii. Cavernous angioma
      iii. Plexiform angioma (venous angioma)

Bergstrand, Olivecrona, and Tonnis (1936)[20]

1. Angioma cavernosum
2. Angioma racemosum (a grapelike cluster of vessels)
   a. Telangiectasis
   b. Sturge–Weber syndrome (a condition consisting of an angioma of the surface of the brain with calcification of the underlying cortex and an ipsilateral facial nevus)
   c. Angioma racemosum arteriale (a grapelike cluster of vessels exclusively arterial)
   d. Angioma racemosum venosum (a congeries of vessels resembling veins)
   e. Arteriovenous aneurysm (a mass of inextricable vessels resembling arteries and veins)
3. Angiorecticuloma (angioblastoma)
4. Angioglioma (a combination of glial and vascular elements)

Russel. D. S[280-283]

1. Cirsoid aneurysm (lesions generally termed racemose angioma)
2. Capillary haemangioma (angioblastoma)
3. Capillary telangiectasis (telangiectasis)
4. Cavernous haemangioma

Virchow (1863)[343]

1. Cavernous angioma
2. Angioma simplex (telangiectasis)
3. Telangiectatic tumour formation (false angioma)
4. Angioma racemosum)

Bort (1920)[25]

1. Aneurysm (a simple aneurysm of an artery, not an angioma)
2. Serpentine aneurysm (angioma racemosum arteriale or an extensive simple aneurysm)
3. Serpentine angioma (venous or arteriovenous angioma)
4. Arterial racemose angioma (a congeries of arteries and probably veins)
5. Venous racemose angioma (a plexus of veins)
6. Racemose varix (probably similar to the type described below, being composed of a congeries of varices, but no doubt, also includes cavernoma)
7. Varix (a simple dilatation of a vein or a venous anomaly

Benda (1924)[19]

1. Phlebectasia (a diffuse widening of a vein)
2. Varicosity (a diffuse irregular dilatation with circumscribed ampullar or saclike formations)
3. Venous angioma (a circumscribed conglomeration of veins)

Cushing and Eisenhardt (Classification of Angioblastic Meningeal Tumours)[68]

These angioblastic meningeal tumours were put under the meningioma type IV, which was divided into three variants, as follows:

1. Incompletely differentiated, with mitoses (it is a cellular tumour showing histologic evidence of rapid growth)
2. Transitional between the meningothelial type and angioblastoma (it shows transitions toward the meningothelial meningioma)
3. Angioblastoma (capillary or cellular) (it has typical structure of angioblastoma)

Courville and Abbott (1940)[54]

1. Meningeal angioblastoma
2. Transitional angioblastoma
3. Angioblastic meningioma
4. Combined meningotheliomatous angioblastic meningioma

Globus (1937) (Classification of Vascular Meningeal Tumours with Meningioma)[96]

Meningioma piale (pial or vascular meningioma)

1. Haemangioendotheiomatous subtype (angioblastic meningioma also includes angioblastoma situated within the neural parenchyma)
2. Haemangiomatous subtype (angiomatous meningioma)

Noran (1945)[215]

1. Telangiectasis
    a. A collection of dilated capillaries.
    b. The capillaries are separated by normal brain tissue.

2. Rendu–Osler disease
    a. Multiple telangiectasis of the skin, the mucous membranes, and various internal organs.
    b. Only occasionally it involves the nervous system.
3. Varix or varicosity
    a. One or several relatively large dilated vessels of regular contour.
    b. The vessels contain thin walls comprising an endothelial lining and a layer of hyalinised connective tissue.
    c. Cerebral tissue separates the varicose vessels.
    d. The varix may be situated within the brain or the meninges.
    e. It may rupture to produce intracerebral haemorrhage.
4. Sinus pericranii
    a. A midline vascular tumour of the scalp or the forehead.
    b. It communicates with the superior sagittal sinus.
    c. Occasionally, there may be an associated intracranial angiomatous lesion.
5. Cavernous angioma or cavernoma
    a. Closely packed cavernous spaces, situated adjacent to one another without intervening neural tissue.
    b. The cavernous walls are thin, being composed of an endothelial lining and a layer of hyaline connective tissue.
6. Venous (racemose) angioma
    a. A congeries of entangled vessels often extending from the brain surface into the underlying parenchyma
    b. The mural structure of most of the vessels resembles that of veins.
    c. The vessels are separated by degenerated parenchyma.
7. Arteriovenous (racemose) angioma
    a. Similar to venous angioma except that vessels resembling arteries are prominent.
    b. The walls of the arterial vessels are composed of a fairly well-developed muscular media and an internal elastic membrane.
8. Angiomatous meningioma
    a. A plexus of enlarged vessels restricted principally to the leptomeninges.
    b. The vessels consist of arteries, veins, cavernous spaces, or capillaries.
9. Sturge–Weber disease
    a. Atrophy and calcification of the cortex of a part or all of one cerebral hemisphere.
    b. The involved cortex is often covered with an angiomatous meningioma.
    c. There may be a homolateral port-wine nevus of the face.
    d. The atrophic cortex shows parenchymal devastation, glial repair, and vascular calcification (no angioma).
10. Angioblastoma
    a. It occurs most commonly in the cerebellum.
    b. It is often cystic (a nodule in a cyst wall).
    c. Structurally, it consists of numerous capillaries separated by proliferating cells, producing embryonic vascular spaces.
    d. There is an interlacing network of reticulum throughout the tumour.
11. von Hippel–Lindau disease
    a. Angioblastoma of both the retina and the nervous system (essential lesions).
    b. There are often associated visceral lesions, such as cystic disease of the kidney, the pancreas, and the liver.
12. Angioblastic meningioma
    a. It grossly resembles the more common types of meningioma.

b. It is often invasive, manifesting rapid growth.
c. Morphologically, it is similar to other forms of angioblastoma.

13. Angioglioma
    a. A nodule in a cyst wall or a solid tumour.
    b. It contains visible calcium deposits.
    c. It is composed of glial and vascular elements.
    d. There are numerous thick-walled vessels, which are often calcified and are embedded in glial tissue (usually fibrous astrocytes).
14. Arterial (racemose) angioma
    a. A tangled collection of coiled vessels.
    b. All the vessels must display arterial structure.

The results of his study suggest that the following classification is more closely correlated with the types of vascular structure (gross and microscopic) than the other possible arrangements.

Pathological Classification of the Intracranial Vascular Tumours and Malformations

1. Angiomatous lesions (consisting of adult vascular elements)
    a. Parenchymal angioma
        i. Telangiectasis (capillary lesion), Rendu–Osler disease
        ii. Parenchymal varix or varicosity (single or multiple)
        iii. Cavernous angioma or cavernoma
        iv. Venous (racemose) angioma
        v. Arteriovenous (racemose) angioma
        vi. Arterial (racemose) angioma
    b. Meningeal angioma
        i. Angiomatous meningioma
        ii. Meningeal varix or varicosity: leptomeningeal varix, dural varix, sinus pericranii associated with intracranial angioma (?)
        iii. Sturge–Weber disease associated with angioma of the meninges
2. Angioblastic lesions (composed of embryonic vascular elements)
    a. Parenchymal angioblastoma
        i. Lindau's disease (von Hippel–Lindau disease)
3. Miscellaneous vascular lesions
    a. Sinus pericranii that is mainly extracranial
    b. Sturge–Weber disease without angiomatous lesions

Bergstrand19 cited in Olivecrona and Ladenheim (1957)[229]

'The arteriovenous aneurysm may be defined as an abnormal, direct communication between arterial and venous channels without the interposition of a capillary system. Among the many etiologic classifications suggested, a separation of this entity into congenital and acquired forms appears to best facilitate description (Classification).

Table 1.1 Classification

Aetiology	Pathology
1. Acquired	1. Cavernous
2. Congenital	Racemose
a. Anomalous arteriovenous	a. Telangiectasia
b. Angiomatous arteriovenous	b. Sturge–Weber
	c. Venous racemose
	d. Arterial racemose
	e. Angiomatous arteriovenous

Newton and Cronqvist (1969)[209]

Table 1.2 Intracranial arteriovenous malformations

	Supratentorial	Infratentorial
Pure dural	6	9
Mixed dural-pial (cerebral or cerebellar)	16	4
Pure pial (cerebral or cerebellar)	81	13
Total	103	26

Table 1.3 Extent of angiographic opacification of external carotid artery

Type of angiography performed	Location of arteriovenous malformations	
	Supratentorial	Infratentorial
Selective external carotid	34	10
Common carotid	42	5
Internal carotid (external carotid not opacified)	26	3
Vertebral (carotid not opacified)	1	8
Total	103	26

Table 1.4 Extent of meningeal arterial supply

		External carotid artery (middle meningeal)						Internal carotid artery (meningeal branch)		Vertebral artery (posterior meningeal branch)	
		Anterior branch		Posterior branch		Occipital					
		R	L	R	L	R	L	R	L	R	L
Pure dural	Supratentorial (6 cases)	1/3	3/5	1/3	2/5	0/3	1/5	2/4	2/6	0/0	0/2
	Infratentorial (9 cases)	1/7	0/7	5/7	4/7	4/7	4/7	5/7	2/7	1/3	2/3
Mixed pial-dural	Supratentorial (16 cases)	7/15	4/11	7/15	6/11	3/15	1/11	1/15	1/13	0/1	0/11
	Infratentorial (4 cases)	0/1	0/2	2/2	1/2	2/2	1/2	0/3	2/3	0/2	0/3.

Note: Numerator = patients with demonstrated meningeal contribution; denominator = patients in whom the vessel was opacified.

McCormick (1966)[180&181]

Vascular malformations (congenital malformations of intracranial blood vessels, excluding berry aneurysms) consist of the following:

1. Telangiectasias (including some cases of Sturge–Weber syndrome)
2. Varix (including some vein of Galen malformations)
3. Cavernous malformation ('angioma')
4. Arteriovenous malformation ('angioma')
5. Venous malformation ('angioma') (including some cases of Sturge–Weber syndrome)

2

Development of Cerebral Arteries and Veins

A brief description of the development of cerebral arteries and veins, based on the work of D. H. Padget, is given. This is intended as a quick reference to the reader who wishes to refresh his or her knowledge of the basic concepts of embryology.

Summary of the Development of the Normal Aterial System in the Brain

The primitive neural tube consists of a capillary plexus situated in the pial layer. This venous plexus drains into the superficially situated dural venous network by way of short dorsal venous channels. The adult cerebral venous system evolves from this basic pattern.

By 5-mm stage, the dural venous network is divisible into anterior, middle, and posterior dural plexuses, each of these drained by a single channel into the primary head vein. The latter is continued as the anterior cardinal vein.

By 14-mm stage, the segmental drainage of the neural tube is well established. Each of the spinal segments is drained by a pair of intersegmental veins. Similarly, the brain, which is now divisible into telencephalon, diencephalon, mesencephalon, metencephalon, and myelencephalon, has a pair of pia-arachnoidal veins in each region.

The anterior end of the primary head sinus surrounds the enlarging telencephalon by a dorsal and ventral channel, the precursors of the superior sagittal sinus and tentorial sinus, respectively.

Around the 18–20-mm stage, the otic capsule expands rapidly, stretching the segment of the head sinus between the middle and the posterior dural plexuses. As a substitute, a second channel is formed dorsal to the otic capsule, connecting the stems of the middle and posterior dural plexuses. Figure. 2.1 and 2.2 show the newly formed sigmoid sinus and the primitive transverse sinus.

The development of the choroid plexus at this stage (24 mm) influences the formation of the ventral diencephalic vein, which drains laterally and inferiorly into the tentorial sinus.

The stem of the middle dural plexus situated anteriorly to the otic capsule now becomes the pro-otic sinus and drains into the junction between the transverse and sigmoid sinuses. The supraorbital vein, which hitherto drained into the anterior dural plexus, is now connected to the pro-otic sinus.

The further proliferation of the choroid plexus increases the venous output. The formation of the superior choroidal vein draining into the internal cerebral vein meets this demand (40 mm). The internal cerebral vein at this stage is mainly extracerebral and plays a minor role in the cerebral venous drainage.

The spinal intersegmental veins are connected by the development of a longitudinal anastomotic channel, and this persists in the adult as the vertebral vein. Similar anastomosis occurs between the segmental veins of the brain also. The expansion of the temporal lobe and the backward swing of the torcula stretches the tentorial sinus. This is compensated by a longitudinal channel connecting the pia-arachnoidal veins in the telencephalon, diencephalon, mesencephalon, metencephalon, and myelencephalon. The segment of the channel extending between the diencephalon and mesencephalon drains medially into the internal cerebral vein. This represents the adult basal vein. Frequently, it drains laterally into the transverse sinus. Such a lateral drainage into the transverse sinus is the most commonly seen pattern in both the metencephalon and myelencephalon.

The pro-otic sinus receives two tributaries – the middle meningeal vein laterally and the diencephalic vein medially. The expansion of the otic capsule anteriorly separates the pro-otic sinus from the ventral metencephalic vein (see Figure. 2.1 and 2.2).

The formation of petro-squamosal sinus diverts the pro-otic and middle meningeal drainage into the sigmoid sinus. The ventral metencephalic vein is now represented as the superior petrosal sinus and reaches the junction between the transverse and sigmoid sinuses. Formation of inferior petrosal sinus and cavernous sinus renders the pro-otic sinus atritic.

Between the third month (at 80 mm) and term, the rapid cerebral expansion demands more venous outlets. The internal cerebral vein supplements the function of the basal vein.

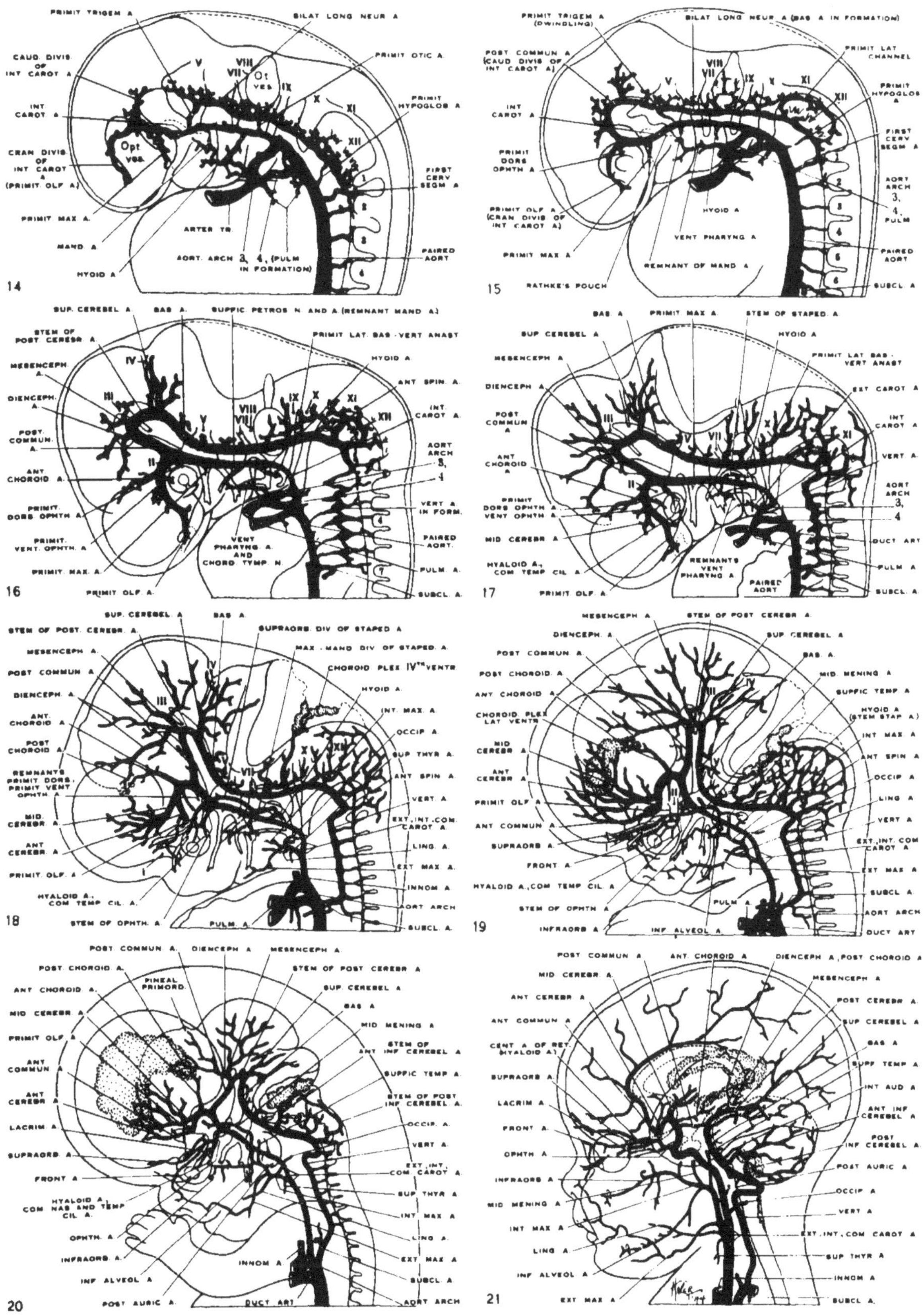

Figure 2.1 Normal development of the arterial system in man (lateral) (Padget).[233-235]

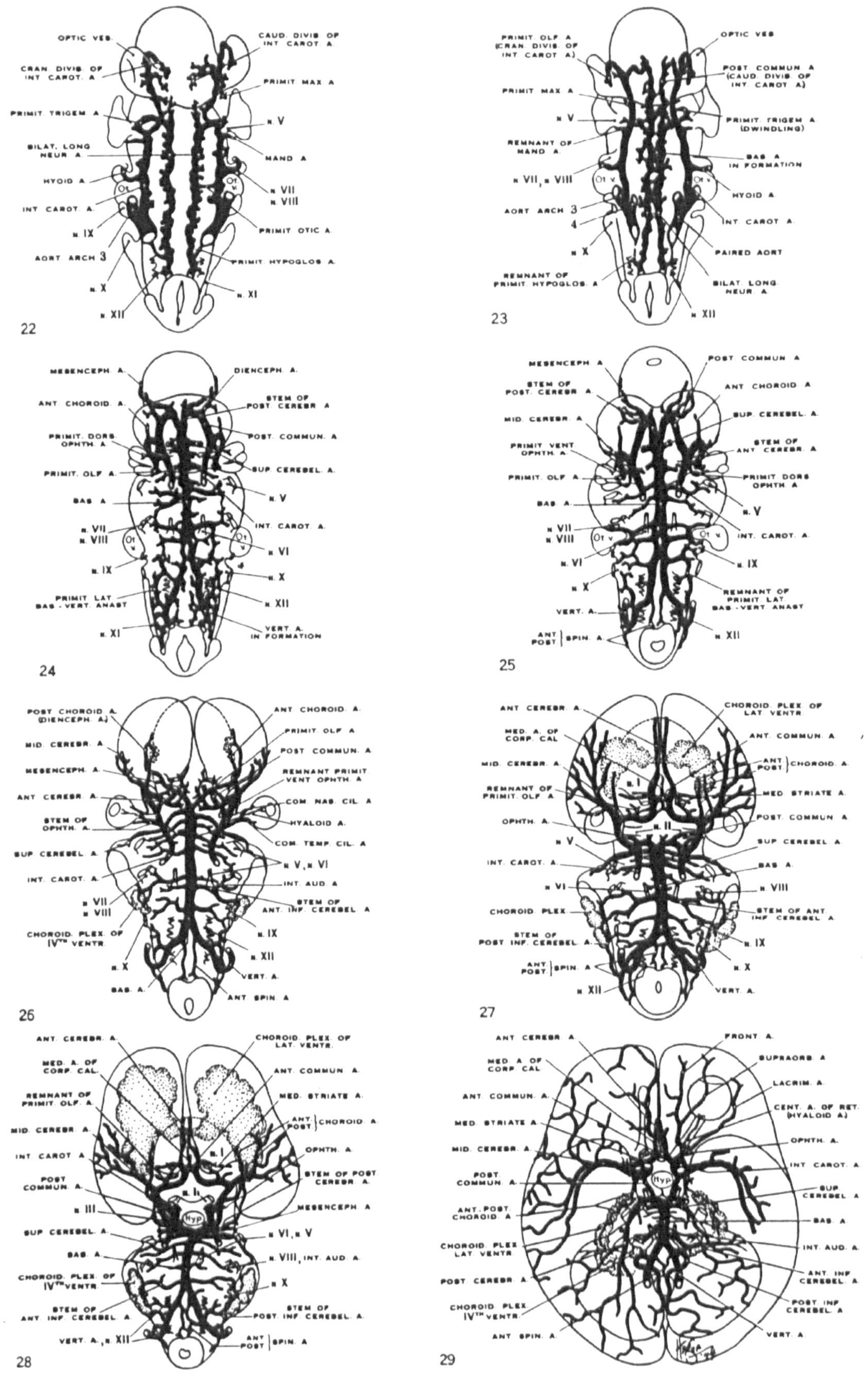

Figure 2.2 Normal development of the arterial system in man (basal) (Padget).[233-235]

The venous drainage of the convexity and the cerebral hemisphere is undertaken by the superior sagittal sinus, formed by the approximation of the marginal veins of each side.

The anterior and middle dural plexuses combine and are retained in the formation of the torcula. The tentorial sinus may occasionally persist and connect the cavernous sinus and the middle cerebral veins. The middle meningeal vein establishes secondary connections with the superior sagittal sinus.

The above description of the development is only a very brief summary. The reader is referred to the original work of Padget for a more detailed exposition.

Development of the Cranial Veins in Man

From the first vascular endothelium, two principal cranial vessels appear around 4 mm – the internal carotid artery and the neural artery.

The internal carotid and neural arteries are connected by four vessels, of which the most cranial channel – the caudal division of the internal carotid artery – persists in the adult as the posterior communicating artery. The trigeminal, stapedial, and hyloglossal disappear soon.

To each of the principal regions of the brain – the telencephalon, diencephalon, mesencephalon, metencephalon, and myelencephalon – vessels arise from this arterial loop.

From the cranial division of the internal carotid artery (the primitive olfactory artery) arise the anterior cerebral and middle cerebral and right choroidal arteries. The olfactory artery is soon rendered inconspicuous and is sometimes retained as a lateral striate branch.

The anterior cerebral and middle cerebral arteries supply the telencephalon. The medial striate artery arises from the anterior cerebral artery.

The anterior choroidal artery, with the posterior choroidal and posterior cerebral arteries, supply the diencephalon, including the choroid plexus.

The mesencephalon is supplied by the mesencephalic artery arising from the caudal division of the internal carotid artery (20 mm). During the further development of the brain, this segment becomes relatively inconspicuous, and the mesencephalic artery is incorporated in the posterior cerebral arterial stem.

The metencephalon is primarily supplied by the superior cerebellar artery at this stage, arising from the basilar artery formed by the fusion of the neural arteries cranially.

The myelencephalon is supplied by the anterior and posterior inferior cerebellar arteries arising from the basilar artery. These represent the persistent transverse segmental branches related to the lower cranial nerves. These branches are often interconnected by long channels, and persistence of these results in variation in the origin of these myelencephalic vessels.

By 40-mm stage, all these vessels can be identified (compare the venous system at this stage) and resemble the adult layout in broad terms.

Few major alterations occur beyond this stage.

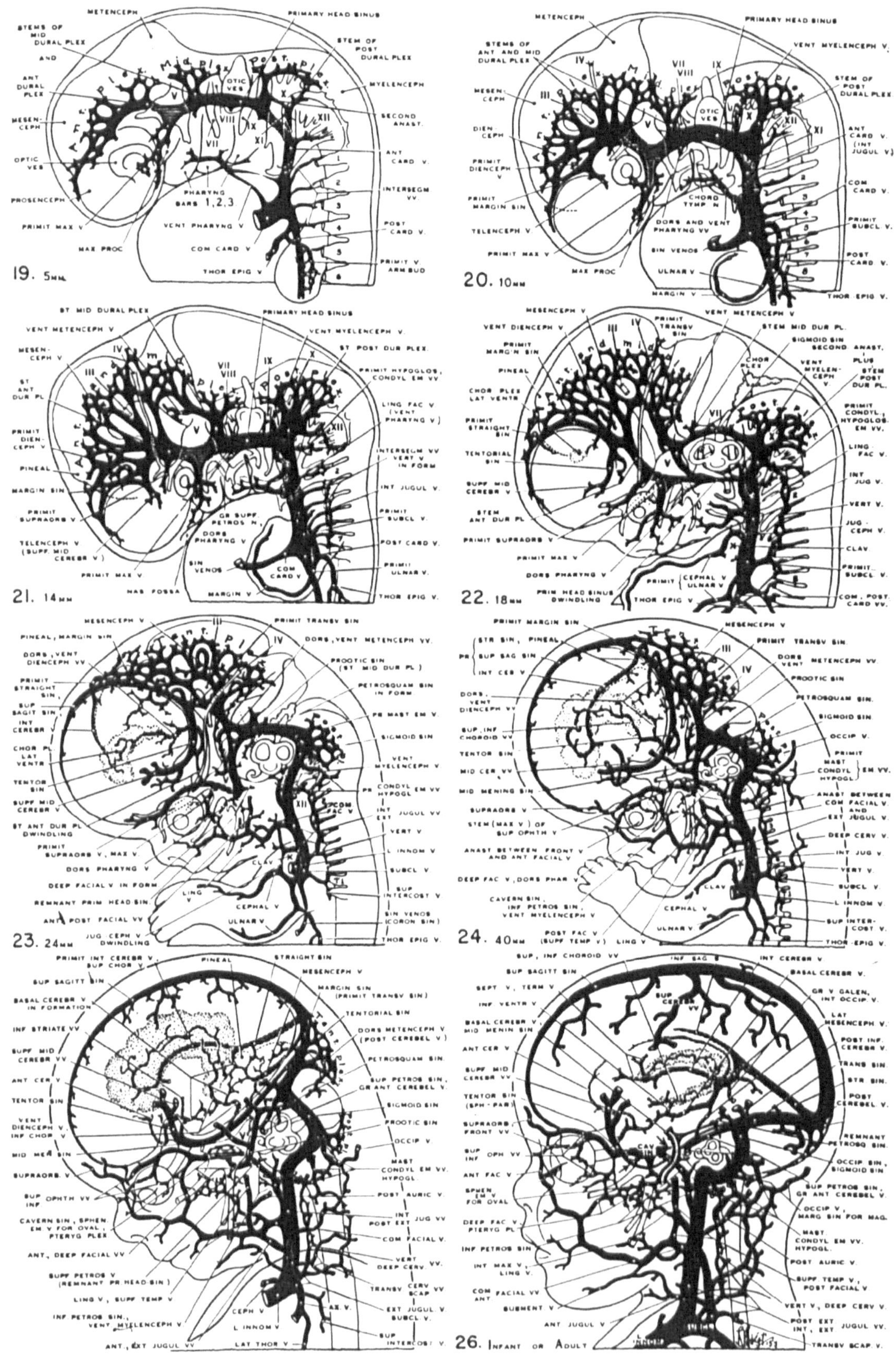

Figure 2.3 Normal development of the venous system in man (lateral) (Padget).[233&235]

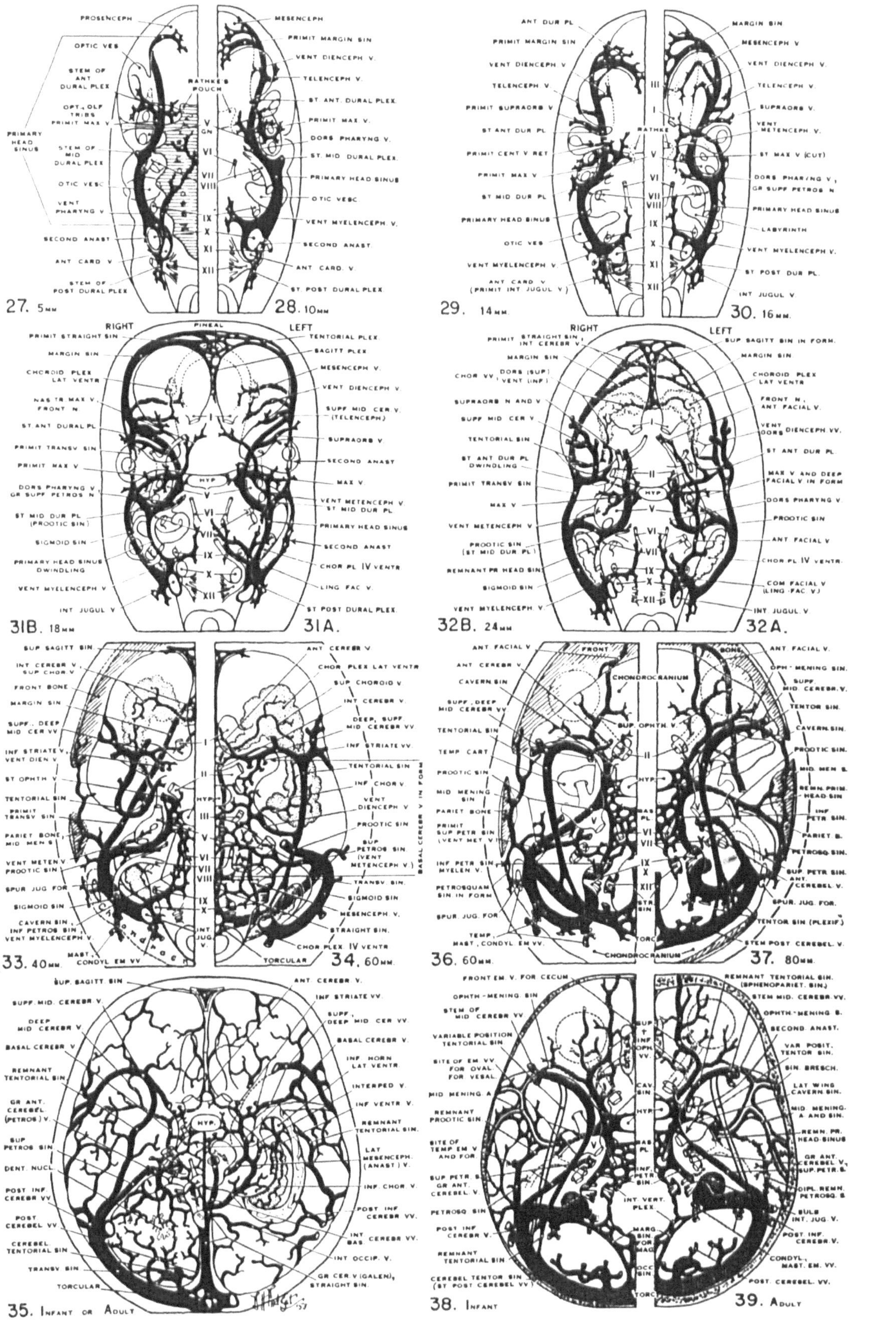

Figure 2.4 Normal development of the venous system in man (basal) (Padget).[233&235]

3

The Strategy

The methodology used during the study is described. The sequence of thoughts that led to the hypothesis that the 'embryonic veins, which normally become atritic and disappear, persist when an arteriovenous fistula occurs' is outlined.

Methodology

The Process of Identification of the Main Arterial Component of the Malformation

A preliminary review of all the angiograms of the patients who were found to have arteriovenous malformation was made. Of the fifty-four cases studied, forty-four cases were selected for a more detailed review. The rest were excluded as the clarity of the radiographs was unsatisfactory for detailed examination. Each of the cases studied contained approximately twenty films.

To begin with, a series of tracings of all the films were made to define the source of the main arterial component feeding the malformation and the course the feeder had taken to reach the site of the lesion. These cases were then grouped according to the main arterial feeder (see Table 3.1).

Identification of the Angiomatous Elements of the Malformation

Each of the radiographs was traced to determine the size and the extent of the arterio-capillary tangle intervening between the feeding artery and the draining vein. The variation in the appearance and site of these angiomatous elements is summarised in Table 3.2.

The Identification of the Venous Elements of the Malformation

Attention was directed to the venous channels leaving the site of the malformation. Tracings of the X-rays were made to define the course taken by these vessels through the brain to reach the dural venous sinuses. The particular dural sinus into which each of these vessels drained was also recorded (see Table 3.3).

At this stage, it became apparent that many of these vessels could not be labelled in normal adult anatomical terms, although there seemed to be a repetitive pattern in many of them.

Regrouping of Cases According to the Similarity of Venous Pattern

Cases found to have similar venous patterns were grouped together. Most of the cases could be put into one of four groups, but about eight cases defied this categorisation so they were set aside. The main arterial feeders of the malformation in each of these venous groupings were defined, and so three forms of categorisation were therefore made possible.

Identification and Matching of the Abnormal Vascular Channels with the Normal Embryonic Vascular Channels

The classical works on the development of the blood vessels of the embryo by Streeter and Padget were studied. During this study, it appeared that many of the early embryonic channels, which normally disappear in the process of development, resembled some of the abnormal vascular channels seen in the tracings of the radiographs. It was possible to match these atritic embryonic channels with the abnormal vessels in a considerable proportion of cases (see Table 3.1).

Regrouping of Cases of Arteriovenous Malformation According to the Arterial Feeder but with Reference to the Sources of These Arteries During Embryonic Development

The developmental process of the arterial system was again studied with reference to the embryonic division of the developing brain. The embryonic sources and segments of the adult cerebral arteries were categorised as follows:

1. Telencephalon
2. Diencephalon
3. Mesencephalon
4. Metencephalon
5. Myelencephalon

Table 3.2 shows that grouping of the cases according to the arteries in each of the embryonic regions corresponded to the grouping of the embryonic venous channels. Compare Table 3.2 and Table 3.2.

Preparation of the New Classification of the Arteriovenous Malformation Based on the Embryological Site of Their Formation

The classical embryological studies were reviewed and interpreted with the aid of some new diagrams. A series of carefully selected tracings of the radiographs were prepared, and a colour code was used to mark out the vessels.

Artery	Red
Adult vein	Blue
Embryonic vein	Green
Arteriocapillary tangle	Yellow

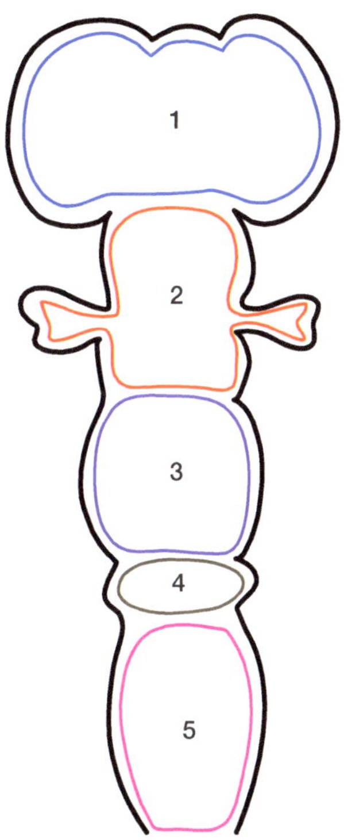

1 Telencephalon **2** Diencephalon **3** Mesencephalon **4** Metencephalon **5** Mylencephalon

Figure 3.1 Colour code to the segments of the brain.

Based on the above findings, a hypothesis that these abnormal vessels seen in arteriovenous malformations represent normal embryonic channels that have failed to regress was suggested.

To establish this concept, a careful study and tracings of the plates of Padget were made. Special attention was given to the course and relationship of the embryonic arteries and veins at 20-, 40-, 80-mm, and term stages of the development.

The actual tracings of the anatomy (in this series) already made from the radiographs were matched up to the hypothetical lesion drawn from the information derived from the interpretation of the embryological study by Padget [190-194]. Many matching examples were found in the series. A search for the previously published radiographs was made to collect examples to complete the validation of the hypothesis.

The grouping of the illustrations was according to the embryonic segment in which it was contended that the malformation started. The more simple patterns in the caudal segment were dealt with first before proceeding to the more intricate cranial patterns.

The hypothetical points at which the embryonic (cerebral) arteries could rupture into the contiguous veins, producing arteriovenous communications, were established. The possible ways in which such embryonic vascular ruptures could prevent the normal process of atresia by continuous distension of the primitive veins were depicted in a series of hypothetical diagrams. The effects of continuing growth and unfolding of the developing brain upon the ultimate anatomy of the cerebral arteriovenous malformation were also included in these diagrams.

Table 3.1 Classification of the Arterio-Venous Malformations based on the pattern of the Venous drainage [C4]

Arterial Feeder	Course and Mode of Termination of the Abnormal Veins		Case Reference
	Backwards and Medially	Int. Cr. V.	
	Upwards, Medially and Backwards	S.S.S.	
	Upwards, Medially and Backwards	Gr. C. V.	
	Downward, Medially and Backwards	Trans. S.	
	Medially and Downwards	Gr. C. V.	
	Laterally and Downwards	Trans. S.	
	Medially and Upwards	Gr. C. V.	
	Laterally and Backwards	Trans. S.	
	Medially and Backwards	Trans. S.	
	Not Known		

Table 3.2 Grouping the Cerebral Arteries according to their situation in the embryo [C5]

The Artery	Embryonic Segment
Anterior Cerebral Artery Middle Cerebral Artery	Telencephalon
Anterior Choroidal Artery Posterior Choroidal Artery Posterior Cerebral Artery	Diencephalon
Mesencephalic Artery	Mesencephalon
Superior Cerebellar Artery	Metencephalon
Anterior Inferior Cerebellar Artery Posterior Inferior Cerebellar Artery	Myelencephalon

Findings

The Arterial Component of the Malformations

In all the cases studied, the main arterial component of the malformation was easily identifiable. The calibre and the tortuosity of these feeding vessels varied considerably. In some cases, the main arterial trunk itself was the feeder. The development of the arterial tree was essentially normal in each case. The formation of the rest of the arterial system was entirely normal in every case.

The Angiomatous Elements of the Malformations

There were considerable variations in the size and situation of these arterio-capillary tangles.

1. Anterior Cerebral Artery Malformations
   In the twelve cases studied, an angioma was present in seven and was absent in the remaining five cases. The location of the angioma varied considerably. The usual sites were subfrontal, frontal, temporal, parietal, and occipital. In some, the angioma was large and in some very small.

2. Anterior Choroidal Artery
   There were three cases in this category, and an angioma was present in each of these. It was situated in the temporal area in all of these. The size of the angioma again varied considerably. Although this arterio-capillary tangle was situated close to the choroid plexus, there was no evidence of the involvement of the latter in any of these.

3. Middle Cerebral Artery Lesions (7 cases)
   In all the cases studied in this group, the arterio-capillary tangle was situated either in the sylvian territory or over the convexity of the cerebral hemisphere. In the sylvian territory it was deeply situated, sometimes extending to the surface. The angioma situated on the cerebral convexity again varied in its location and was generally distributed between the parietal and occipital lobes.

4. Posterior Cerebral Artery (8 cases)
   The angioma was absent in only one case. Of the remaining seven, the angioma was infratentorial in four and supratentorial in three cases. In spite of these variations in the location of the angioma, the other features of the malformation were identical in all these cases.

5. Superior Cerebellar Artery (3 cases)
   The angioma was supratentorial in two of the cases and was infratentorial in one case. The infratentorial angioma had a supratentorial extension also.

   There were no examples of posterior choroidal, anterior inferior or posterior inferior cerebellar artery malformations in the series of cases studied.

The Venous Elements of the Malformations

The venous elements could be divided into two types:

1. The dural venous sinuses
   The ultimate venous drainage in all the cases studied was into one of the three major venous sinuses of the brain, namely, the superior sagittal, transverse, and the internal cerebral vein. The location and the development of these dural sinuses were normal in all. In some cases more than one sinus was involved.

2. The abnormal venous channels
   The course and direction of the venous channels draining from the angioma to the dural sinuses varied to a large extent. In most cases they could not be identified in terms of normal adult anatomy. On closer examination, in many instances these abnormal channels were repeated. Their course and direction resembled certain embryonic channels (the venous channels which normally undergo atresia in the process of development).

   a. Anterior Cerebral Artery
      The venous channels were of two types:
      i. A superficial group. These channels were situated close to the medial surface of the cerebral hemisphere, and their direction was always backwards and superiorly into the superior sagittal sinus.
      ii. There was another set of venous channels situated deep in the substance of the hemisphere. These channels were directed backwards and medially, and they drained into either the great cerebral vein or the internal cerebral vein. In many of the cases the dilatation of the internal cerebral vein was enormous and could be interpreted as dilatations of the vein of Galen.

   b. Anterior Choroidal Artery
      The venous channels in this group either drained medially into the internal cerebral vein or laterally into the transverse sinus. Their course and direction were, therefore, either backwards, upwards, and medially, or backwards, upwards, and laterally.

c. The Middle Cerebral Artery
The pattern of the venous drainage for the middle cerebral artery lesions was more difficult to define. In some, it coursed downwards and laterally into the transverse sinus, and in others, medially into the great cerebral vein or superficially into the superior sagittal sinus. Various combinations of the above types were also seen. In one case, the drainage occurred by independent channels into each of the three sinuses.

d. Posterior Cerebral Artery Lesions
The venous drainage in this group was always medially, upwards, and backwards into the great cerebral vein.

e. Superior Cerebellar Artery Lesions
The venous channels drained into the transverse sinus in all the cases. The point of drainage into the transverse sinus varied. In one case it was near the torcula, and in the others near the sigmoid end.

It thus became clear at this point that the development of the arterial feeders and the dural venous sinuses were normal in every case. The variations seem to arise mainly with regard to the site of the angioma and the course and direction of the abnormal venous channels extending between the angioma and the dural venous sinuses.

Regrouping of Cases According to the Similarity of Venous Pattern

When an attempt was made to regroup the lesions of similar-looking venous channels together, the following classification emerged:

1. The anterior cerebral artery and middle cerebral artery lesions had comparable abnormal venous channels.
2. Similarly, anterior choroidal artery and posterior cerebral artery lesions had similar-looking venous channels.
3. The venous drainage of the superior cerebellar artery had a pattern of its own.

Identification and Matching of the Abnormal Venous Channels with the Normal Embryonic Venous Channels

Some of the venous channels in the above groups were found to resemble the embryonic venous channels, as described by Padget [192&194].

1. Anterior Cerebral and Middle Cerebral Arteries
   a. The superficial venous channels of both anterior cerebral and middle cerebral artery lesions could be compared with the venous tributaries of the marginal sinus (primitive superior sagittal sinus). Some of its tributaries, which were situated in the frontal regions of the embryo, around the 20-mm stage, were found to be shifted into the parietal and occipital areas at 80 mm, following the backward swing of the superior sagittal sinus. It seemed that a similar process could account for the variations seen in this group.
   b. The venous channels arising from the malformations situated deep in the cerebral hemisphere and draining medially had features comparable to that of the basal veins and anterior terminal vein in the embryo. The venous channels draining laterally could be compared with the primitive tentorial sinus.
2. Posterior Cerebral Artery
The resemblance between the embryonic venous channels was more easily seen in this group. The venous channels related to the posterior cerebral artery resembled the configuration of the dorsal diencephalic vein between 20- and 60-mm stage. Similarly, the ventral diencephalic vein and the vascular channels in relation to the anterior choroidal artery lesions were comparable.

Classification of the Cases When Arterial Feeders Are Grouped with Relation to Their Situation in the Embryonic Segment

The principal cerebral arteries were grouped in relation to the segment of the developing brain. It was then possible to place them in five categories:

1. Telencephalic vessels Anterior cerebral, middle cerebral
2. Diencephalic
3. Mesencephalic artery A branch of the posterior cerebral
4. Metencephalic artery Superior cerebellar arteries
5. Myelencephalon Inferior cerebellar arteries

By comparing Charts 4 and 5, it will be noted that malformations whose arterial feeders are from the same segment of the primitive brain have similar abnormal venous channels.

Hypothesis

1. The state of development of the arterial system is quite advanced by the time an arteriovenous fistula occurs. Therefore, the arterial component of an arteriovenous fistula is not greatly affected.
2. Arteriovenous shunts do not occur normally in the human brain, and therefore, arteriovenous malformations found in adults must be the result of pathological rupture between embryonic arteries and veins.
3. In the embryo, the development of the cerebral venous system follows after that of the arterial system. The anatomical abnormalities are more severe in the venous channels because they have not developed fully at the time the arterial system breaks into the venous system and the fistula is formed.
4. Each embryonic segment has its own particular pattern of veins, and the patterns are specific for each of the segments.
5. The occurrence of a fistula in an embryonic segment will prevent the normal process of atresia in the venous channels of that segment. The persistence of these normally atritic vessels in the extrauterine period is responsible for the complex anatomical configuration of arteriovenous malformations.
6. When an arteriovenous rupture occurs in an area of the brain that itself undergoes a very complicated developmental process, the anatomy of the arteriovenous anomaly will be correspondingly complex. The site and size of the arteriovenous rupture and the period of embryonic life at which it occurs will condition the final anatomical picture of the lesion in adult life.
7. All the arteriovenous fistulae can be grouped in terms of the embryological site of formation.
8. The basic anatomical features of the malformation are specific to each segment. The pattern is easily conceived in the spinal cord. This is attributable to the simplicity of structure. The complex mode of development of the brain obscures the fundamental layout.
9. The anatomical and radiological aspects of the malformation in each segment can be predicted.

Pathogenesis

The Angioma

The vascular system arises from the primitive mesenchyme. Some parts of the system differentiate from the endothelium directly, whilst the remaining re-form as extensions of these primary vessels.

Sabin[284] reported on the sequence of development of the vascular system, on the basis of the studies of the living chick blastoderm by injecting dyes into the vascular tree. The earliest injection was possible at the ninth somite stage by puncturing the aorta directly, but when the vitelline vein was used, there was no dye seen in the aorta. The vessels of the neural tube, though connected with the aorta, could only be injected partially even when the direct aortic injections were made. The failure to demonstrate the neural vessels was due to two factors – first, since the lumen was filled with fluid which was not circulating and the vessels had blind terminations, the dye injected into the aorta could not permeate into the channels. Second, the circulation had not yet started to facilitate the flow of the contents in the vessel.

Sabin's experiments also showed that although a heartbeat occurred around the tenth somite stage, a definite evidence of circulation was seen only at the sixteenth somite stage. It appeared, therefore, that the development of the arteries preceded that of the veins. The appearances of the latter were closely followed by that of the circulation (see Figure 3.2.)

It will be noted that the arteries in the reconstruction of this chick embryo are very advanced, compared with the veins.

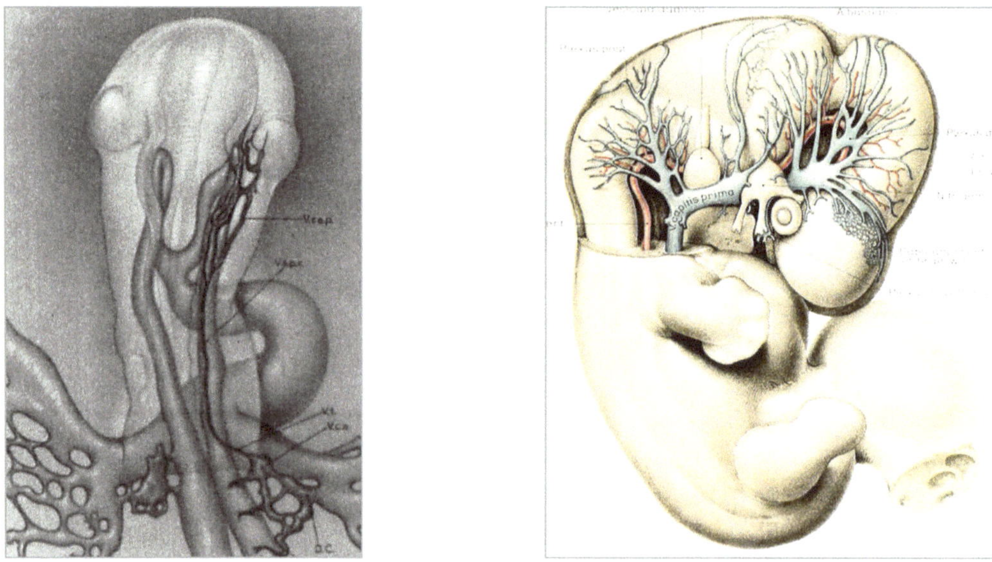

Figure 3.2 The vascular system in the chick (Sabin)[284] (AP).

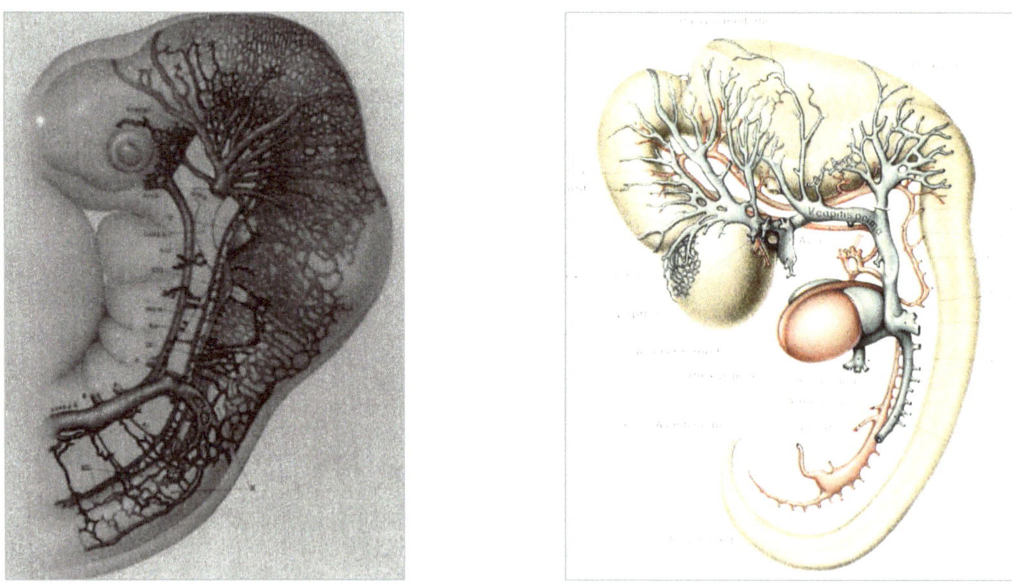

Figure 3.3 The vascular system in the chick (Sabin)[284] (lateral).

Although it is difficult to repeat the injection techniques in the human foetus, similar inferences could be drawn from the work of Padget[233-235]. Compare Figure 3.4a and b.

The cranial arterial system at 5-mm stage consists of the primitive internal carotid artery, which supplies the forebrain by its cranial and caudal divisions. By 40-mm stage (Fig 3.4)[236], the arterial pattern resembles that of the adult closely, except for the preponderance of the cerebellar hemisphere. Further changes in the development are related to the more rapid growth of the forebrain. There are no gross structural changes seen after this stage.

Arterio-Capillary Tangle or Angioma

Pfeifer[246] described the fundamental morphological characters of the mammalian brain and claimed that it was possible to distinguish between arteries and veins. But Campbell[37] pointed out that Pfeifer, in fact, had mistaken arteries for veins and vice versa. Therefore, this concept that there are normally numerous arteriovenous anastomoses of the brain appears inconsistent.

Scharrer[286] again produced further experimental evidence to support Campbell's views. She injected the vessels with starch solution, whose particles were small enough to pass through the arteries and veins but were too large to enter the capillary system. She demonstrated by this injection experiment that there were no normal existing fistulae between the arteries and the veins.

However, the concept that there exist normally arteriovenous fistulae in the early stages of the human brain was used to explain the presence of these angiomatous lesions in the brain by Kaplan[147]. He contended that these shunts would normally be replaced by an intervening capillary network. In the absence of this interposition of the capillary system, the arteries open

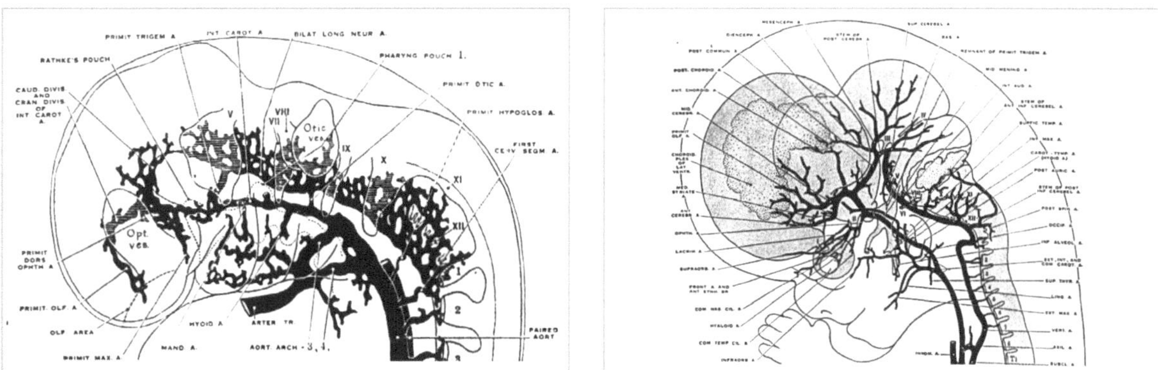

Figure 3.4 The arterial system in the human brain. Top picture at 4mm, bottom at 40mm (Padget).[234]

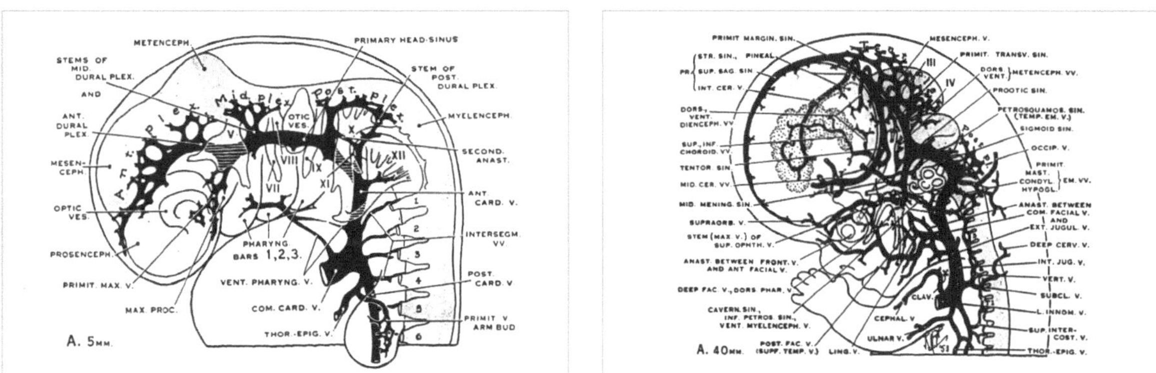

Figure 3.5 Venous system of the Brain. Top picture at 5mm, bottom at 40mm (Padget).[233&235]

directly into large sinusoids, producing changes such as progressive dilatation, phlebosclerosis, or occasional rupture in the veins. Similarly, Dandy[59] classified the lesions into two types:

1. Persisting foetal shunts – the angioma
2. Congenital veins connecting artery and vein

Whilst he recognised that a persistent foetal vein connected to the artery was an essential feature of this condition, he interpreted those lesions with an angioma as a different entity. He felt that the angioma was a greatly exaggerated capillary plexus formed by the shunt of arterial blood into the thin-walled capillaries which represented persistent foetal shunts. This concept of foetal capillary shunt influenced the subsequent thinking of mechanisms of formation of arteriovenous fistula a great deal.

There is, so far, no evidence to support the existence of primitive arteriovenous shunts in the normal embryo (Reid[267-270]). Although the primitive vascular system consists of vascular spaces lined by endothelium, definite pial vessels begin to form as early as 14-mm stage.

But if it is assumed that such a connection exists normally, then one should have expected to see, in every case, malformations involving almost the entire vascular system of the brain. At the site where Kaplan[145] and others postulated the lesions to occur, the vascular system was represented mainly by endothelial sinusoids. The normal development of the venous channels from these sinusoids in the presence of an abnormally large influx of blood appears improbable. It was exceptional in the present study to see instances where the developmental aberration had involved more than the localised segment of the arterial system.

Arteriovenous shunts which normally produce circulatory disturbances seldom involve more than one or two principal branches of the cerebral vascular system. So if there are multiple vascular shunts in the embryo, the circulatory overload must be proportionately enormous on the foetal heart. The embryo is unlikely to survive such a circulatory state (Carroll[39] Cronqvist[56] Davidoff[60] De Haan[62], Glatt[95], Holden[125] Hook[136&137] Laplace[159&160], Lehman[163] Levine[164] Perret[244&245]). The fact that many cases are recognised in adult life indicates that in addition to massive shunts, which are probably fatal in the womb, there must exist many instances where the lesion is confined to a very small segment of the vascular system, and where the overall circulatory disturbance is generalised, only a segment of the system will remain abnormal (Corrin[52] Elkin[75&76] Fincher[79&80] Hernandez[121] Lindegaard[166] McGuire[182&183] Shumacker[302] Siverman[303]). It is not possible to state categorically that arteriovenous fistulae do not occur very early in the development soon after onset of the circulation. But such a lesion is unlikely to be compatible with normal intrauterine life and probably ends in the death of the foetus.

Therefore, the concept that the angiomatous lesions seen represent persistence of segmental foetal arteriovenous shunts seems improbable (Lussenhop[173-175]).

The Development of the Venous System

Figure 3.5 is reproduced from the work of Padget[233] to indicate the development of the venous system.

The development of the venous system lags behind that of the arterial system, and at 40-mm stage, the arterial system was nearly representative of the adult pattern (Fig 3.3), whilst the venous pattern was very primitive.

The theory of persistent foetal fistula perhaps stems from the misconception that the developmental process of the vascular system is an unfolding of the primitive channels into the adult pattern followed later by the development of the neural tissues and that, with the further development of the brain, only a few of the shunts persist into the adult life.

There is, at any stage, a system fully adequate to cope with the existing structures. The changes are produced secondary to changing environmental influences and not as a primary process anticipating subsequent changes that are likely to happen. It seems illogical to assume that a vascular system for any part of the embryo is laid out before the particular structure has appeared on the scene. If, for any reason, the development of the embryo is arrested at any stage, the existing vascular system would be fully capable of functioning in that context. The pattern seen in the adult is not the finished model developed in stages, but is the sum total of the influences of various environmental factors that have operated during the entire period of the development. This essential embryological principle is termed as 'integrative development' (Streeter[314-315]).

Streeter classified these changes into three types with reference to the venous system in particular:

1. Passive migration
   Changes in the surrounding structures alter the position of the walls of the veins due to traction or flexion.
2. Spontaneous migration
   The flow of blood from a channel is directed to adjacent channel or channels. There is, here, only a change in the direction of blood flow whilst both the channels are already present.
3. Replacement channel
   The venous channels are changed in both position and direction.

Chapman[43] and Clark[47] studied the growth potential of the vascular endothelium in the digital webs of the tadpole and found that the vascular differentiation could be classified into two stages – before and after the commencement of the circulation.

In the first stage the endothelium puts forth a vascular system comprising mainly of the capillary system. This process occurs independently of the circulation; when the development of the circulation was deliberately arrested by excising the heart, the vascular plexus failed to evolve further. This passive primary development of the vascular system was thought, both by Clark and Chapman, to be due to hereditary factors.

For the second stage to occur, circulation was essential in their experiments. The mechanical effects of circulation on the capillary plexuses were considered an essential stimulus for the further differentiation of the vascular system.

The influence of mechanical factors on the development of the circulatory system was more graphically put forth by Thoma[323&324] in the form of physical laws (Thoma's laws):

1. Increase or decrease in the size of a vessel is regulated by the rate of the blood flow.
2. Increase or decrease in the length of a vessel is governed by the tension exerted on the vessel wall in a longitudinal direction by the tissue and organs outside of the vessel.
3. Increase or decrease in the thickness of the vessel wall is dependent upon the blood pressure.
4. New formation of capillaries depends upon increase of pressure in the capillary area.

Whilst such a clear distinction between hereditary and mechanical factors controlling the development of the vascular system is perhaps an oversimplification of the process, it is certainly possible to appreciate the influence of the physical properties of circulatory fluid on the vascular channels.

The same postulations can be restated more simply that the vascular system constantly adjusts to provide a most efficient machinery possible to the rapidly changing needs of the nervous system.

Pathogenesis of the Fistula

Developmental Changes in the Arterial Component of the Malformation

The nervous system develops from the neural tube formed by the folding of the neural plate. The cavity so enclosed forms the neural canal. The wall of the tube differentiates into three concentric zones, namely,

1. The ependymal layer
2. The cellular mantle
3. The fibrous marginal layer

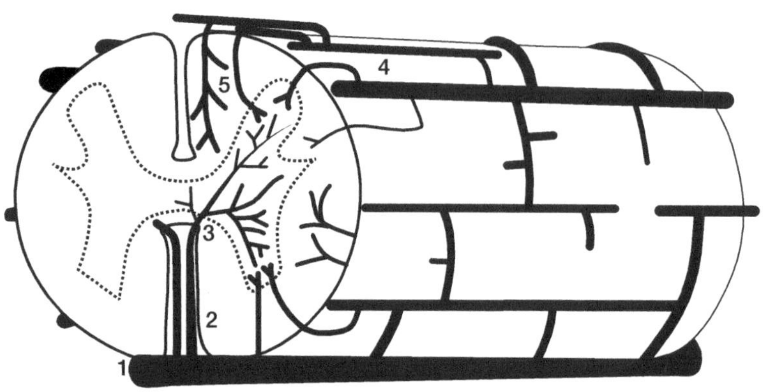

1 Anterior Spinal Artery
2 Anterior Sulcal Artery
3 Sulco-Commissusral (Paracentral) Artery
4 Postero-Lateral Artery
5 Dorsal Fissural and Interfunicular Artery

Figure 3.6 Schematic drawing of spinal cord arteries (DI Chiro).[66]

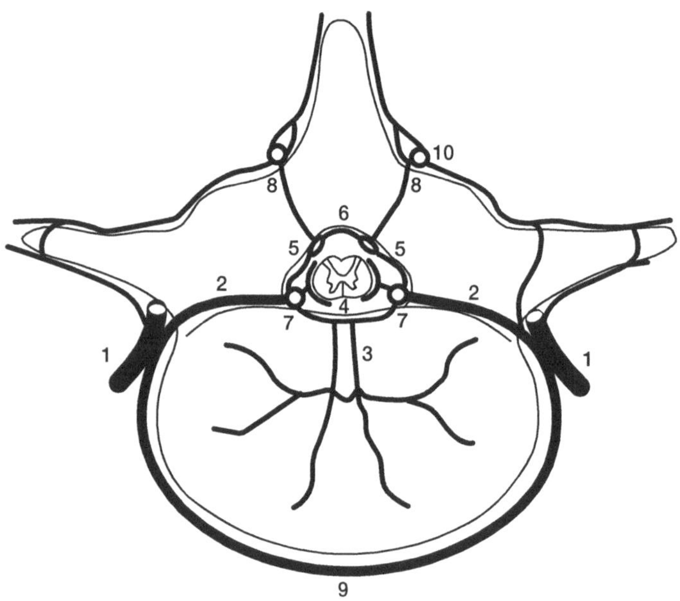

1 Lumbar Vein
2 Intervertebral Vein
3 Basivertebral Vein
4 Anterior Transverse Branch
5 Lateral Transverse Branch
6 Posterior Transverse Branch
7 Longitudinal Internal Vertebral Ligament
8 Branch Perforating Yellow Ligament
9 Anterior External Vertebral Plexus
10 Posterior External Vertebral Plexus

Figure 3.7 Schematic drawing of veins of the vertebral column (Krueger).[156]

From this evolves the basic nervous system consisting of central roof and floor plates. Included between them are the alar and basal plates.

Each segment consists of a pair of dorsal and ventral nerve roots and a pair of segmental arteries and veins accompanying these nerves. Each segmental vein has a pial tributary. These pial veins are interconnected by a pair of longitudinal channels, one on either side of the midline (see Figure 3.6, Figure 3.7, Figure 3.8 & Figure 3.9). In addition, these longitudinal veins are again secondarily interconnected across the midline.

Modifications in the Arterial System

Although both arteries and veins develop from the same endothelium, the arterial system differentiates faster than the veins. (Torr[327]) So by about 20-mm stage the arterial system very closely resembles the adult pattern. When an arteriovenous fistula occurs, the arterial system is unlikely to undergo major changes, as it is nearly adequate for most circulatory changes that are likely to occur at the 20-mm stage. The following are the two changes that are significant in relation to the present study:

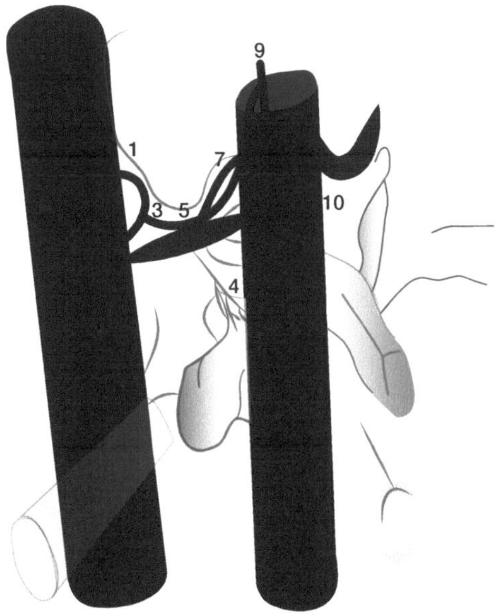

1 Aorta
2 Intercostal (or Lumbar, or Iliolumbar) Artery
3 Ventral Branch
4 Dorsal Branch
5 Muscle Branch
6 Spino-Medullary Branch
7 Branch of Posterior Canal
8 Branch of Anterior Canal
9 Anterior Radicular Artery
10 Posterior Radicular Artery
11 Anterior Spinal Artery
12 Posterolateral Spinal Artery

Figure 3.8 Segmental arteral supply of the spinal cord (DI Chiro).[66]

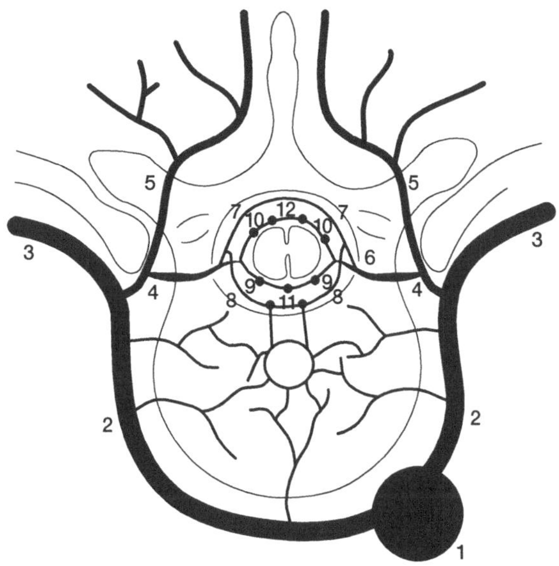

1 Aorta
2 Intercostal (or Lumbar, or Iliolumbar) Artery
3 Ventral Branch
4 Dorsal Branch
5 Muscle Branch
6 Spino-Medullary Branch
7 Branch of Posterior Canal
8 Branch of Anterior Canal
9 Anterior Radicular Artery
10 Posterior Radicular Artery
11 Anterior Spinal Artery
12 Posterolateral Spinal Artery

Figure 3.9 Schematic drawing of the arteries of the spinal segment (Krueger).[156]

The Development of the Arteriovenous Fistula

Following the establishment of the circulation, the vascular system differentiates further from the network of capillary plexus. Vessels that are most ideally situated persist, whilst the rest disappear.

For an arteriovenous fistula to occur at this stage, two essential conditions need to be specified. First, the artery and the vein involved in the lesion must be in close proximity, close enough to have their walls in contact with each other, at least at some point in their course. Second, there has to occur a breach in the walls between them to produce a fistula. Scharrer[286] compared the vascular pattern of the masupilea and the placentilea. In the former, the artery and the vein always met at the surface of the brain before entering the cerebral tissue. They remain paired throughout their course until they end in terminal loops, but there is no anastomosis between them. In contrast, in the placentilea the arteries and the veins enter the brain separately. The arteries give off their branches at narrow angles, and the veins receive their tributaries at right angles.

Padget[233-235] elaborated these concepts, with particular reference to the human nervous system. At about 14-mm stage the primitive veins are seen passing transversely through the pia-arachnoid to join the primitive dural channels. These channels are connected by longitudinal anastomosing channels. These, in turn, are connected with the corresponding veins across the midline. Thus, an intricate chessboard-like venous network is formed. During this period, the arterial system is continuously shifted away from the neural tube, thus occupying an intermediate position

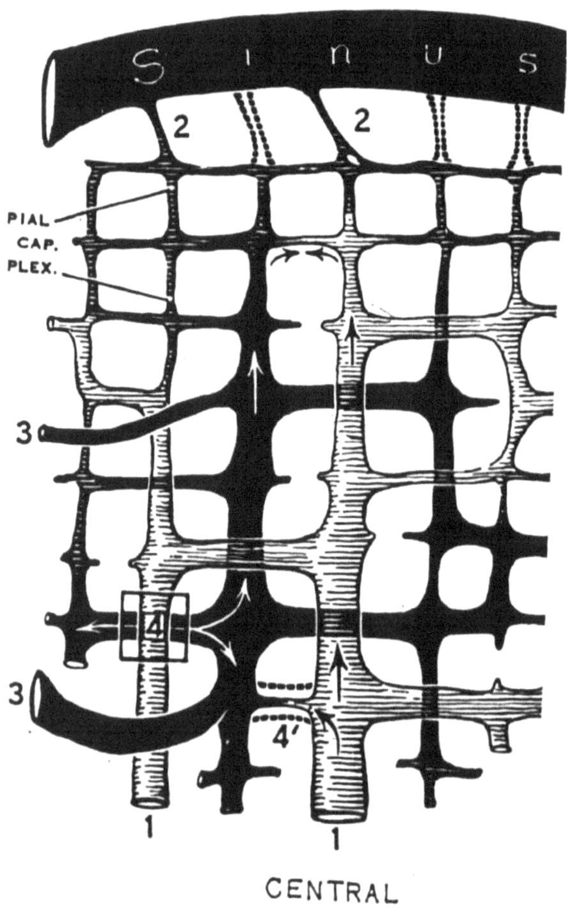

Figure 3.10 The pial arteries and veins crossing at the right angles (diagonally) at 40 mm.

between the neural tube and the dural sinuses. The pial veins lie between the arteries and the wall of the neural tube. These pial veins also cross at approximately right angles (see Figure 3.10).

Padget put forth two possible mechanisms by which the arteriovenous fistula can occur:

1. The retained endothelium connections at the juxtaposed crossings may lead to an arteriovenous fistula. If there are persisting endothelial connections between these vessels, there is bound to be a shunt of blood as soon as the circulation starts, that is, around the 4-mm stage. The effects of such a fistula on the survival of the foetus have already been mentioned. Since these pial arteries and veins occupy their characteristic position only after 20-mm stage, it is difficult to justify the presence of patent endothelial connections which start conducting the blood suddenly at 20-mm stage to produce localised lesions, although the circulation has been established for a much longer period.

   It is more likely that during the development of the vascular system, some areas of the vessel walls are imperfectly formed, creating potential weak spots. If, by any chance, a similar weak area of the venous system comes to light adjacent to the arterial imperfection, the chances of a fistula is likely (Bailey[13]).

2. Padget also felt that the right-angled crossings of the arteries and veins normally acted as a deterrent to the formation of an arteriovenous fistula, as the area of contact between the vessels was minimal in this situation. She contended that there is an alteration in these right-angled crossings – the surface area of contact is proportionately increased and thus increases the chances of a fistula. But this hypothesis cannot be substantiated. It is possible to show by mathematical reasoning that, in

fact, an increase in the surface area reduces the risks of a breach in the adjoining walls.

The proximation of the vessels starts around the 20-mm stage and is complete around 40-mm stage. At this stage the arterial system is very similar to that of the adult configuration, and the venous channels are more definable (though primitive in their anatomical layout). The pattern of malformation in the adult very often corresponds to the layout at this stage than that of any of the earlier stages. Since the evidence in the adult strongly indicates that these fistulae probably occur from this stage onwards, it is reasonable to suppose that these right-angled crossings are significant. The exact process involved in the occurrence of a fistula is difficult to determine. There must occur certain factors which increase the pressure on the walls of the arteries at the point where they cross the veins to produce a breach in the wall. These factors should include the lateral pressure of the circulating blood, the elastic properties of the endothelium, the physical properties of flow, and such other factors of hydrodynamics. The mechanics of the shunt are discussed in chapter 14.

Developmental Changes in the Venous System

The modifications that occur in the pattern of drainage to the venous system are governed by

1. The need to provide an efficient drainage to an increasing flow.
2. The need to overcome the inefficiencies created by the structural alterations of the brain.

   The degree of these changes is related to the segment of the brain concerned. These changes are very minimal in the spinal cord, as the segmental pattern is maintained in this section. But the process gets more complicated as more complex cranial segments are involved. The changes that the venous system has to cope with consist of

3. Increasing growth in both lateral and antero-posterior directions.
4. The changes in the axis of the neural tube by the formation of the flextures.

The Similarity of the Venous Pattern in Groups of Cases

At the time when the arteriovenous fistula occurs, the venous system is still undergoing rapid changes. The effects of the circulatory abnormality are seen in these venous channels. The embryo does not produce new channels specifically to cope with this problem. The existing channels are made use of to the best possible advantage. This adjustment occurs according to the normal principles of development. The most easily suitable channel is used. The shortest route to the principal draining sinus is used. When a channel is inadequate to deal with this problem, other alternate routes are used. Thus, the mode of establishment of these abnormal venous channels is predictable.

Identification of the Abnormal Vascular Channels Specific to Each Embryonic Segment

The above-mentioned changes occur in every situation where there is an arteriovenous fistula. The fundamental principles mentioned are modified to suit the availability of the venous channels in the particular segment concerned. It is also modified in relation to the manner of development of that particular segment.

The overall picture produced in each segment is specific, and all the arteriovenous malformations produced in that region have comparable anatomical features.

As mentioned earlier, the degree of intricacy is related to the degree of specialisation.

4

Arteriovenous Malformations of the Spinal Cord

Segmental pattern is fundamental to the development of the embryo. The complex evolution of the brain has its origin from this. The primitive pattern is to a large extent maintained in the adult spinal cord. Each segment, in addition to other elements, consists of a pair of pial arteries and veins, crossing each other in close approximation. An accidental rupture of their walls at the points of their contact could lead to ateriovenous fistula.

The Arterial Component of the Spinal Malformation

Since the segmental pattern of the notochord is preserved in the spinal cord, the developmental alterations of the vascular system are minimal in this section. The segmental arterial supply being in excess of what is required, there is a consolidation of these vessels (see Figure 3.6, Figure 3.7, Figure 3.8 and Figure 4.1).

Houdart, Djinjian, and Hurth[138] observed in their studies that:

1. The arteries, although abnormal in appearance and size, are of normal topography.
2. The arteries opened into the veins directly.
3. The vessels involved in the malformation bear a relationship to the normal vascular system.

The Angiomatous Elements of Spinal Malformation

In the three types of malformation described by Lazorthes[135], the arterial element is definable and normally formed. The location of the malformation appears to be most frequent in the thoraco-lumbar area. The distribution in cervical and dorsal lumbar areas is probably about equal.

The arterio-capillary tangle is not necessarily seen in every case of the spinal malformations. In type 1, as described by Lazorthes, the artery opens into the vein directly. In type 3, what is generally described as an angioma, in fact, consists of dilated venous channels. Type 2 is similar to type 3, except for the size of the lesion. The clarity between artery and vein is less clear here.(Krayenbuhl[153-155])

The Venous Elements of the Spinal Malformation

The size and type of the remaining veins are dependent upon the size of the fistula. Larger lesions tend to have more obviously dilated venous channels as Houdart, Djinjian, and Hurth[138] observed that these venous channels extend along the spinal cord to more than two or three segments and appear to be abnormal. On closer examination, they are in fact normal venous channels that have become more prominent because of the increased flow through them. Thus, the variations, as mentioned by Lazorthes[162], are produced by the same fistula. The differences in appearance are due to variation in the actual degree of shunting (Antoni[9]). If an arteriovenous fistula in the segment of the spinal cord is very small, the segmental vein drains the blood into one of the longitudinal venous channels. In such cases, the lesion appears to be confined to a single segment only. When the fistula is large and when the prospective segmental veins are unable to drain the blood entirely on their own, the veins from adjoining segments are brought into action. The number of segments so involved depends upon

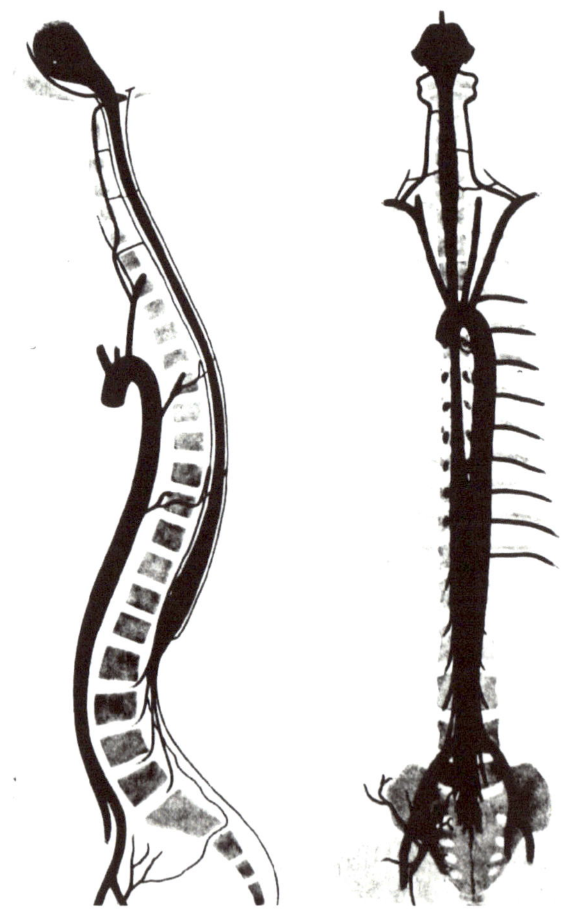

Figure 4.1 Segmental arterial supply modified in the adult (Lazorthes).[162]

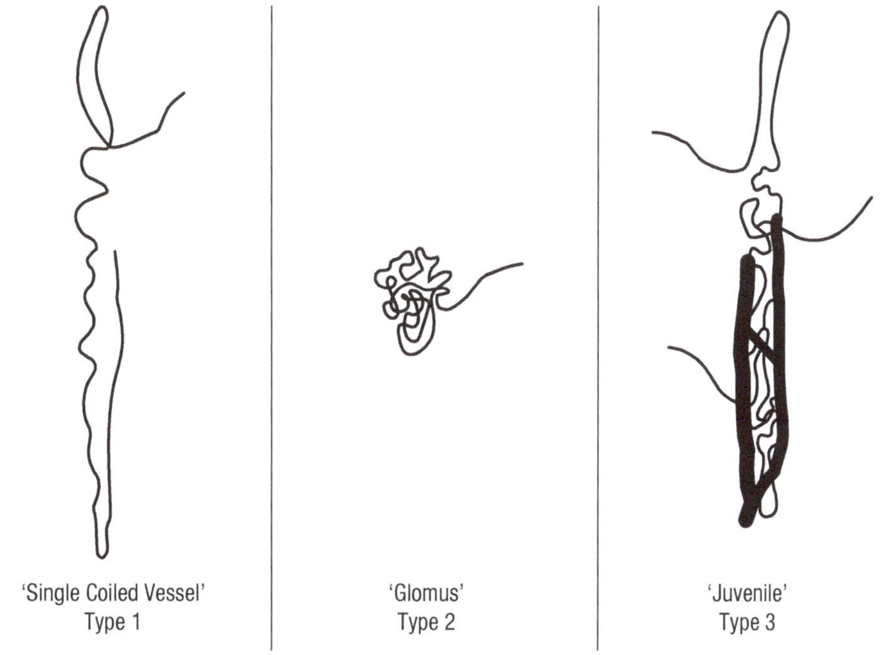

Figure 4.2 Variations in the arterio-venous malformations of the spinal cord.

the size of the fistula and the capacity of the segmental vein to drain the excess flow.

The simplicity of the pattern seen in spinal cord malformations is attributable to the fact that the primary segmental pattern is still maintained here (Brion[30], Gross[104] Herren[122] Hyman[140] Lombardi[170&171] Newman[208].

As one would imagine the anterior part of this tube expanding enormously and folding backwards on itself, the complexity of the pattern is easily appreciated (see Figure 4.6, Figure 4.7 Figure 4.9). The anterior end of the primitive notochord develops three dilatations, namely,

1. The prosencephalon
2. The mesencephalon
3. The rhombencephalon

Further divisions occur in these, and the following five primary segments of the brain are produced (see Figure 4.7)

1. The telencephalon
2. The diencephalon
3. The mesencephalon
4. The metencephalon
5. The myelencephalon

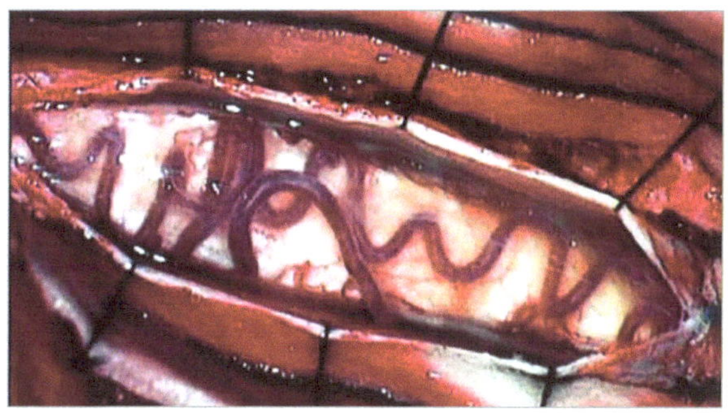

Figure 4.3 Segmental embryonic veins (Ratliff &Conoly).[264]

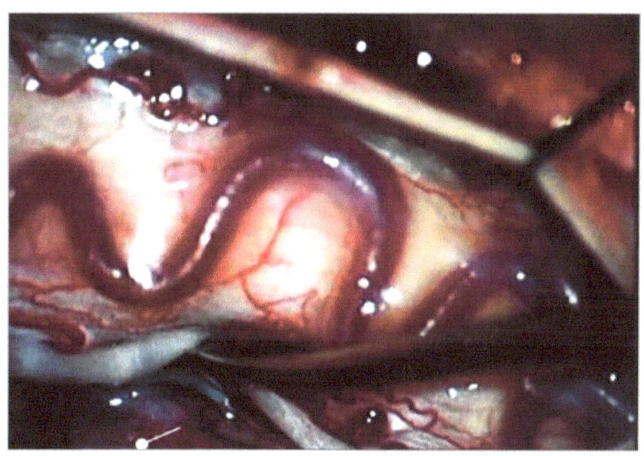

Figure 4.4 Segmental embryonic veins (Ratliff & Conoly).[264]

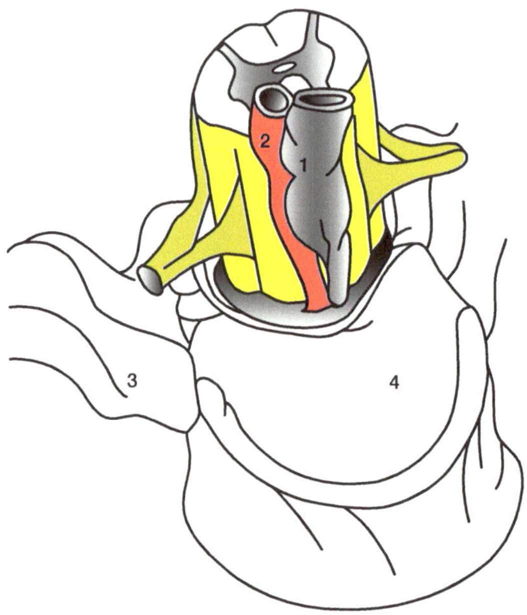

1 Arterial Venous Fatula **2** Arterior Spinal Artery **3** Rib **4** Vertebral Body (Cranial—Anterior Aspect)

Figure 4.5 Spinal Arterio venous fistula (Ratliff and Conoly).[264]

The development of the vascular system also undergoes changes in accordance with these, thereby obscuring the primary segmental pattern to a large extent (see Figure 4.8). It has already been mentioned earlier that the developmental changes with regard to the arterial system are minimal.

The changes produced in the venous system are more dramatic.Figure 4.8, shows diagrammatically the five primary regions of the brain. Each segment has a pair of pia-arachnoidal veins, and they all drain into a lateral channel – the primitive tentorial sinus. The pattern of drainage at this stage in the development of the brain is very similar to that of the spinal system. The most caudal segment, the myelencephalon, connects the cerebral and spinal venous drainage.

Rapid expansion of the telencephalon and the diencephalon increases the venous outflow. The tentorial sinus is unable at this stage to deal with this efficiently. The problem is further accentuated by the backward swing of the brain. The tentorial sinus is stretched, accentuating further the problems of drainage

The telencephalic and the diencephalic segmental veins now drain into a more medially situated venous channel – the basal vein.

The basal vein is formed by the longitudinal anastomosis of these transverse segmental veins – the telencephalic, diencephalic, mesencephalic, metencephalic, and myelencephalic. The medially situated basal vein, being more efficient, replaces the function of the tentorial sinus completely. Further growth and differentiation of the telencephalon and the diencephalon, in particular, the development of the basal nuclear mass, creates further problems in drainage. The basal vein now is unable to cope with this excess demand. Therefore, a more medially placed internal cerebral vein develops and functions as an accessory to the basal vein with the growth of the telencephalon.

The expansion of the cerebral cortex produces further problems in the drainage. The veins on the surface of the telencephalon now require an alternate channel for the drainage, as the medially situated basal and internal cerebral veins are too deep to be efficient. The superior sagittal sinus takes over this function. In this

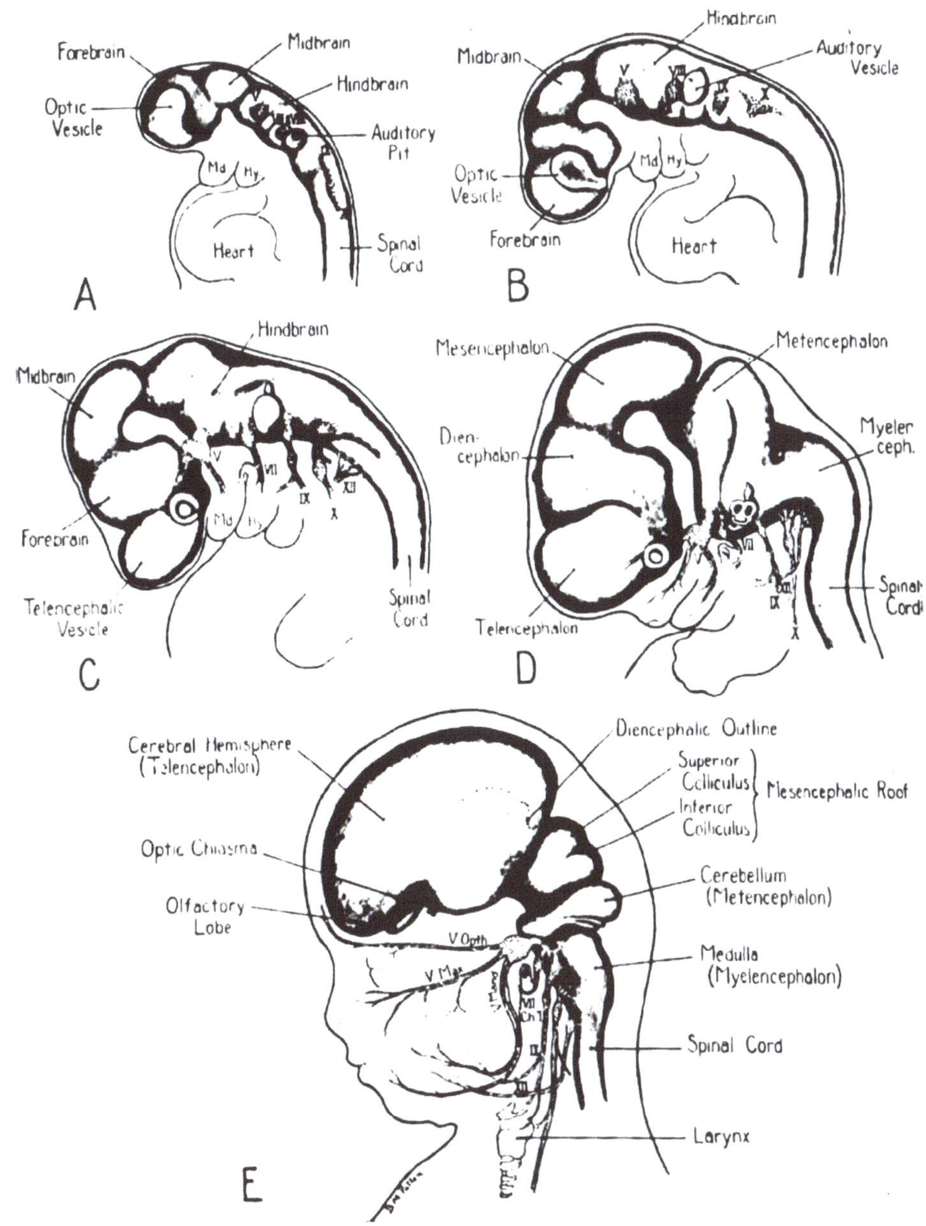

Figure 4.6 Brain developed by bulges and bends in the neural tube (Arey).[10]

diagram the superior sagittal sinus is shown laterally to indicate the surface drainage of the telencephalon. It was found difficult to represent the sinus in its natural relationship without compromising the clarity of the diagrams.

The Effects of Arteriovenous Fistula on the Normal Developmental Process

The entire sequence of normal developmental alterations seen in the vascular system (in the venous system particularly) is essentially dependent upon the quantity of blood that has to be dealt with in the various regions of the neural tube. The alterations are naturally more extensive where this problem is most severe. The introduction of an arteriovenous fistula merely exaggerates the need for circulatory adjustment. The process is perhaps accelerated so that some of the channels are brought into action earlier than the usual period. This probably accounts for the persistence of certain embryonic appearances and connections in certain recognised adult channels, where the abnormal circulatory demands have not permitted the channels to reach their maturity.

It is essential to recognise that the embryo does not produce any new channels to deal with the problem. The adjustment is brought about as efficiently as possible in the available system. In this process, certain channels normally destined to disappear may be used. They are often seen as abnormal vessels. This failure of atresia is mainly responsible for the complexity of the pattern seen in the postnatal period (Vidyasagar[334]).

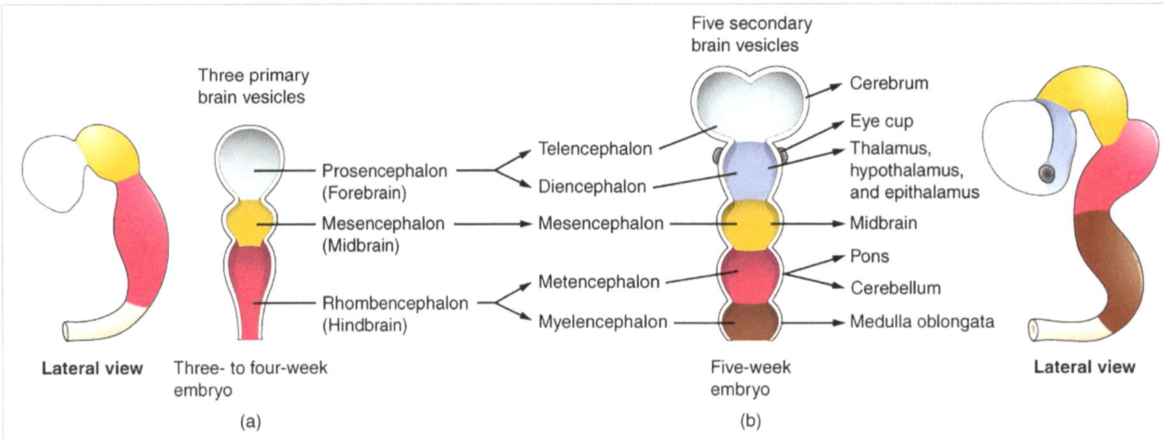

Figure 4.7 Development of Human Brain (Dev. Neurology).

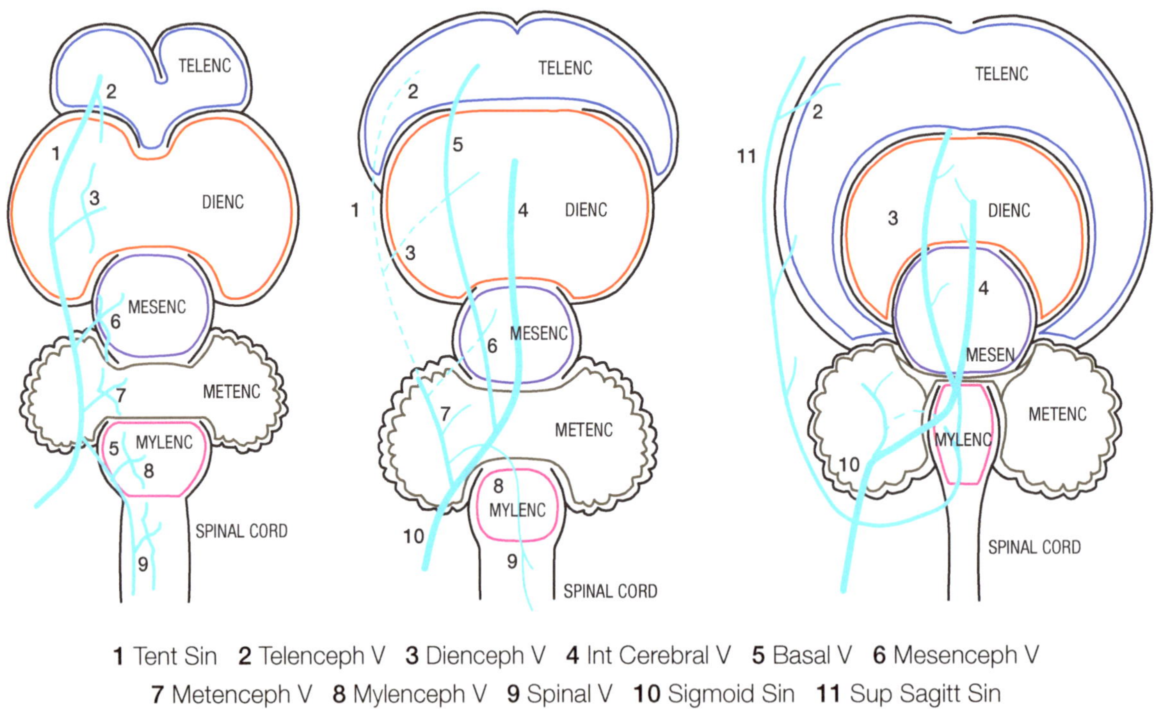

Figure 4.8 Development of cerebral venous system.

5

Myelencephalic Abnormalities

The caudal slope of the embryonic hindbrain constitutes the myelencephalon. This segment develops into the medulla oblongata. Anterior and posterior inferior cerebellar arteries represent the early pial arteries. The dorsal and ventral myelencephalic veins represent the corresponding pial veins. These persist in the adult if an arteriovenous fistula occurs in this segment.

The Myelencephalon forms the junction between the spinal cord and the brain. It is represented by the medulla oblongata in the adult. This segment of the brain is only slightly more specialised than the spinal cord, so the basic pattern of the vascular system is very similar to that of the spinal cord (Castellano[42], Ciminello[45], Evans[77]).

The Arterial Components of the Myelencephalon

There are two arteries in this segment of the brain, and these are represented in the adult as anterior and posterior inferior cerebellar arteries (Zingesser[356] Verbiest[332&333]. Schultz[293], Seljeskog[296], Shenkin[299], Moody[201], Mount[202]).

The Arteriovenous Fistula

Like all pia-arachnoidal vessels, the myelencephalic arteries cross the ventral myelencephalic veins at approximately right angles. The arteriovenous fistula in this situation is possible (Figure 5.1 & Figure 5.2).

The Venous Elements of the Myelencephalon

The developmental changes in the myelencephalon consist mainly of the consolidation of the notochordal segments. The ventral nerve roots are, therefore, brought closer. The alterations in the venous system match this process. The segmental veins are reduced in number, and the single ventral metencephalic vein (the vagal vein)

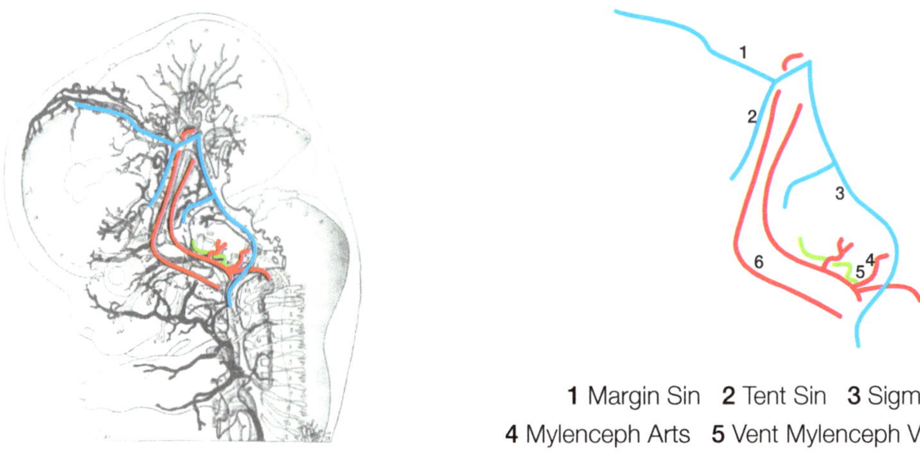

Figure 5.1 Myelencephalic vein draining into the transverse sinus (lateral).

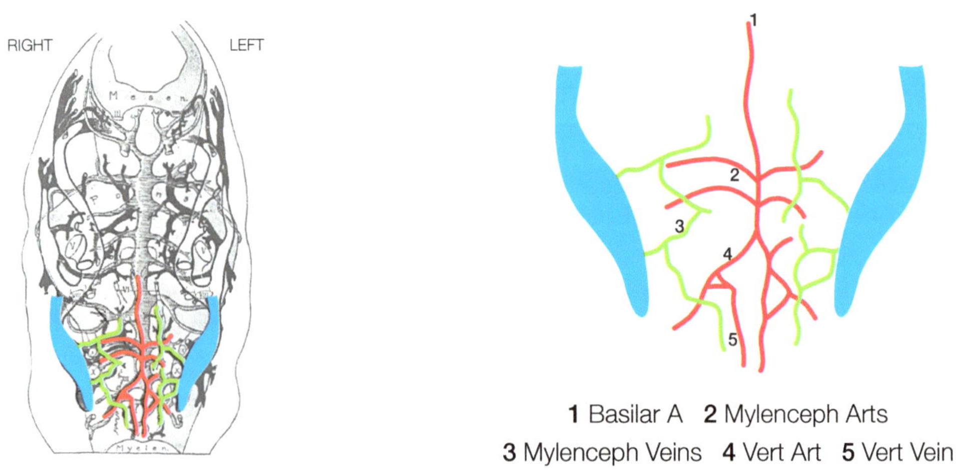

Figure 5.2 Myelencephalic vein draining into the transverse sinus (basal).

represents this change. As in the spinal cord, it makes longitudinal connections with the adjoining segmental veins cranially and the anterior spinal vein caudally. Since the afferent elements (sensory elements) of the vagal and hypoglossal nerves are not prominent in man, the dorsal nerve roots and their veins tend to disappear (Figure 4.8).

Regrouping of Cases According to the Similarity of Venous Pattern

This was the only case reported in the literature, and therefore, it was not possible to compare the venous drainage in this group of malformation.

Identification and Matching of Abnormal Vascular Channels with Normal Embryonic Vascular Channels

The blood shunted into the venous system can find its way either caudally into the spinal vein or cranially into the ventral metencephalic vein. The latter is probably a more direct route, as it is better developed to meet the demand. In the adult, the persisting ventral myelencephalic vein should then be coursing upwards and laterally to reach the superior petrosal sinus.

Grouping of the Arteries According to the Situation in the Embryo

Both anterior inferior and posterior inferior cerebellar arteries supply the region of the myelencephalon. Therefore, the malformations whose arterial components arise from these arteries should have similar features.

New Classification of Arteriovenous Malformations Based on the Embryological Site of Their Formation

The arteriovenous malformations arising from these inferior cerebellar arteries would normally be grouped with Posterior Cerebral artery lesions under the common title 'Posterior Fossa Arteriovenous Malformations'. The anatomical features of the lesion of these two groups are similar in many respects, but the differences are sufficiently distinct to group them separately. The venous channels are directed upwards and laterally and drain into the junction of transverse and sigmoid sinuses or into the sigmoid sinus itself (compare with metencephalic veins).

The Theoretically Possible Anatomical Configuration of Myelencephalic Arteriovenous Malformation

Figure 5.3–Fig 5.10 show the theoretically possible anatomical configuration of the myelencephalic arteriovenous malformation. The changes for purposes of convenience are divided into four stages: 20 mm, 40 mm, 80 mm, and the adult (Vidyasagar[339]).

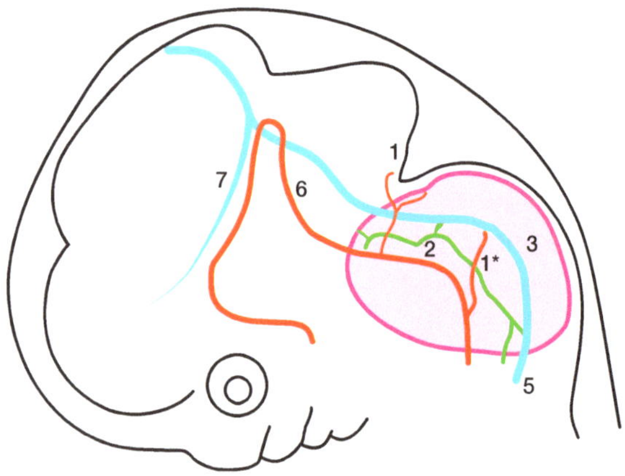

Figure 5.3 The Mylencephalic vein draining into the Transverse Sinus at 20mm (Lateral).

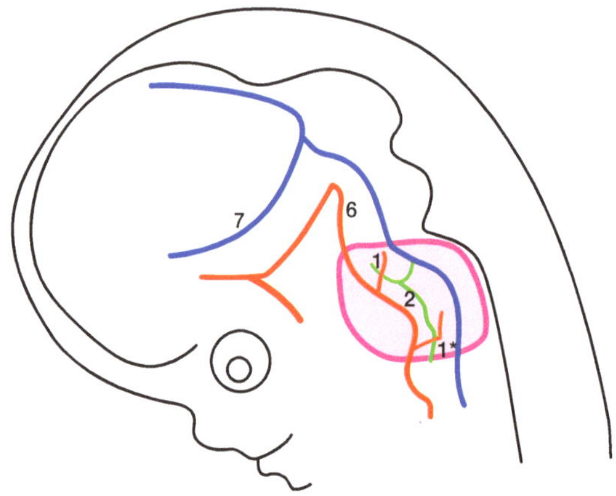

Figure 5.4 The Mylencephalic vein draining into the Transverse Sinus at 40mm (Lateral).

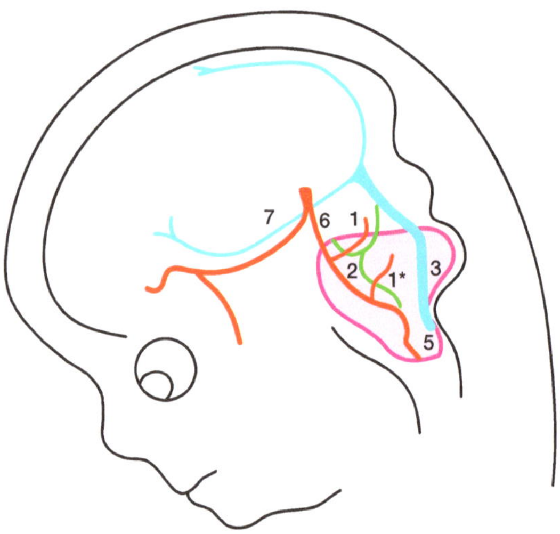

Figure 5.5 The Mylencephalic vein draining into the Transverse Sinus at 80mm (Lateral).

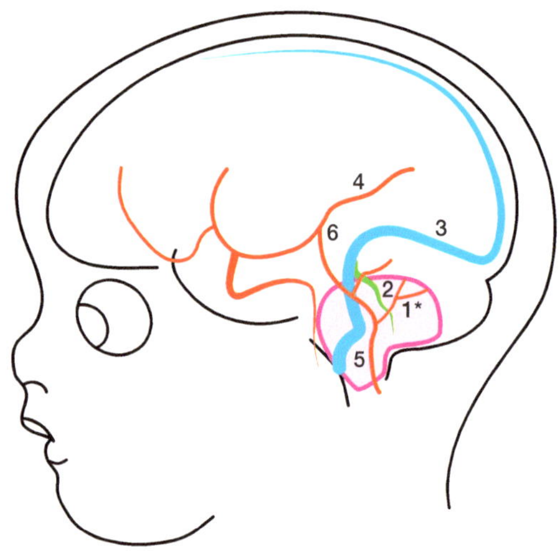

Figure 5.6 The Mylencephalic vein draining into the Transverse Sinus in an adult (Lateral).

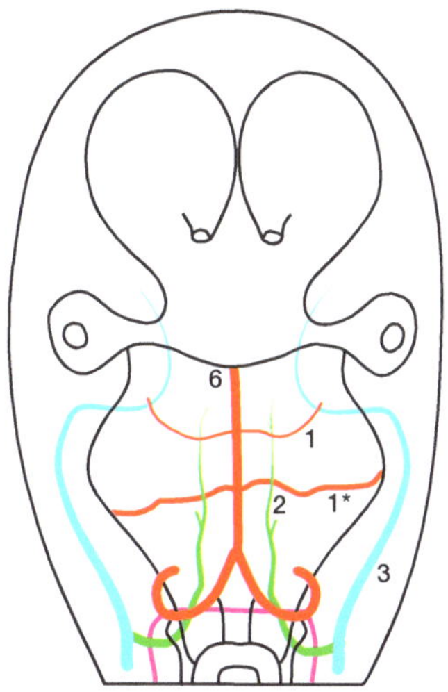

Figure 5.7 The Mylencephalic vein draining into the Transverse Sinus at 20mm (Basal).

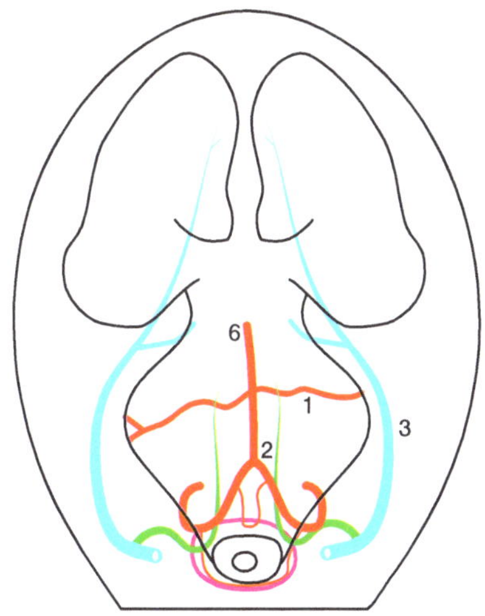

Figure 5.8 The Mylencephalic vein draining into the Transverse Sinus at 40mm (Basal).

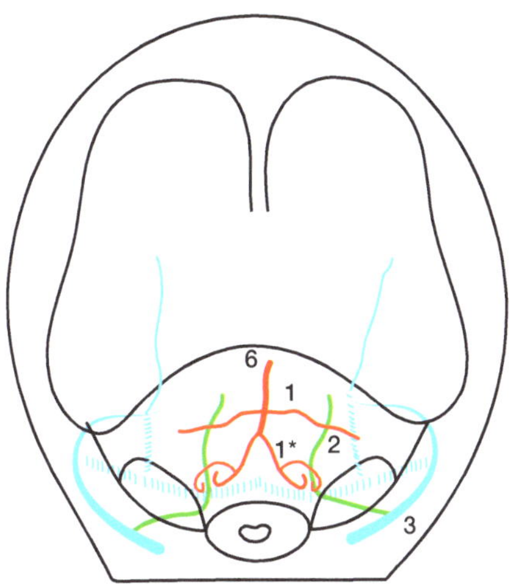

Figure 5.9 The Mylencephalic vein draining into the Transverse Sinus at 80mm (Basal).

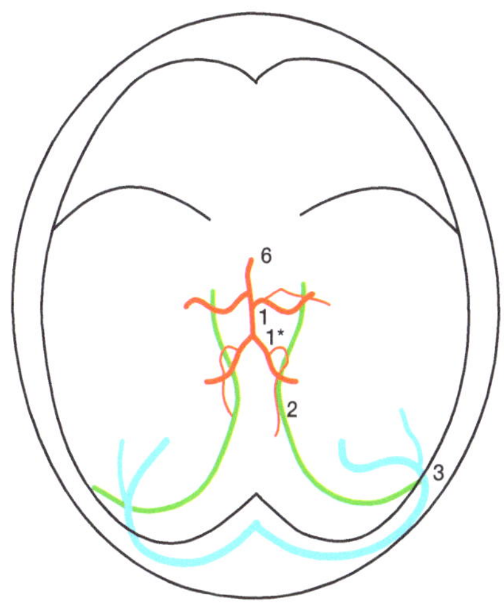

Figure 5.10 The Mylencephalic vein draining into the Transverse Sinus in an adult (Basal).

1 Ant Inf Cerebellar A **1*** Post Inf Cerebellar A **2** Vent Mylenceph V
3 Trans Sin **4** Post Cerebellar A **5** Sigmoid Sin **6** Basilar **7** Tent Sin

Examples

Figure 5.11, and Figure 5.12 are examples for myelencephalic arteriovenous malformation. The arterial feeder is from the right anterior inferior cerebellar artery. The venous drainage is lateral and upwards into the superior petrosal sinus. Although in theory the occurrence of an arteriovenous fistula should be as frequent here as anywhere else in the nervous system, for some unknown reason this seems to be an extremely rare phenomenon. The first case was reported by Mount in 1965. It is possible that the difficulties in identifying the anterior cerebellar artery in posterior fossa angiograms are responsible for this.

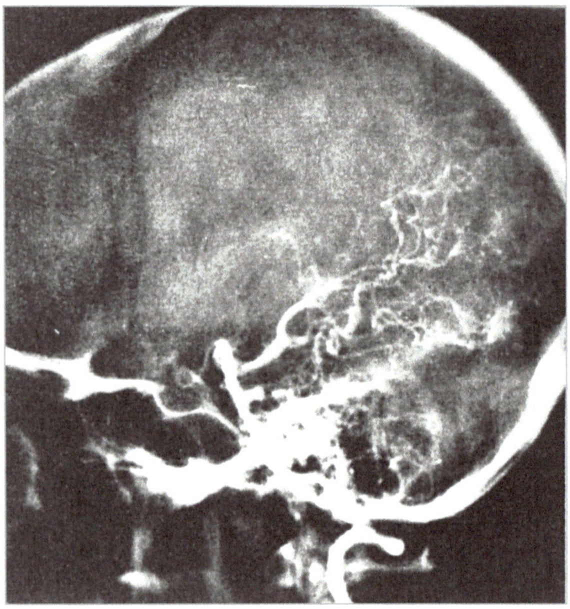

Figure 5.11 The myelencephalic arterio-venous maleformation. Arterial feeder from anterior inferior cerebellar artery (lateral).

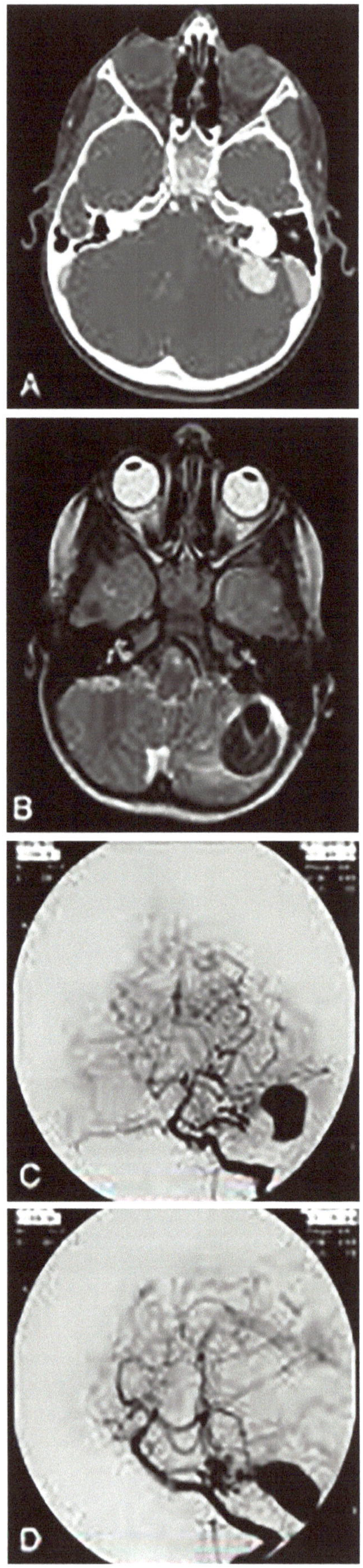

Figure 5.12 Mylencephalic AVM Lateral drainage (Neurosurgery Focus 2335, American Association of Neurological Surgeons).

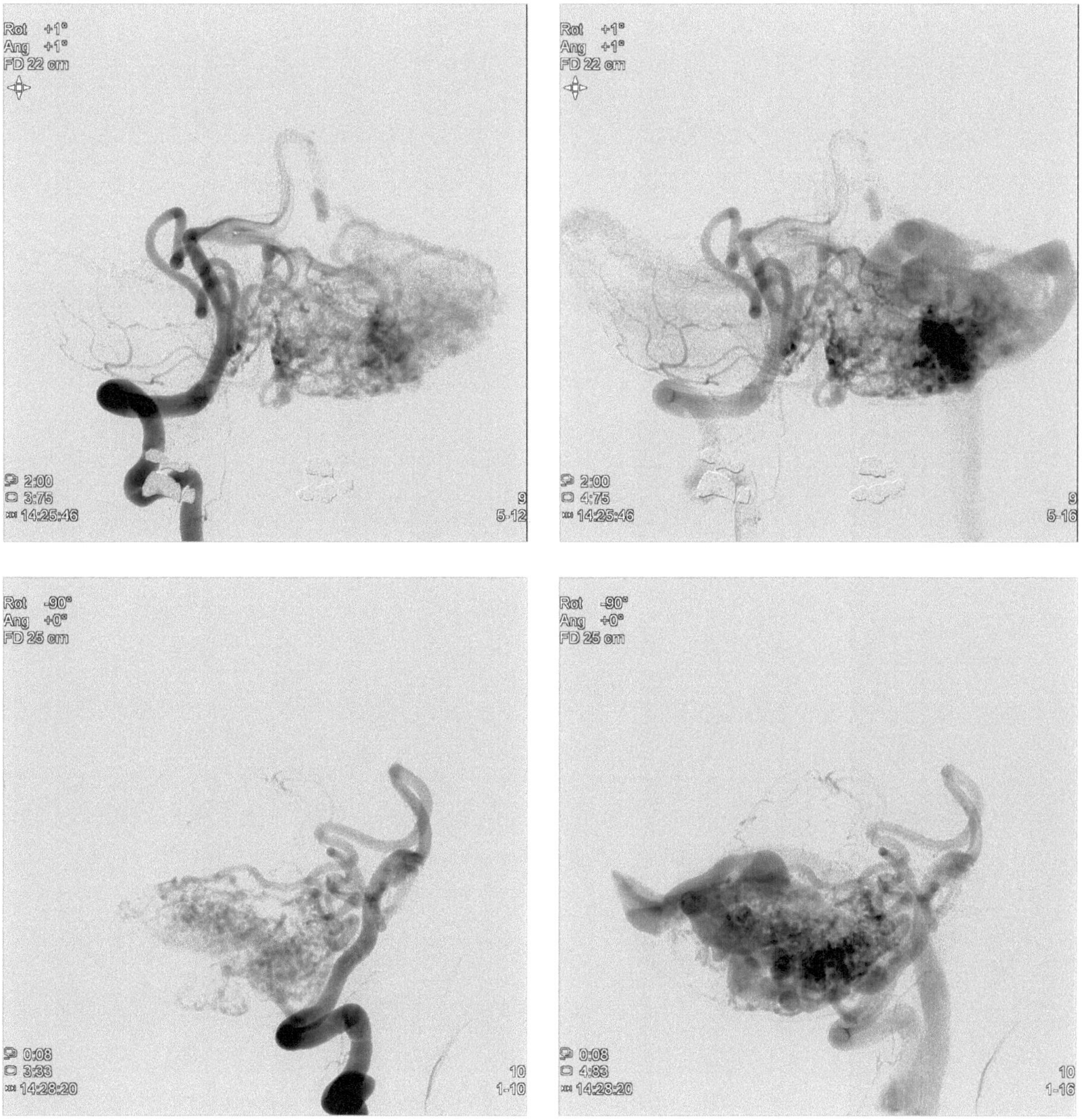

Figure 5.13 Mylencephalic AVM. Lateral drainage into Transverse Sinus (Golkar).[100]

6

Metencephalic Abnormalities

The dorsal part of the embryonic midbrain represents the metencephalon. Cerebellum and pons are derived from this segment. The superior cerebellar artery and dorsal and ventral metencephalic veins represent the corresponding pial arteries and veins respectively. The latter persist in the adult as arterialised venous channels in the event of ateriovenous fistula in this area of the developing brain.

The metencephalon is the segment of the brain extending between the myelencephalon and the mesencephalon. In the adult it is represented by the pons and cerebellum. The segmental pattern of the primitive notochord can still be appreciated in this segment of the brain. As in the case of the myelencephalon, there is consolidation of the primitive segment. The development of the cerebellar hemispheres from the dorsal regions is the only significant developmental process seen.

The Arterial Components of the Metencephalon

The primitive metencephalon is supplied by a pair of metencephalic arteries arising from the primitive arterial ring. In the adult they are represented by the superior cerebellar arteries.

The Arteriovenous Fistula

The superior cerebellar artery crosses the pia-arachnoidal veins of the metencephalon, represented by the dorsal and ventral metencephalic veins. An arteriovenous fistula occurs between these vessels at the points of their intersection.

The Venous Elements of the Metencephalon

The dorsal and ventral metencephalic veins course laterally to join the transverse sinus. The dorsal metencephalic vein joins the dural sinus near its torcula end, and the ventral metencephalic vein is the principal vein and drains most parts of the metencephalon, except the caudal and dorsal areas, which occur in the later stages of development. These are then drained by the dorsal metencephalic vein. The ventral metencephalic vein is situated in the anterior aspect of the cerebellum and courses laterally and downwards to drain into the junction of the pro-otic sinus with the transverse sinus.

The great anterior cerebellar vein and the stem of the superior petrosal sinus represent in the adult the ventral metencephalic vein and the segment of the pro-otic sinus into which it joins.

Grouping of Cases According to the Similarity of the Venous Pattern

There are two types of abnormal vascular channels that can be seen in this region:

1. A channel coursing upwards, backwards, and medially into the transverse sinus near the torcula end.
2. The venous channel travelling laterally and upwards to reach the junction between the transverse and the sigmoid sinuses.

In the present series examples of both types were found.

Matching of the Abnormal Vascular Channels with Normal Embryonic Vascular Channels

The channels draining medially into the torcula region represent the dorsal metencephalic vein, whilst those draining laterally into the transverse sinus represent the ventral metencephalic vein.

Grouping of Arteries According to Their Situation in the Embryo

The proximity of the posterior cerebellar artery and the inferior cerebellar artery to the superior cerebellar artery, in the adult, often leads to the categorisation of the latter with the rest under the term 'posterior fossa lesion'. In embryological terms they belong to different regions. The metencephalic arteries of the embryo are represented by the superior cerebellar arteries alone (see Metencephalic and Diencephalic).

The New Classification Based on the Embryological Site of Their Formation

Generally, the malformation arising from the superior cerebellar artery is classified under posterior fossa lesions. The anatomical features are distinct and should be classified as metencephalic abnormalities, in view of their situation in the embryo.

The Possible Anatomical Configurations of the Metencephalic Arteriovenous Malformations

Figure 6.1 - Figure 6.8 show the possible anatomical variations of the metencephalic arteriovenous malformation. The changes are represented as usual in four stages, namely, 20 mm, 40 mm, 80 mm, and the adult, according to the standard code used. The vessels in green represent the embryonic pia-arachnoidal veins (Vidyasagar[334&339]).

Examples

Ventral Metencephalic Vein Malformations

Figure 6.9 shows the ventral metencephalic arteriovenous malformations in which the persistent ventral metencephalic vein is draining

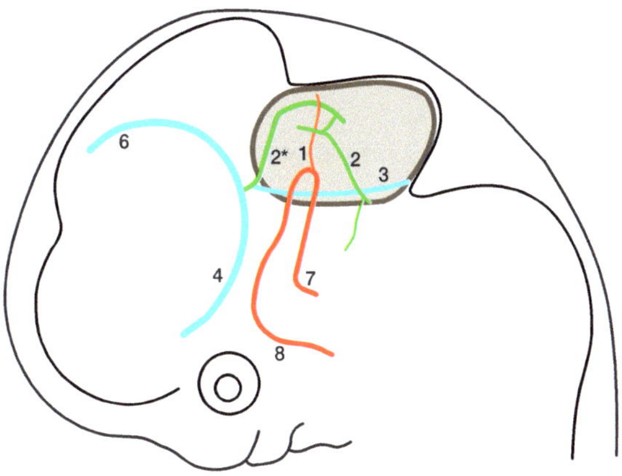

Figure 6.1 Dorsal and ventral metencephalic veins draining into the transverse sinus at 20mm (lateral).

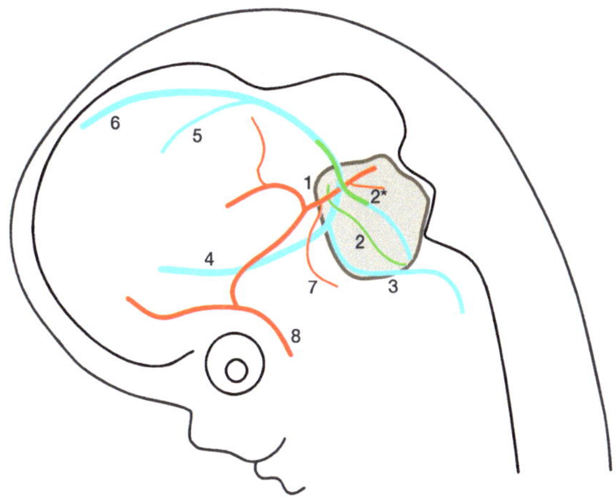

Figure 6.2 Dorsal and ventral metencephalic veins draining into the transverse sinus at 40mm (lateral).

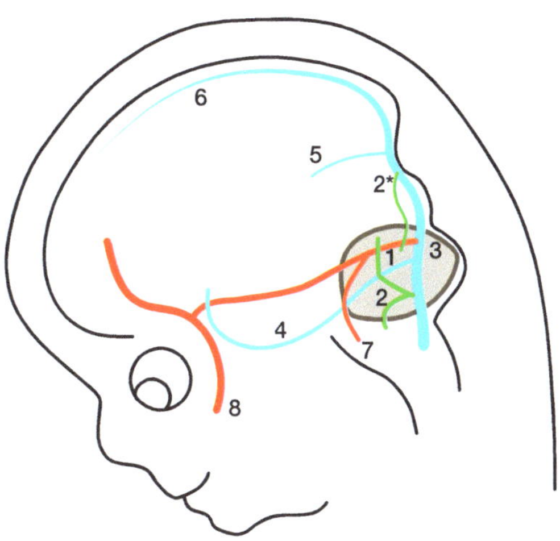

Figure 6.3 Dorsal and ventral metencephalic veins draining into the transverse sinus at 80mm (lateral).

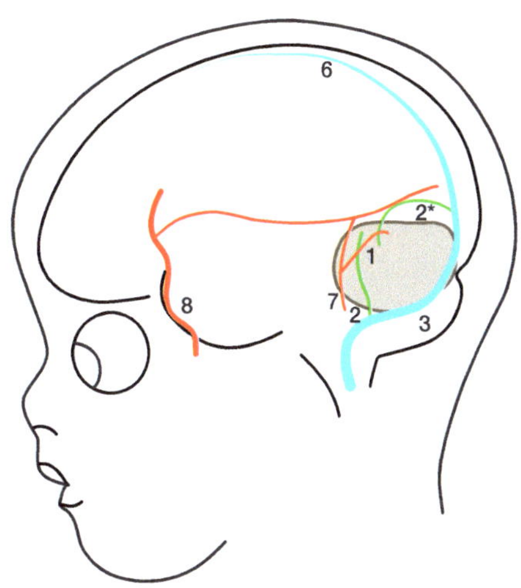

Figure 6.4 Dorsal and ventral metencephalic veins draining into the transverse sinus in the adult (lateral).

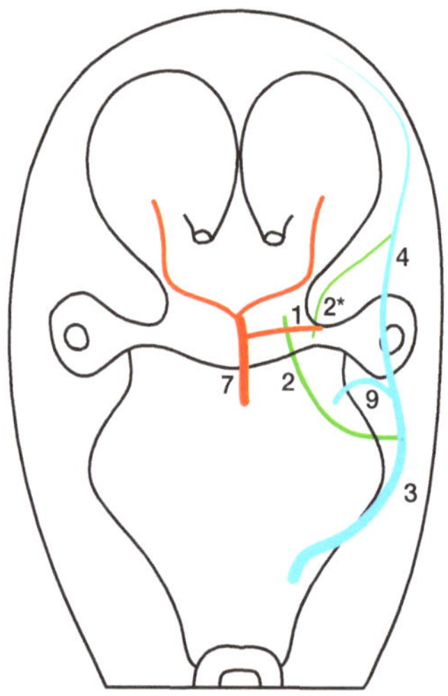

Figure 6.5 Dorsal and ventral metencephalic veins draining into the transverse sinus at 20mm (basal).

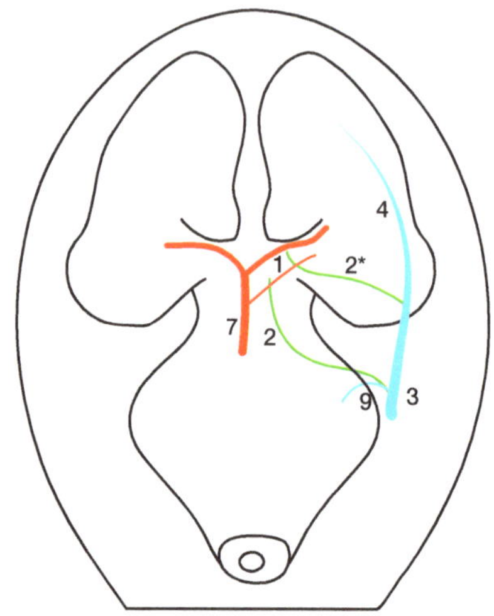

Figure 6.6 Dorsal and ventral metencephalic veins draining into the transverse sinus at 40mm (basal).

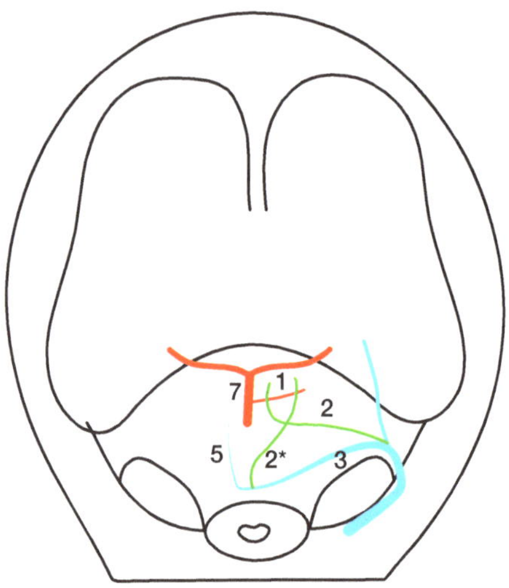

Figure 6.7 Dorsal and ventral metencephalic veins draining into the transverse sinus at 80mm (basal).

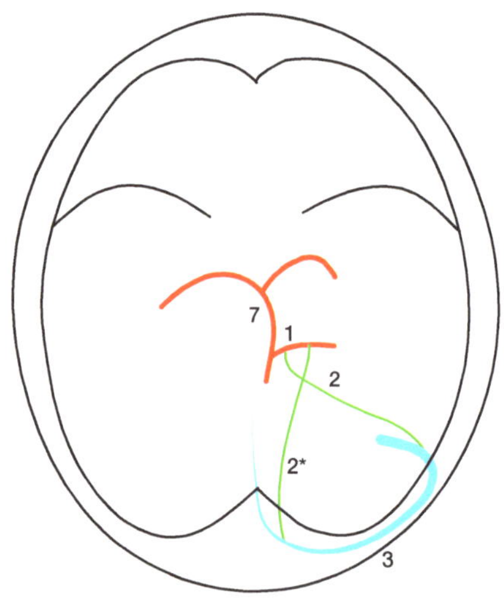

Figure 6.8 Dorsal and ventral metencephalic veins draining into the transverse sinus in the adult (basal).

1 Sup Cerebellar A **2** Vent Metenceph V **2*** Dorsal Metenceph V **3** Trans Sin
4 Tent Sin **5** Int Cereb V **6** Sup Sagitt Sin **7** Basilar A **8** Int Carotid A **9** Pro-Otic Sin

into the transverse sinus. The course of the venous channel is downwards and lateral, and the opacification of the transverse sinus confirms its mode of termination.

It was mentioned earlier that the ventral metencephalic vein joins the junction between the pro-otic sinus and the transverse sinus. The pro-otic sinus primarily functions as a drainage of the orbito-ophthalmic veins. The expansion of the otic capsule produces regression of the middle segment of the pro-otic sinus. The drainage of the orbito-ophthalmic veins is then taken over by the inferior petrosal sinus. The caudal end of the pro-otic sinus by secondary anastomosis reaches the sigmoid sinus. The ventral metencephalic vein (the superior petrosal sinus) drains into the junction between the sigmoid and transverse sinuses. Huang[139]

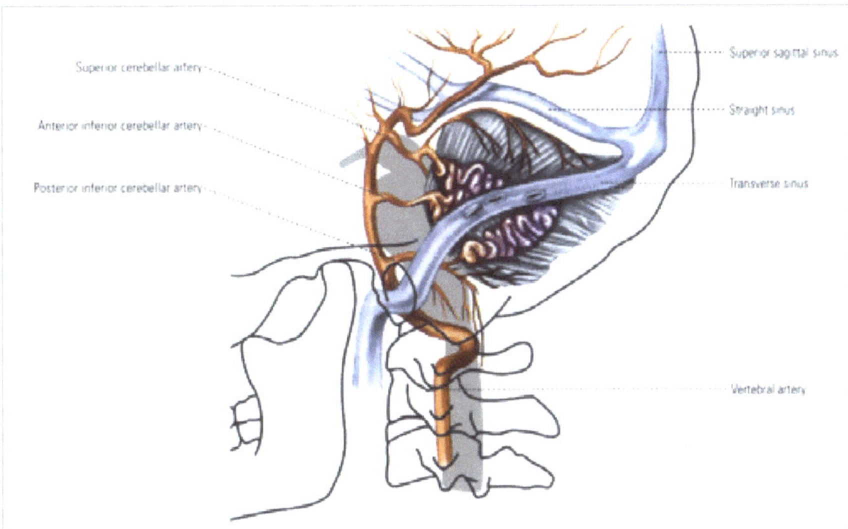

Figure 6.9 An arteriovenous malformation over the left cerebellar hmisphere. Feeding arteries come from the major intracranial branches of the basilar and vertebral arteries (Kempe's operative Neurosurgery).

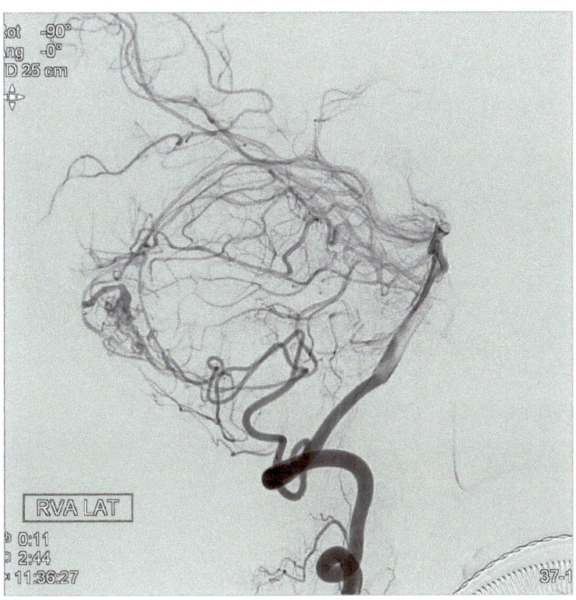

Figure 6.10 Superior Cerebellar Artery feeder (Golkar).[100]

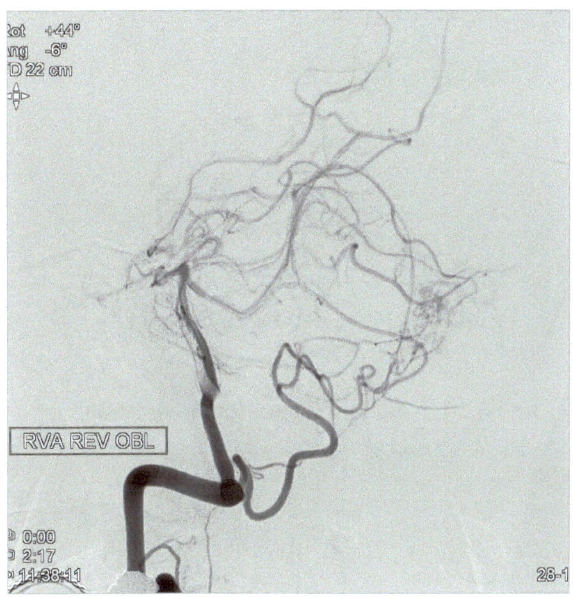

Figure 6.11 Superior Cerebellar Artery feeder. Lateral Venous drainage (Golkar).[100]

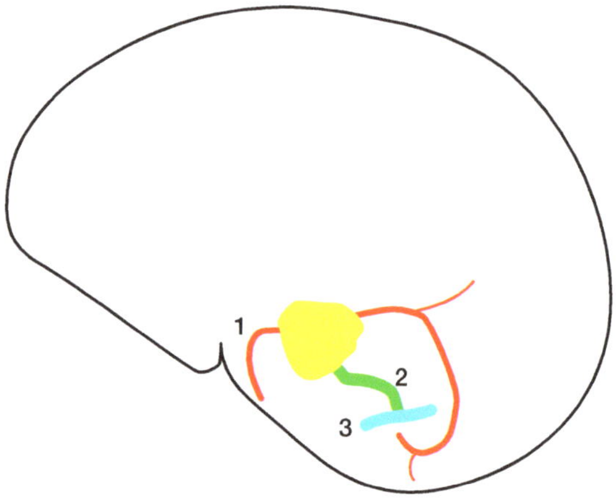

1 Sup Cerebellar A
2 V Metenceph V **3** Trans Sin

Figure 6.12 Superior Cerebellar Artery feeder. Lateral Venous drainage (Lateral view).

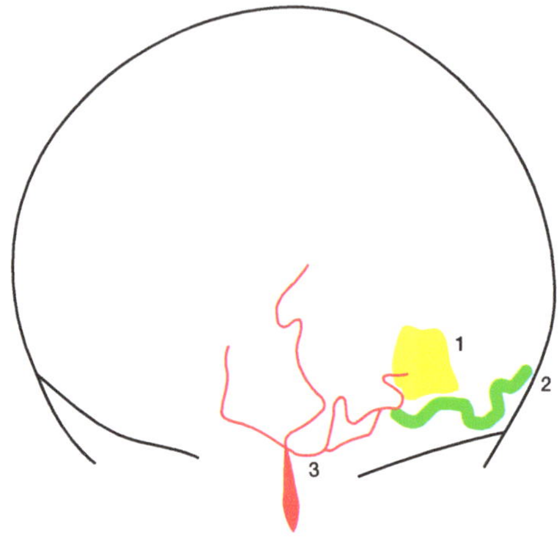

1 Angioma **2** Vent Metenceph
3 Sup Cerebel A

Figure 6.13 Superior Cerebellar Artery feeder. Lateral Venous drainage (AP View).

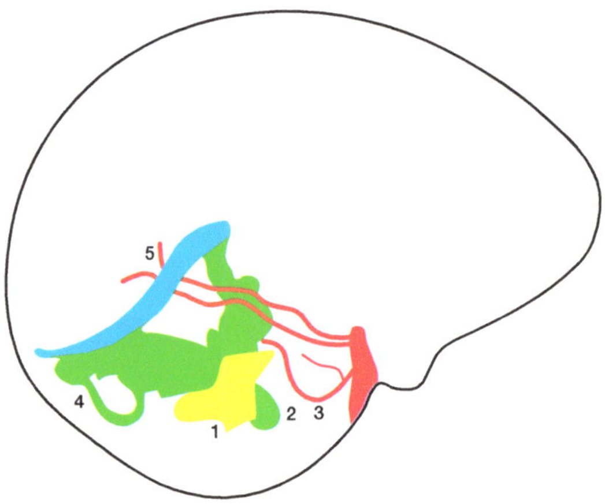

1 Angioma **2** Trans Sin **3** Sup Cerebel A
4 Dors Metenceph V **5** STR Sinus

Figure 6.14 Superior Cerebellar Artery feeder. Medial Venous drainage (Lateral view).

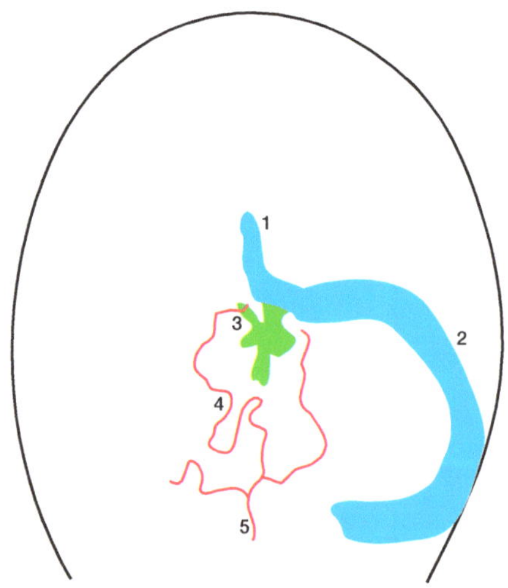

1 GR Cerebral V **2** Trans Sin **3** Dors Metenceph V
4 Sup Cerebellar A **5** Baskar A

Figure 6.15 Dorsal Metencphalic V Lateral drainage (Lateral).

In the above example, the normal adult anatomical configuration of the superior petrosal sinus is not clear because of the arrest in the normal developmental changes within the ventral metencephalic vein. The primary embryonic characters can be seen clearly in this example.

The superior petrosal sinus in the adult vein has secondary connections with the cavernous sinus. It can be argued, therefore, that the blood shunted from the fistula could find its way anteriorly and medially towards the cavernous sinus, but this situation is less likely to occur since the connection between the superior petrosal and cavernous sinuses is a secondary post-natal process. The primary connection between the cavernous sinus and the pro-otic sinus is medial and ventral to the otic capsule, whilst the post-natal channel is lateral and dorsal to the capsule.

Figures 6.12 - 14 are examples of Metencephalic AVMS. (The original radiographs were not suitable for reproduction).

Dorsal Metencephalic Vein Malformations

Figure 6.15 show an example where the dorsal metencephalic vein has persisted. The dorsal metencephalic vein (posterior cerebellar veins) meets in loops and joins the infratentorial sinus. This, in turn, joins the transverse sinus through a single trunk near the torcula. The loop of vessel near the medial end of the transverse sinus indicates the final termination of the dorsal metencephalic vein. The opacification of the straight sinus is probably retrograde.

The venous phase of the angiograms shows the opacification of the transverse sinus better than that of the straight sinus. If the blood is shunted into the transverse sinus near the torcula, it is not difficult to imagine the possibility of a retrograde filling in the straight sinus. At the time this shunting is likely to have occurred in the embryo, the function of the internal cerebral vein is still very minor, and therefore, the volume of blood flowing towards the torcula is unlikely to be more than the abnormally shunted stream flowing in the opposite direction.

The basal vein around the 80-mm stage is still in the process of formation and establishing connections with the internal cerebral vein. The retrograde flow can occur in this channel also. The course and direction of this channel for this example resemble the basal vein in the process of formation. The persistence of the embryonic features is related to the retrograde flow from the fistula, which has prevented its usual stages of development by creating abnormal circulatory conditions. The dilated and tortuous nature of this vein is similar to that of the varicose veins seen in other parts of the vascular system (extracranially), subjected to similar abnormal circulatory conditions.

In this section of the brain the primary lateral drainage of the pia-arachnoidal veins into the transverse sinus, being efficient, is retained in the adult. Therefore, when an arteriovenous fistula occurs, the same mode of drainage is maintained. Thus, the malformations arising from the metencephalic arteries shunt the blood primarily into the transverse sinus. It reaches the sinus either at the sigmoid end or at the torcula end, depending upon whether the ventral metencephalic or the dorsal metencephalic vein is involved in the lesion, respectively.

Occasionally, the drainage from the ventral metencephalic vein can get diverted into the internal cerebral vein via the anastomosis with the mesencephalic vein. But the primary lateral drainage of the dorsal metencephalic vein persists as a rule.

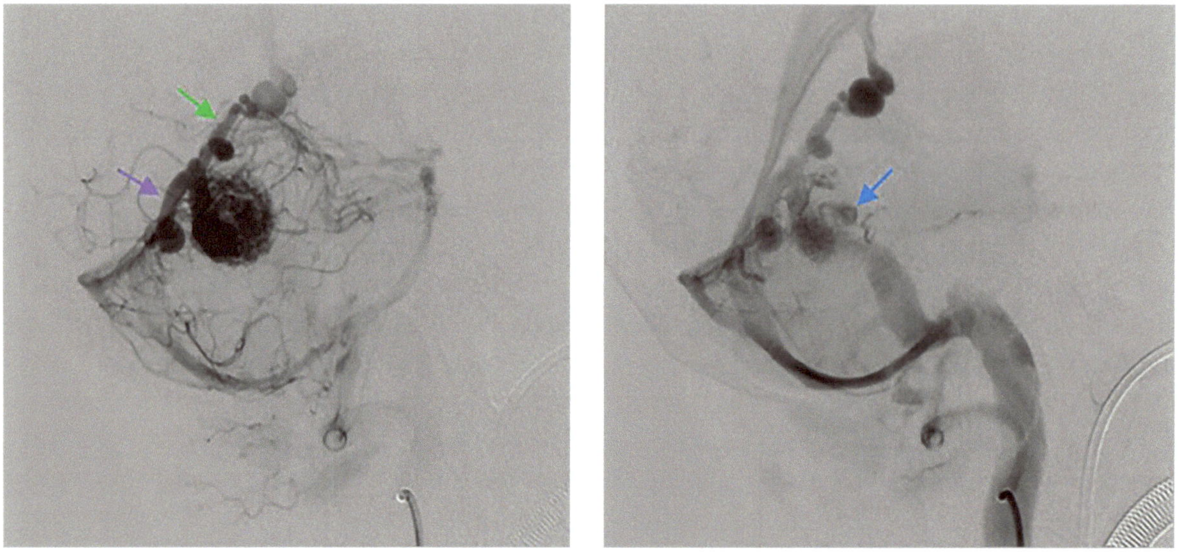

Figure 6.16 Dorsal Metencephalic venous drainage (Radiopedia).

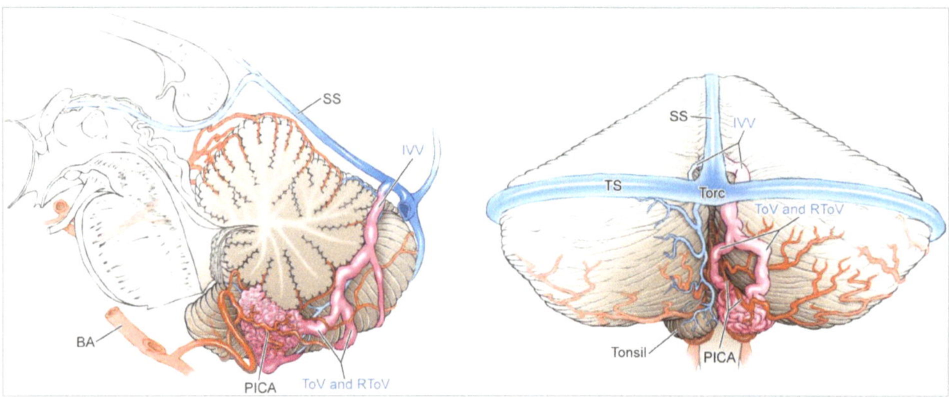

Figure 6.17 FDorsal Metencephalic Venous drainage (Kempe's Operative Neurosurgery).

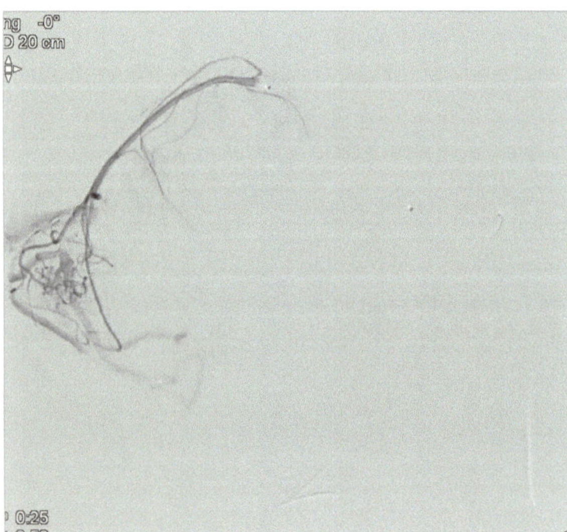

Figure 6.18 Dorsal Metencephalic Venous Drainage (Golkar).[100]

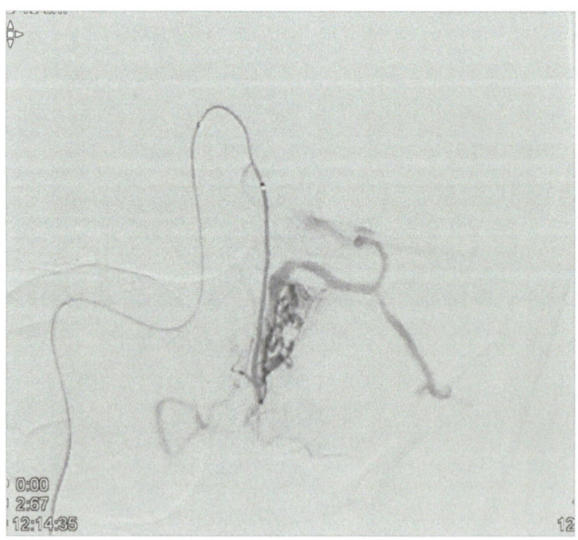

Figure 6.19 Dorsal Metencephalic venous drainage (Golkar).[100]

7

Mesencephalic Abnormalities

The primitive mesencephalon develops into the midbrain and aqueduct. The segmental pial vessels, namely, mesencephalic artery and vein, are represented in the arteriovenous fistulae of this region. In the adult the mesencephalic artery is often inconspicuous as it is incorporated into the stem of the posterior cerebral artery.

The mesencephalon is the part of the brain extending between the diencephalon cranially and the metencephalon caudally. It represents the midbrain in the adult. During the early stages of development, this segment of the brain constitutes a large proportion of the primitive brain. The rate of growth in this section being slower when compared with that in the rest of the neural tube in the adult, the midbrain enclosing the aqueduct (the remnant of a once large cavity of the mesencephalic vesicle) is inconspicuous.

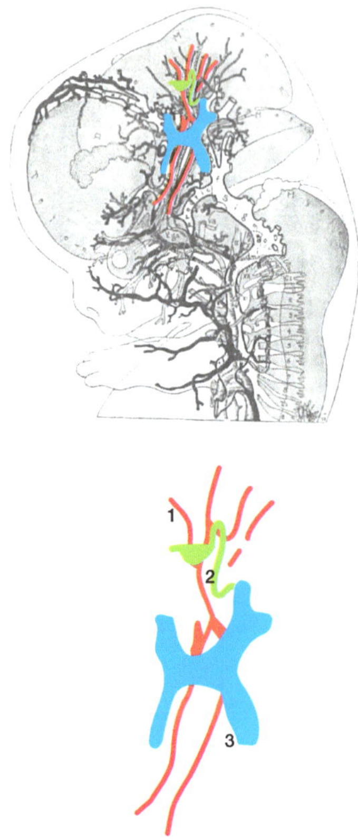

Figure 7.1 Mesencephalic vessels.

The Arterial Components of the Mesencephalon

The mesencephalic arteries arise independently from the primitive cerebro-arterial ring (see Figure 7.1 and Figue 7.2). During the process of development, this is incorporated in the stem of the adjoining diencephalic (the posterior cerebral) artery. These mesencephalic arteries in the adult are often represented as branches of the posterior cerebral artery.

The Angiomatous Elements in the Mesencephalon

Figure 7.1 and Figure 7.2 show the characteristic relationship between the mesencephalic arteries and the basal veins. These cross each other at right angles. There are chances of an arteriovenous fistula occurring at these intersections.

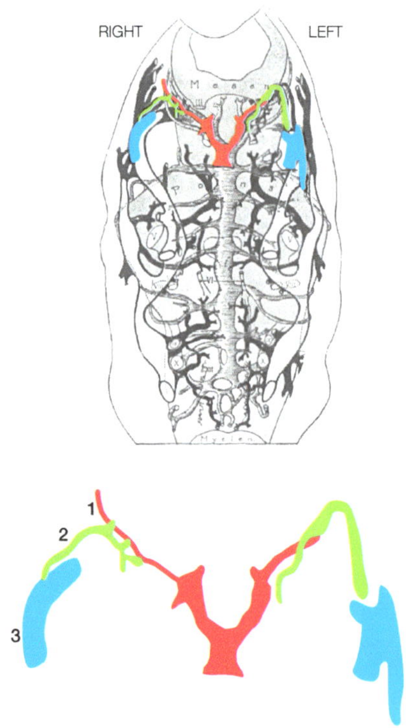

Figure 7.2 Mesencephalic vessels.

1 Mesenceph A **2** Mesenceph V **3** Tran Sin

The Venous Elements of the Malformation

The mesencephalic vein primarily courses laterally and downwards to reach the transverse sinus. Although this is often very conspicuous in the early stages of development, subsequent developmental alterations tend to produce atritic changes in this vessel. This draining territory is often taken over by the adjoining diencephalic veins. Sometimes this vein in the region of the lateral mesencephalic sulcus establishes an anastomosis between the great anterior cerebellar vein and the basal vein. This anastomosing vein, namely, the lateral mesencephalic vein, represents the drainage of the basal vein into the petrosal sinus seen in the lower primates (Hedon 1888[119]; Hochstetter (1938[124]; Bedford 1934[18]). The persistence of this channel may divert the blood thus into the superior petrosal sinus.

Regrouping According to the Similarity of Venous Pattern

In mesencephalic malformations, venous channels course around the region of the midbrain and drain medially into the great cerebral vein. Frequently, the diencephalic vein takes over the drainage, and the above-mentioned feature, typical of the mesencephalic lesion, is obscured. Occasionally, the venous drainage could occur laterally into the transverse sinus.

Matching of the Abnormal Venous Channels with Normal Mesencephalic Veins

Although in theory an arteriovenous fistula in the midbrain ought to occur as frequently as elsewhere, in practice this does not appear to be so.

The pia-arachnoidal vein initially drains laterally into the transverse sinus to be later diverted medially by the development of the basal vein.

There are two possible explanations:

1. Since in this region the degree of specialisation and the rate of growth are less compared with the rest of the brain, there is correspondingly a diminished need for the formation of new vessels. This probably decreases the chances of an arteriovenous fistula occurring.
2. The mesencephalic pia-arachnoidal vein initially drains into the transverse sinus to be diverted later medially with the development of the basal vein. Since this feature is similar to those of the diencephalic vein, still distinguishing one from the other is often very difficult.

Regrouping of the Adult Mesencephalic Arteries with Reference to the Embryonic Region

Incorporation of the mesencephalic artery with the posterior cerebral artery renders the malformations of this region to be grouped as under those belonging to the posterior cerebral artery lesion.

Classification Based on the Embryological Site of Formation

It is, therefore, clear from the above findings that although the mesencephalic vascular system is independent in the early stages of development, the subsequent secondary alterations make it difficult to recognise it as a different entity in many instances. Identification of the mesencephalic artery in adult angiograms is not always easy.

Theoretically Possible Variations

Figure 7.3–Figure 7.10 illustrate the theoretical interpretation of the vascular faults that represent the manner in which the mesencephalic vein may persist into the adult life in the presence of an arteriovenous fistula (Vidyasagar[337&339]).

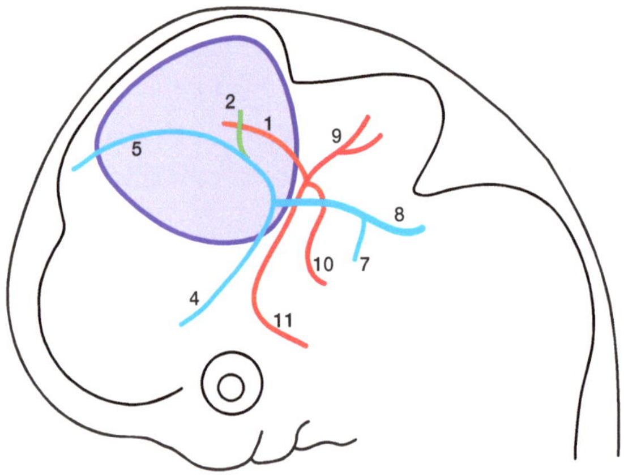

Figure 7.3 Mesencephalic vein draining into the junction between the tentorial and transverse sinus at 20mm (Lateral).

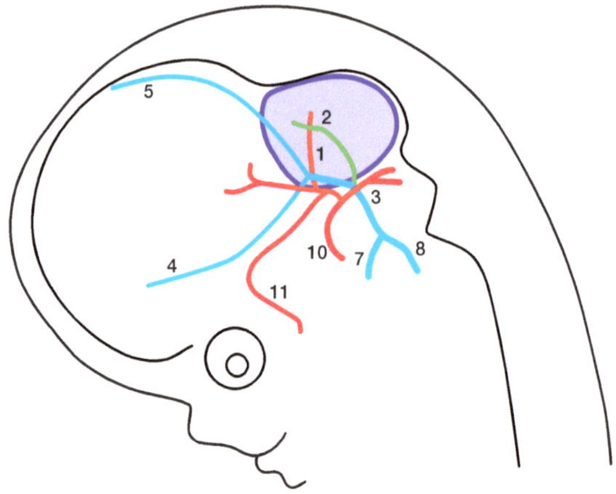

Figure 7.4 Mesencephalic vein draining into the junction between the tentorial and transverse sinus at 40mm (Lateral).

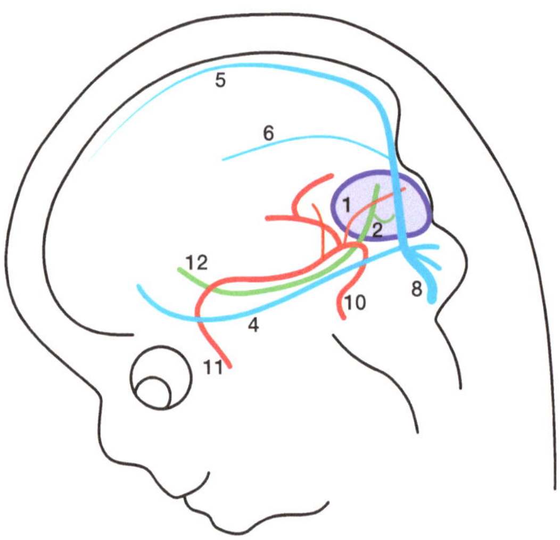

Figure 7.5 Mesencephalic vein draining into the transverse sinus at 80mm (Lateral).

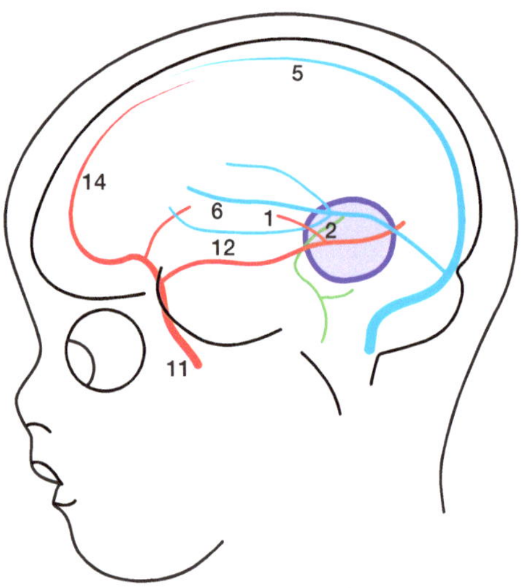

Figure 7.6 Mesencephalic vein draining into the great cerebral vein in the adult (Lateral).

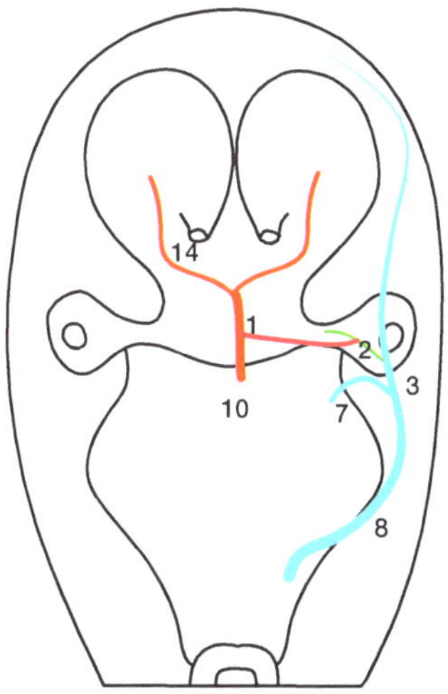

Figure 7.7 Mesencephalic vein draining into the junction between the tentorial and transverse sinus at 20mm (Basal).

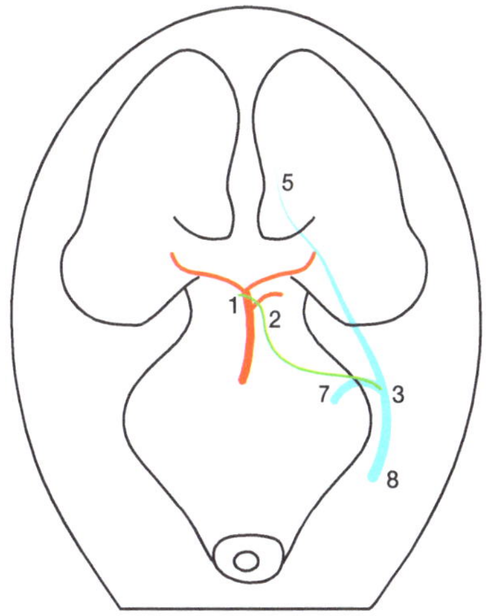

Figure 7.8 Mesencephalic vein draining into the junction between the tentorial and transverse sinus at 40mm (Basal).

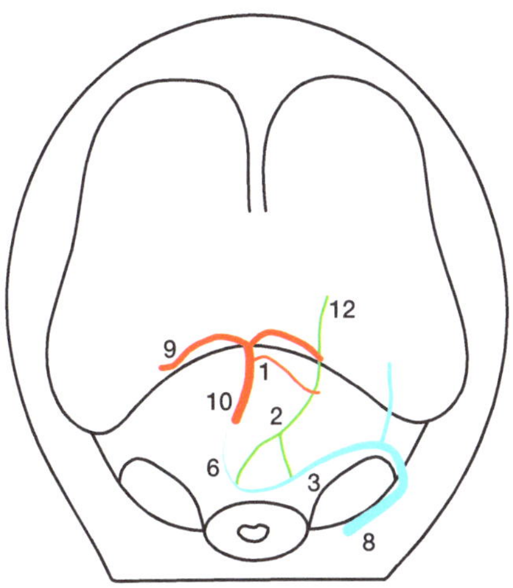

Figure 7.9 Mesencephalic vein draining into the transverse sinus at 80mm (Basal).

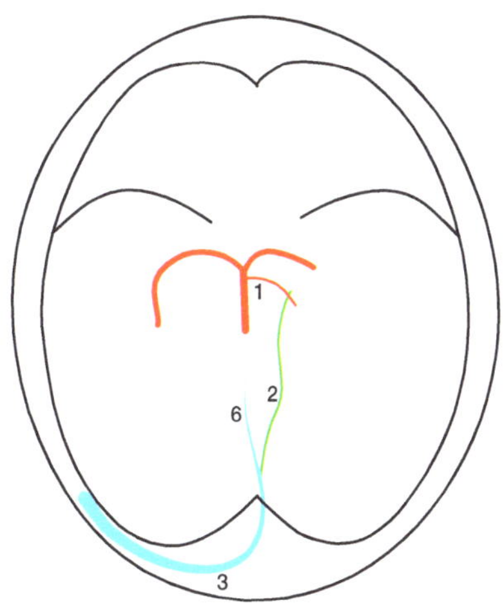

Figure 7.10 Mesencephalic vein draining into the cerebral vein in the adult (Basal).

1 Mesenceph A **2** Mesenceph V **3** Tran Sin **4** Tentorial Sin **5** Sup Sagitt Sin
6 Int Cerebral V **7** Pro-Otic S **8** Sigmoid Sin **9** Post Cerebral A **10** Basilar A
11 Int Carotid A **12** Basal V **13** Inf Sagitt Sin **14** Ant Cerebral A **15** Int Carotid A

Examples

No example was found in the present series to indicate the anatomical features of this lesion clearly. Therefore, Figure 7.13 are borrowed from the work of Alpers and Forster[6] to illustrate the hypothesis. The same standard colour code is also used here. It will be noted that in the original descriptions, vessels numbered 4–7 are labelled as aberrant arteries show the course and direction of these arteries encircling the midbrain. These vessels represent the mesencephalic arteries.

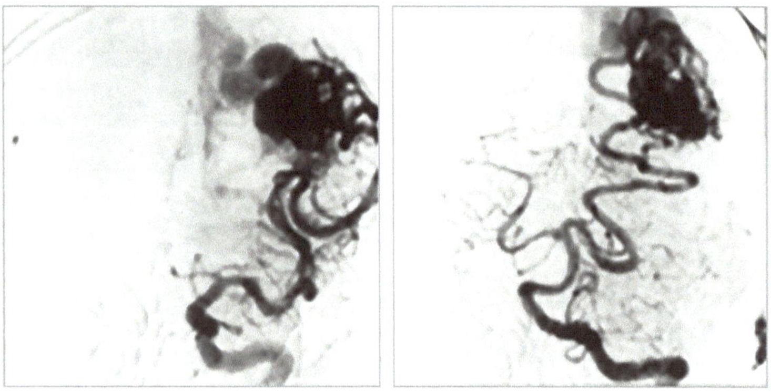

Figure 7.11 Mesencephalic vein draining into the great cerebral vein Radiopedia.

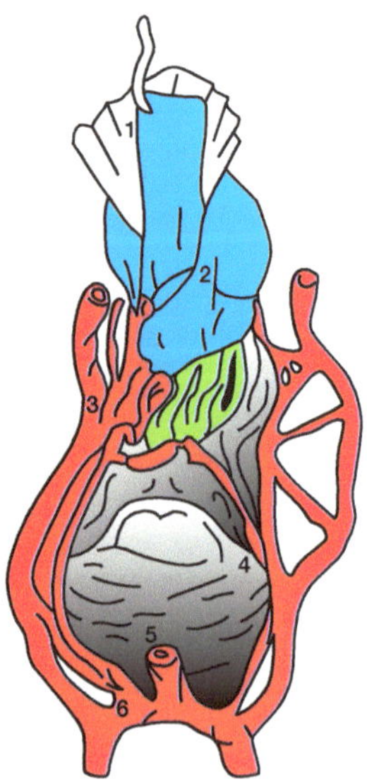

1 Straight Sin **2** Vein of Galen **3** Post Ceres A
4 Mesenceph A **5** Basilar A **6** Post Comm A

Figure 7.12 To be provided as above (Alpers &Forster[6]).

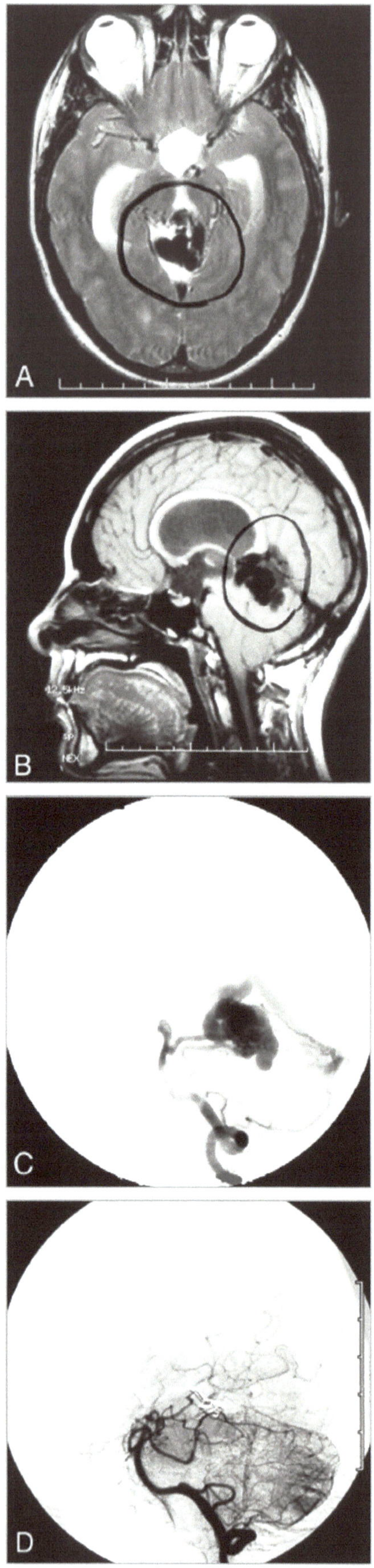

The dilatation of the vein of Galen is clearly seen, but the mesencephalic veins are not very conspicuous. The segments of the vessel marked Green on the overlay represent this vein draining into the internal cerebral vein. It can also be observed that in the original description this was just mentioned as an angiomatous plexus of vessels. It is probably relevant to include the original description of the authors at this point: 'The basilar artery divided normally into two posterior cerebral arteries, but a branch from each posterior cerebral vessel could be followed coursing around the mesencephalon, sending branches into the aneurysm. On the tectum of the midbrain lay a large maze of vessels connected with the posterior cerebral artery, sending many branches into the wall of the aneurysm.' The maze of the vessels on the tectum represents the persisting mesencephalic veins. This example indicates very clearly how the mesencephalic malformations are difficult to recognise as a different entity and get grouped under those arising from the posterior cerebral artery.

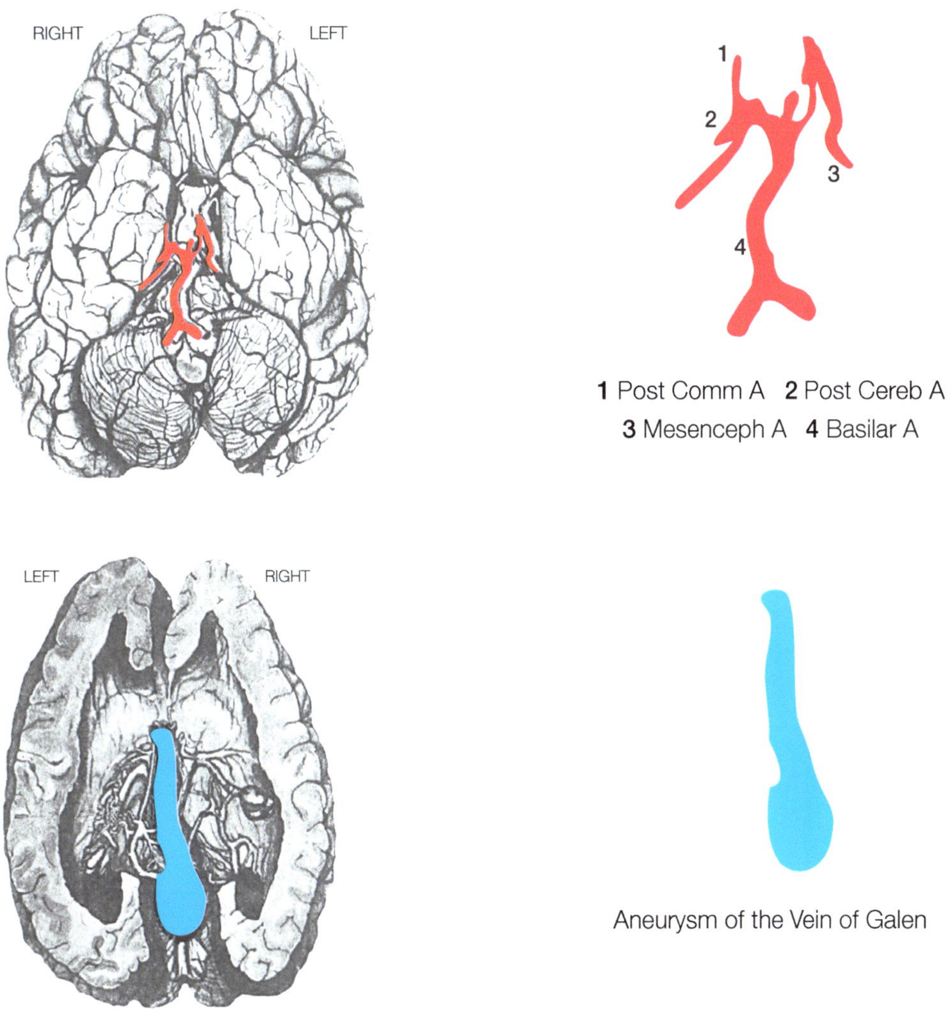

Figure 7.13 Mesencephalic AVM (Alpers and Forster[6]).

8

Diencephalic Abnormalities

Diencephalon develops into thalamus, hypothalamus, Geniculate bodies, pineal gland, mamillary bodies, and Choroid plexuses. The anterior choroidal artery, the posterior choroidal artery, and posterior cerebral arteries represent the segmental pial arteries in the adult. Dorsal and ventral diencephalic veins persist in the adult in the arteriovenous malformations of this area.

The pattern of blood supply seen so far in the myelencephalon, the metencephalon, and the mesencephalon is not very different from that of the spinal cord, as they retain the segmental pattern to a large extent. The development of the diencephalon has certain special features. It is essentially developed from the dorsal elements of the primitive notochord. The ventral elements are not represented (see Figure 8.1 and Figure 8.2). These figures indicate diagrammatically the two existing theories on the development of the diencephalon. The variations in the two figures mainly consist of the degree of incorporation of the alar plates into the formation of the rest of the midbrain. The reader is referred to the original description by Arey (1965)[10] for a more detailed discussion on the subject.

The diencephalic abnormalities have been divided into two sections:

1. Posterior Cerebral Artery Dorsal
2. Posterior Choroidal Artery Diencephalic vein

Posterior Cerebral Artery Dorsal

The Arterial Components of the Malformation

There are two arteries involved in the malformations of this section. They are as follows:

1. Posterior cerebral artery
2. Posterior choroidal artery

Figure 8.3 Figure 8.4, which are the photographic reproductions from the work of Padget, show the vascular system of the diencephalon.

Both the posterior cerebral and the posterior choroidal arteries are crossed by the dorsal diencephalic vein before draining into the tentorial sinus.

During the further stages of the development, the posterior choroidal artery is incorporated into the posterior cerebral artery.

The Angiomatous Elements of the Malformation

The angiomatous elements in this lesion tend to vary a great deal, both in size and situation (see Charts 4 and 2). In seven cases the angioma was situated in the supratentorial region and in two cases in the infratentorial region. It was absent in one case. These variations indicate the confusion created when these malformations are classified according to the site of the angioma. It will be made clear in the following discussion how the location of the angioma itself is not relevant to the classification of these malformations.

The Venous Elements of the Malformations

The venous channels in these lesions mainly consisted of two types. The most frequent pattern was a channel coursing upwards, backwards, and medially into the great cerebral vein. Occasionally, there were channels draining laterally into the tentorial sinus.

Regrouping of Cases According to the Similarity of Venous Pattern

The abnormal venous channels in this group are generally directed upwards and medially into the great cerebral vein. This is the most frequently seen pattern. Occasionally, the vein could drain laterally into the transverse sinus.

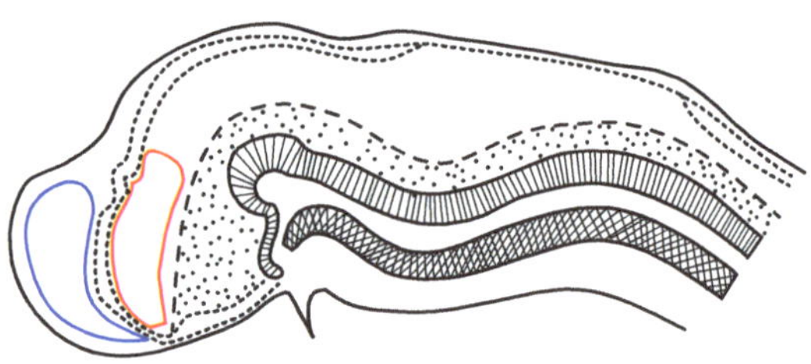

Figure 8.1 Formation of telencephalon and diencephalon from the alar plates (Arey)[10] (concept A).

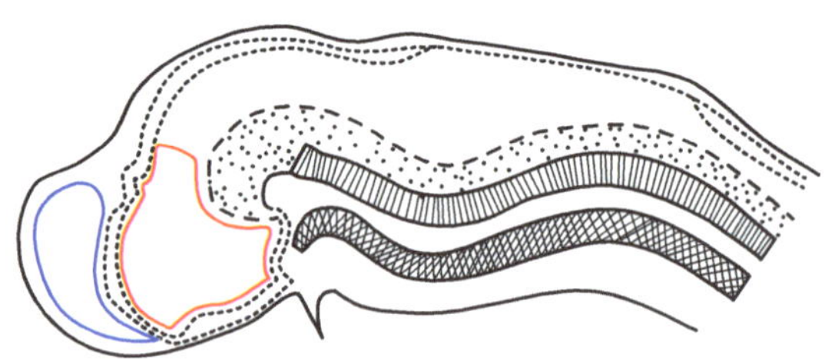

Figure 8.2 Formation of telencephalon and diencephalon from the alar plates (Arey)[10] (concept B).

Matching of the Abnormal Vascular Channels with the Normal Embryonic Channels

The abnormal venous channels could be matched with the two of the diencephalic pia-arachnoidal veins, namely, the dorsal and ventral diencephalic veins. The comparison was easy with reference to the dorsal diencephalic veins, whilst the similarities between the ventral diencephalic vein and the venous channels were less clear. These cases could be classified into two sections with reference to the pia-arachnoidal vein involved.

Regrouping of the Arterial Elements with Reference to Embryonic Features

The malformations arising from the posterior cerebral and posterior choroidal arteries were classified into one section where the persistent venous channels represented the dorsal diencephalic vein. The malformations involving the anterior choroidal artery had venous channels comparable to those of the ventral diencephalic vein.

The New Classification Based on the Embryological Site of the Malformation

Both the posterior cerebral and the posterior choroidal arteries belong to the diencephalic segment of the developing brain. The dorsal diencephalic vein crosses both these arteries at approximately right angles (Vidyasagar[337]) (see Figure 8.3 and Figure 8.4).

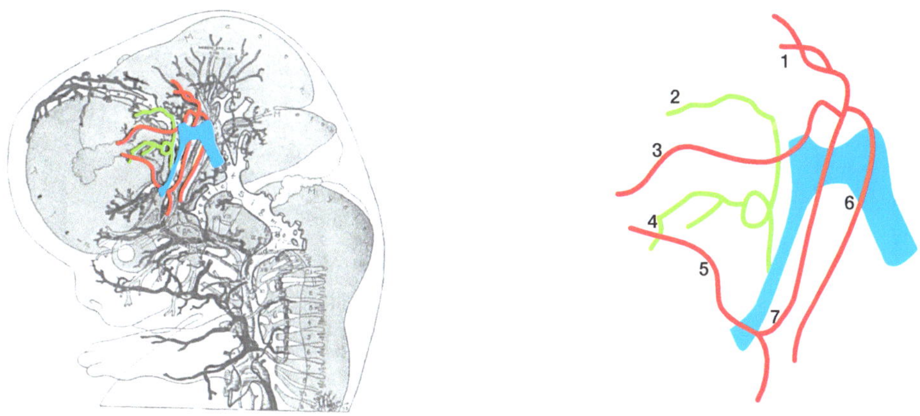

Figure 8.3 Dorsal and ventral diencephalic veins draining into the tentorial sinus at 23mm (Lateral).

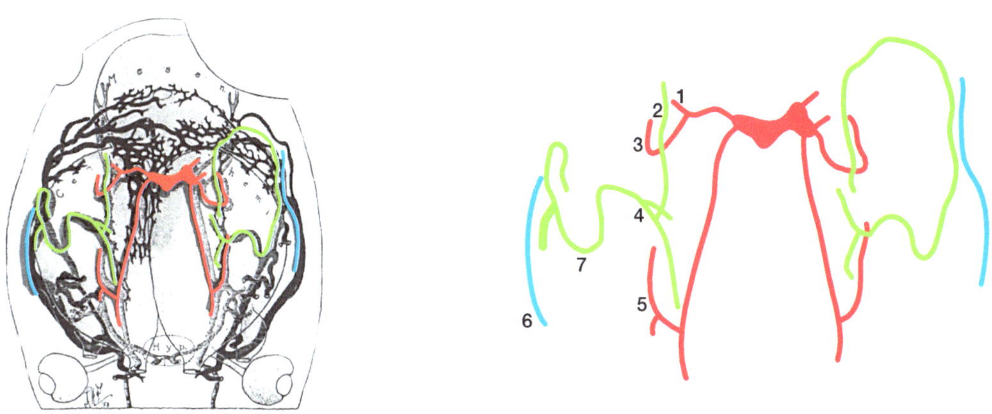

Figure 8.4 Dorsal and ventral diencephalic veins draining into the tentorial sinus at 23mm (Frontal).

1 Post Cerebral A **2** Dors Dienceph V **3** Post Choroid A
4 Vent Dienceph V **5** Ant Choroid A **6** Transv Sin **7** Tent Sin

The Hypothesis

Figure 8.5–Figure 8.12 indicate the theoretical interpretation of the manner in which the dorsal diencephalic vein may persist into adult life in the presence of an arteriovenous fistula. For the purposes of convenience, the changes are divided into four stages: 20 mm, 40 mm, 80 mm, and the adult. The vessels marked Green indicate the course and direction of the persistent dorsal diencephalic vein. It can be appreciated from these diagrams the manner in which the embryonic vessels change their course and direction in accordance with the structural changes in the developing brain and anatomical changes in the vascular system. In Figure 8.6 the dorsal diencephalic vein has a course downwards and laterally into the tentorial sinus, but in Figure 8.7 the course is changed to upwards, backwards, and medially into the internal cerebral vein. The medial direction of the vein is due to the development of the basal vein which diverts the flow into the internal cerebral vein. These changes can be more easily seen in figures.

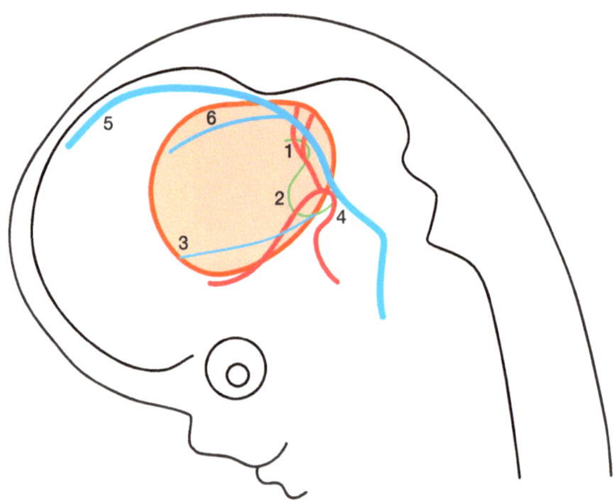

Figure 8.5 Dorsal diencephalic vein draining into the tentorial sinus at 20mm (Lateral).

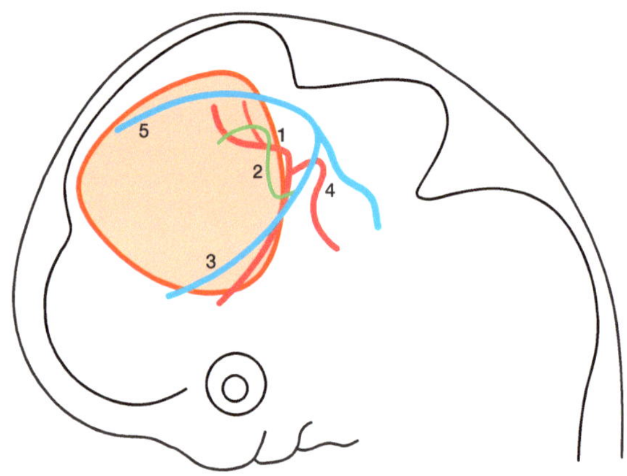

Figure 8.6 Dorsal diencephalic vein draining into the tentorial sinus at 40mm (Lateral).

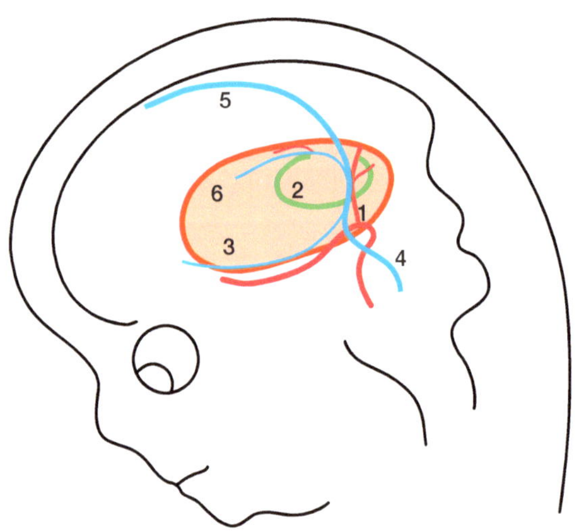

Figure 8.7 Dorsal diencephalic vein draining into the tentorial sinus at 80mm (Lateral).

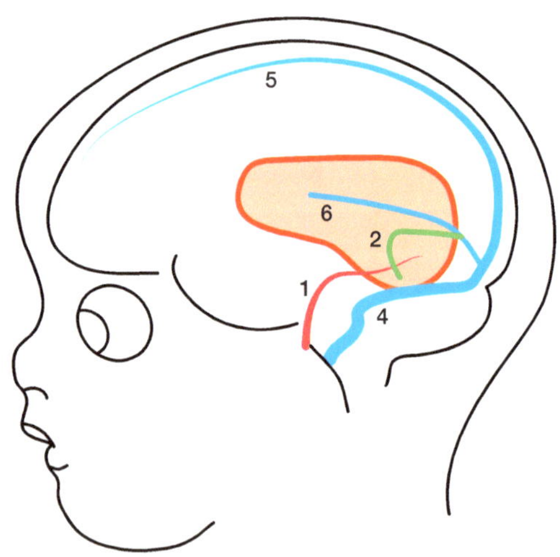

Figure 8.8 Dorsal diencephalic vein draining into the tentorial sinus in the adult (Lateral).

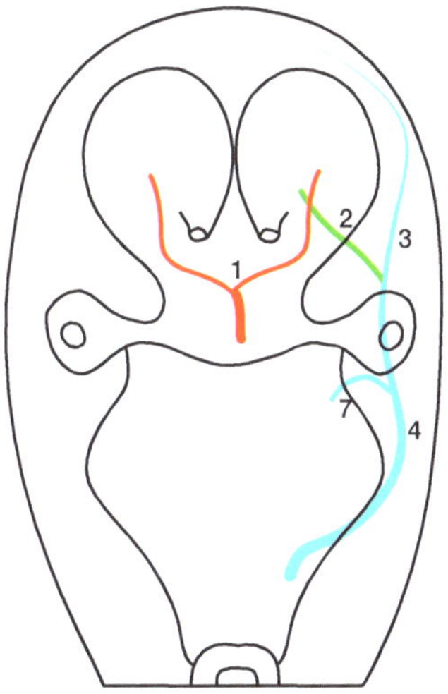

Figure 8.9 Dorsal diencephalic vein draining into the tentorial sinus at 20mm (Basal).

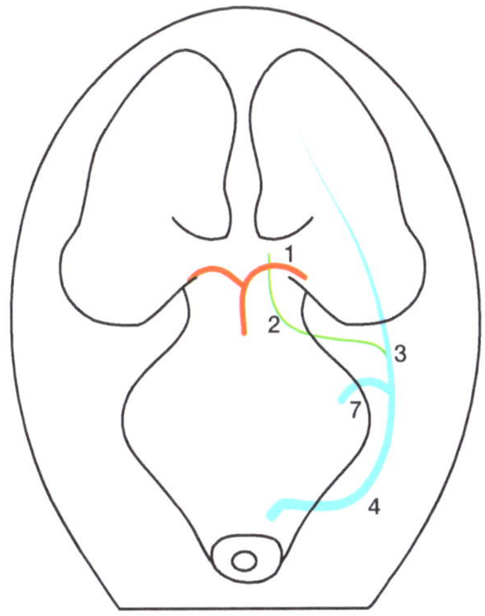

Figure 8.10 Dorsal diencephalic vein draining into the tentorial sinus at 40mm (Basal).

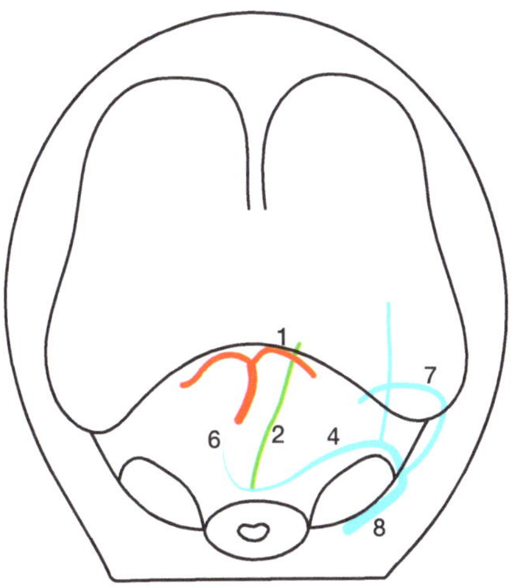

Figure 8.11 Dorsal diencephalic vein draining into the tentorial sinus at 80mm (Basal).

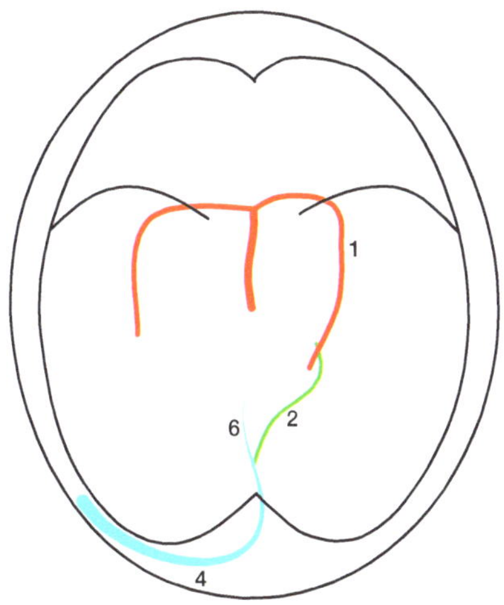

Figure 8.12 Dorsal diencephalic vein draining into the tentorial sinus in the adult (Basal).

1 Post Cerebral A **2** Dors Dienceph V **3** Tent Sin **4** Trans Sin
5 Sup Sagitt Sin **6** Int Cerebral V **7** Pro-Otic Sin **8** Sigmoid Sin

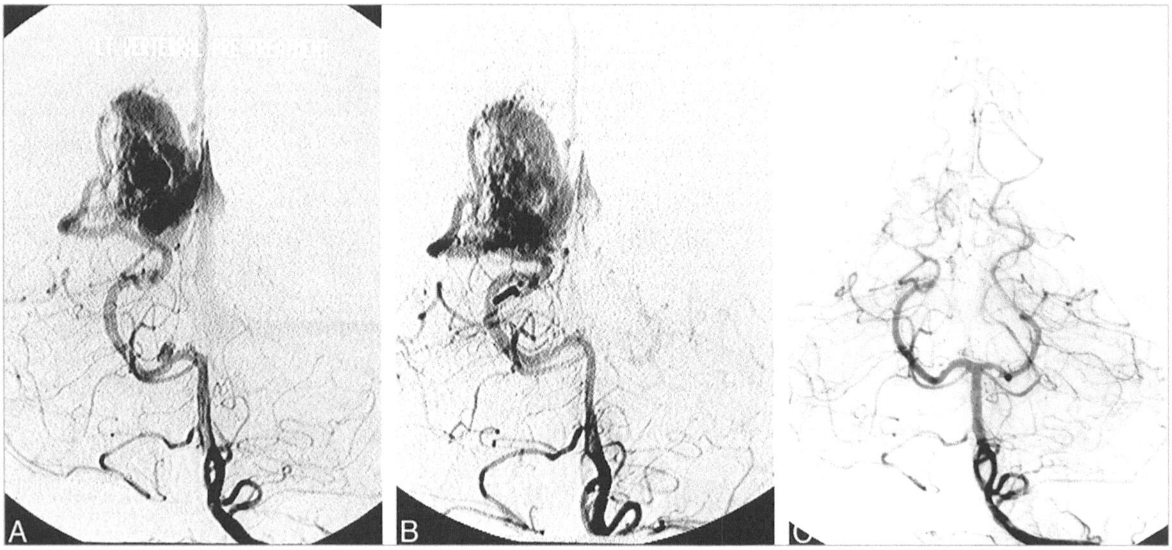

Figure 8.13 Arteriovenous malformation is produced by the left posterior cerebral artery (Radiopedia).

Figure 8.14 to Figure 8.16 show an example where the arteriovenous malformation is produced by the left posterior cerebral artery. The arterio-capillary tangle is situated in the supratentorial region. The venous drainage is through a channel that is directed upwards, backwards, and medially into the internal cerebral vein. It is easy to appreciate that the course and direction taken by this vessel resemble those of the dorsal diencephalic vein, as represented in the preceding hypothetical diagrams.

Figure 8.17 to Figure 8.20 show further examples where the course and direction of the adjoining vein are similar to those seen in an earlier example. There is, of course, variations in the size of this channel, and this is related to the size of the shunt (see Chapter 14).

Figure 8.21 to Figure 8.28 show further examples of diencephalic malformations where the dorsal diencephalic vein has persisted. It can again be noted that the anatomical features of these vessels are similar to those seen before in this section. The arterio-capillary tangle (the angioma) is situated infratentorially in both these sets of examples. Except for these, the examples cited in this section are similar to those seen earlier. These indicate the disparity that exists in the location of the angioma and the problems that arise when a classification is attempted, taking the location of the angioma as the main criterion.

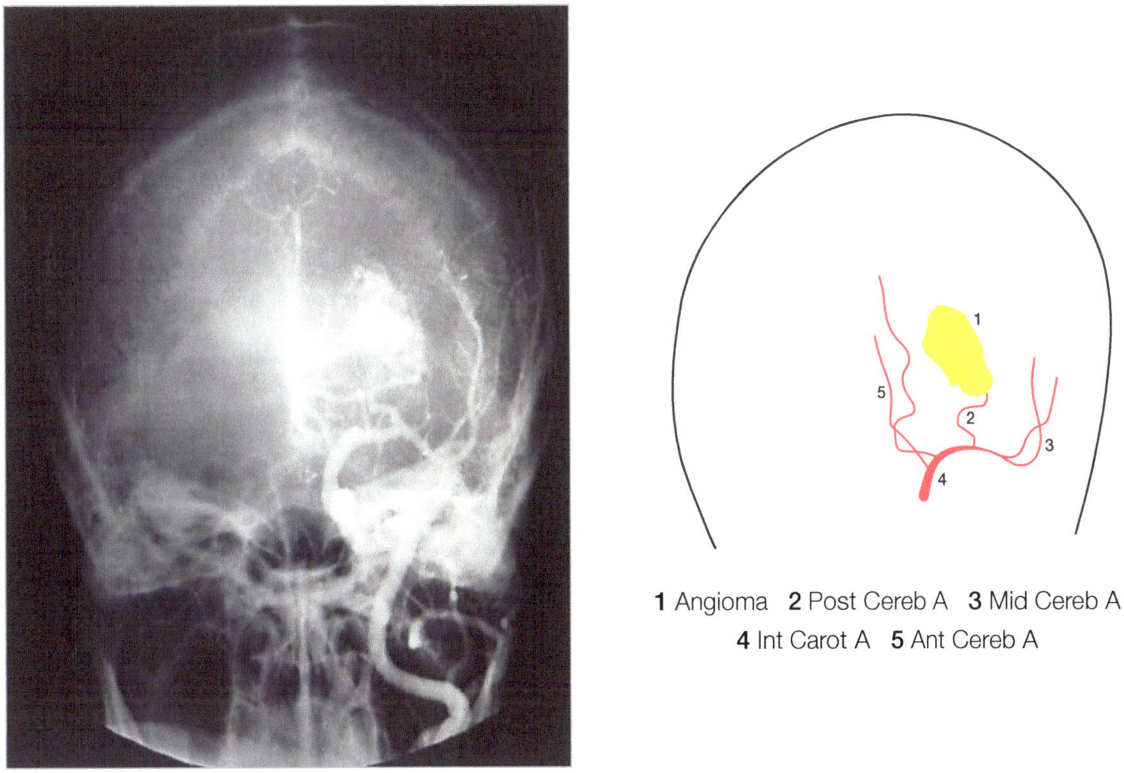

Figure 8.14 Diencephalic Arterior-Venous Malformation. Arterial Contribution from (L) posterior cerebral artery. (L) Carotid Angiogram (AP) Arterial (Radiopedia).

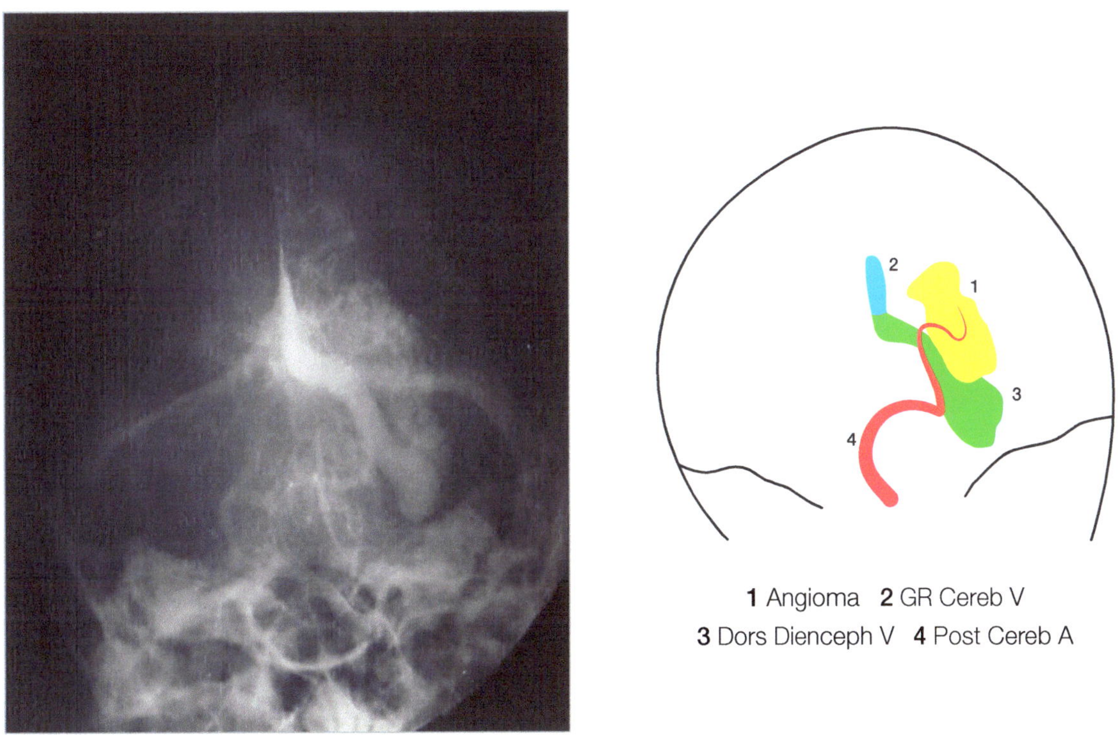

Figure 8.15 Diencephalic arterio-venous malformation. Dorsal diencephalic vein draining into the great cerebral vein (ap) (Late Arterial).

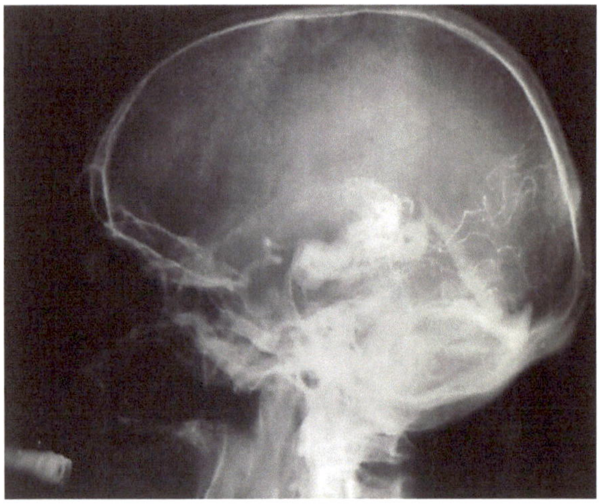

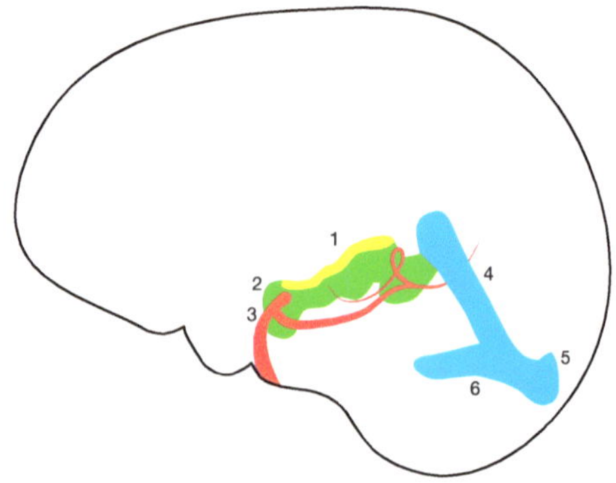

1 Angioma **2** Dors Dienceph V **3** L Post Cereb A
4 STR Sinus **5** Torcula **6** Trans Sinus

Figure 8.16 Diencephalic arterio-venous malformation arterial contribution from (L) posterior cerebral artery (ap) (Compare with Figure 8.15).

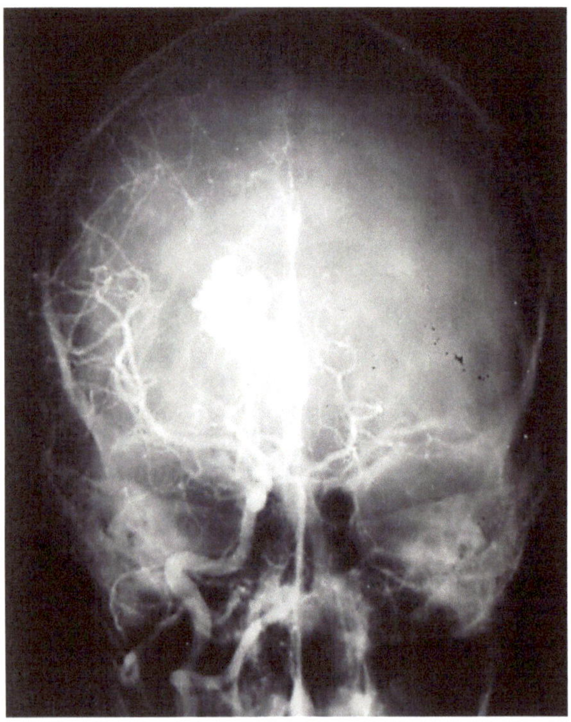

Figure 8.17 Diencephalic arterio-venous malformation. Arterial contribution from (L) posterior cerebral artery (ap) (Arterial).

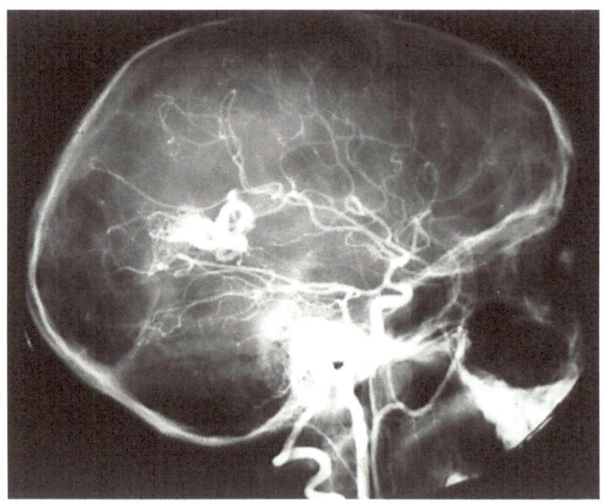

Figure 8.18 Diencephalic arterio-venous malformation arterial contribution from (L) posterior cerebral artery (Lateral) (Arterial).

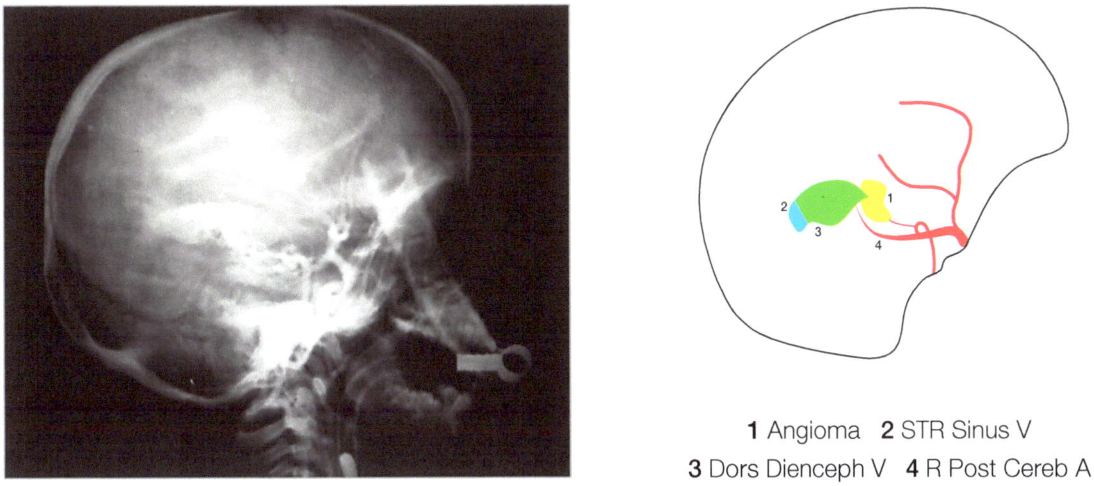

Figure 8.19 Diencephalic arterio-venous malformation. Arterial contribution from (R) posterior cerebral artery. Dorsal diencephalic vein draining into the great cerebral vein (Lateral).

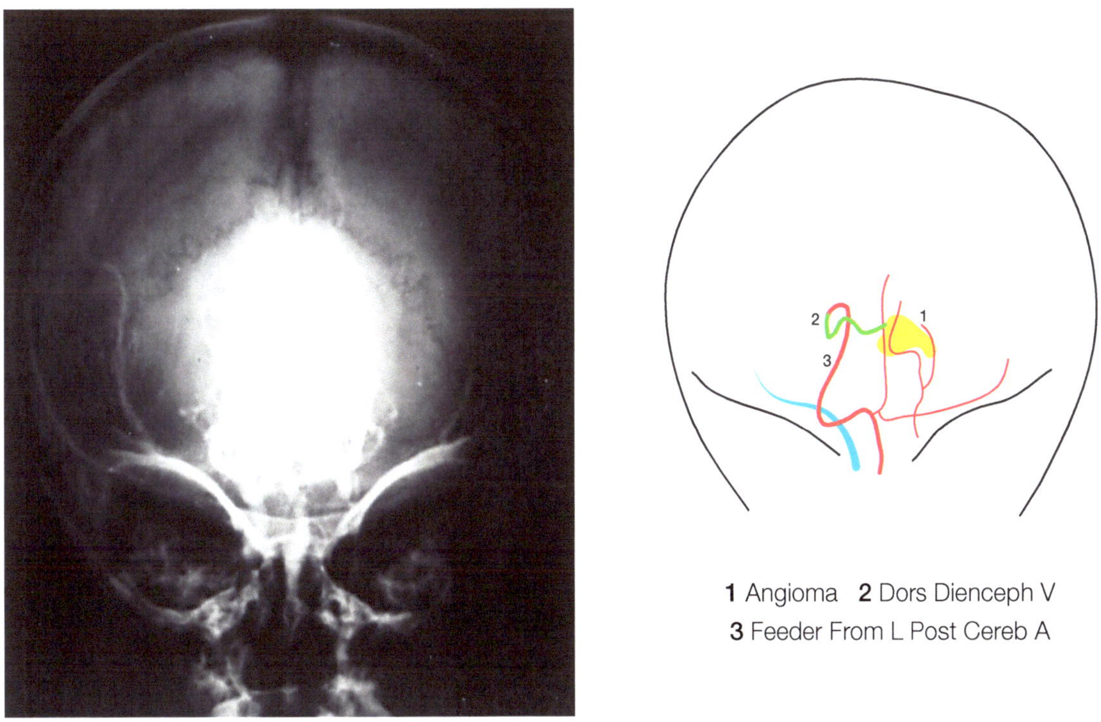

Figure 8.20 Diencephalic arterio-venous malformation. Arterial contribution from (R) posterior cerebral artery. Dorsal diencephalic vein draining into the great cerebral vein (AP).

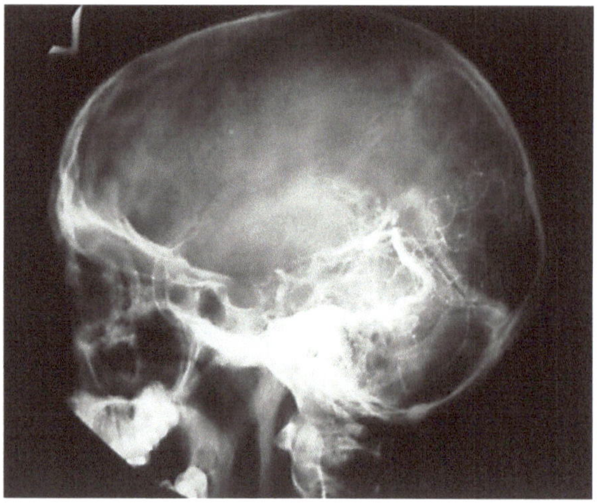

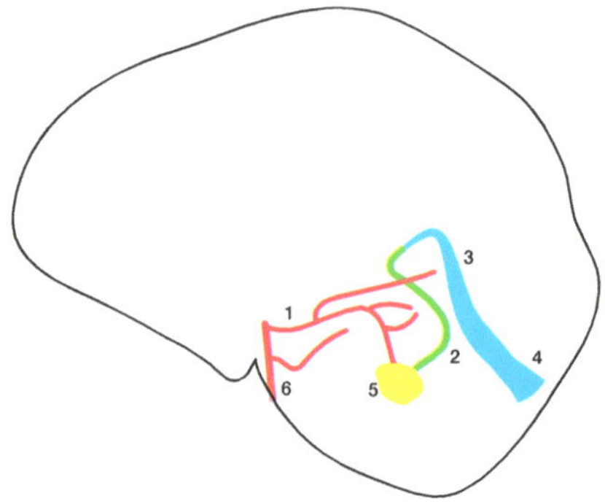

1 Post Cereb A **2** Dors Dienceph V **3** St Sin
4 Torcula **5** Angioma **6** Basilar A

Figure 8.21 Diencephalic arterio-venous malformation. Arterial contribution from (R) posterior cerebral artery. Dorsal diencephalic vein draining into the great cerebral vein (Lateral) (Early Arterial).

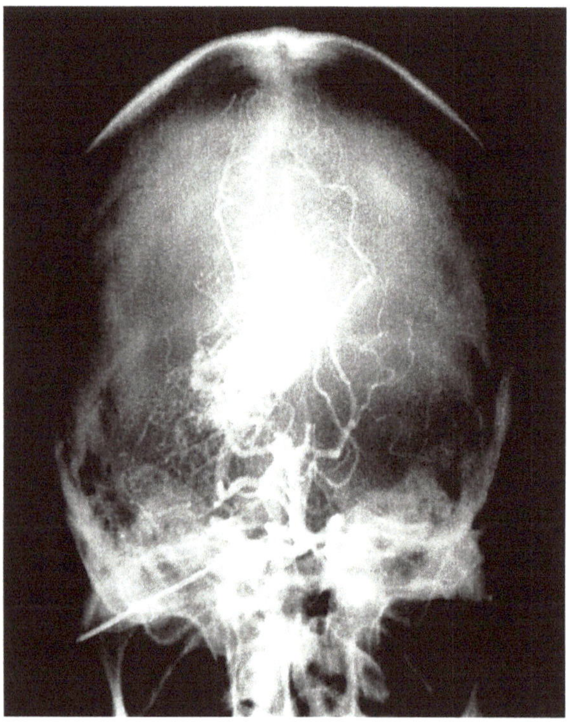

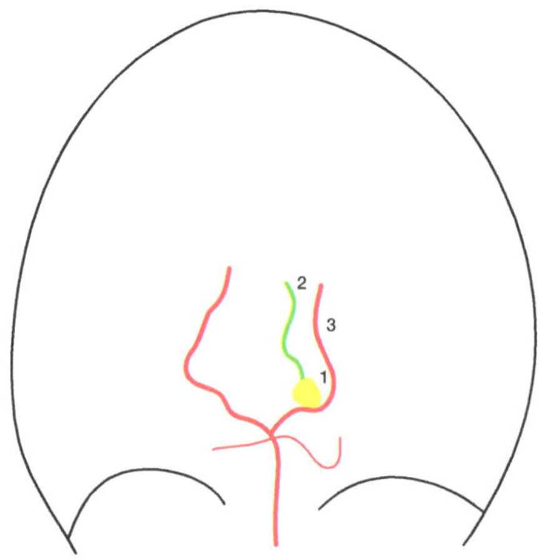

1 Angioma **2** Dors Dienceph V
3 Feeder From L Post Cereb A

Figure 8.22 Diencephalic arterio-venous malformatoin. Arterial contribution from (R) posterior cerebral artery. Dorsal diencephalic vein draining into the great cerebral vein (AP).

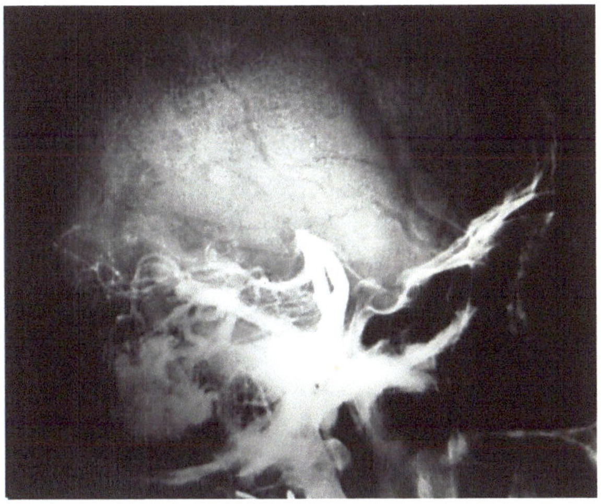

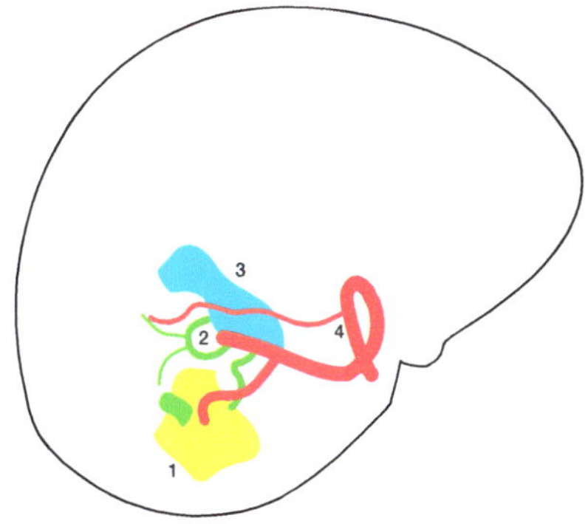

1 Angioma **2** Dors Dienceph V
3 GR Cereb V **4** Post Cereb A

Figure 8.23 Diencephalic arterio-venous malformation.
(R) Posterior cerebral artery feeder. Infra-tentorial angioma (AP).

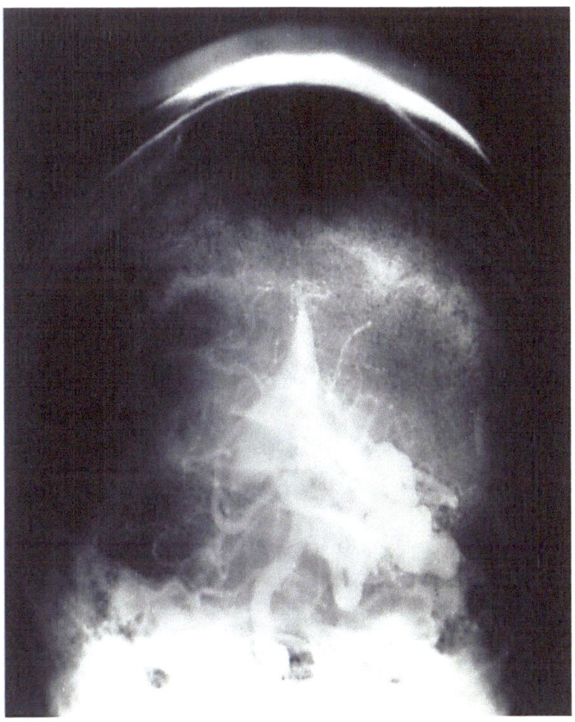

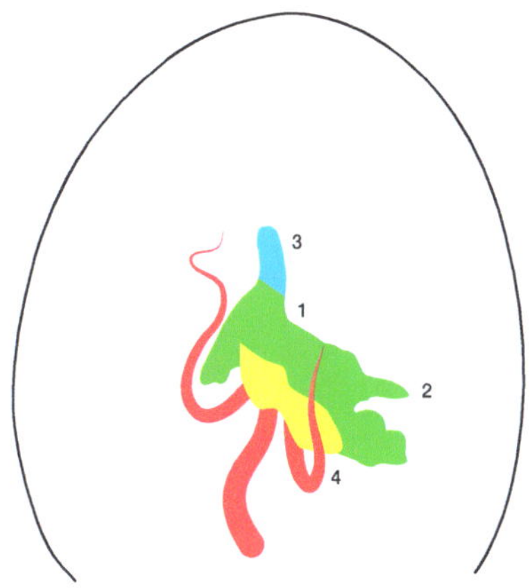

1 Angioma Shift **2** Dors Dienceph V
3 GR Cereb V **4** Post Cereb A

Figure 8.24 (R) Diencephalic arterio-venous malformation.
(R) Posterior cerebral artery feeder. Infra-tentorial angioma (Lateral).

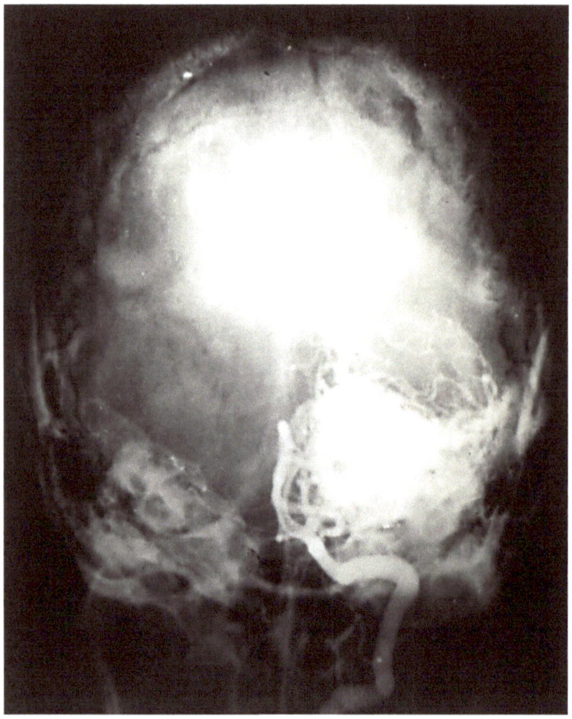

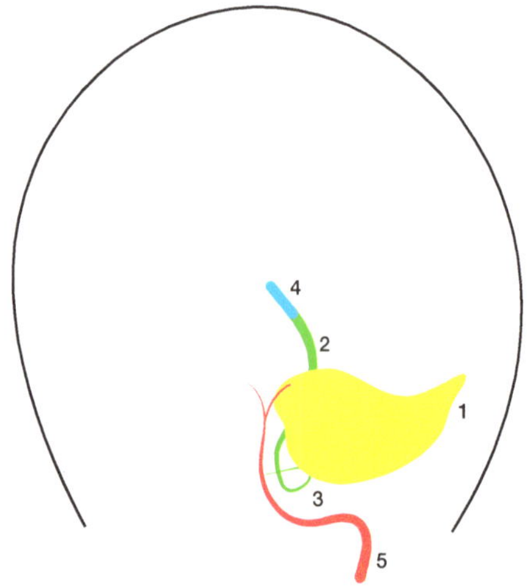

1 Angioma **2** Dors Dienceph V **3** Post Cereb A
4 GR Cereb V **5** L Verteb A

Figure 8.25 (R) Diencephalic arterio-venous malformation. (R) Posterior cerebral artery feeder. Infra-tentorial angioma (AP).

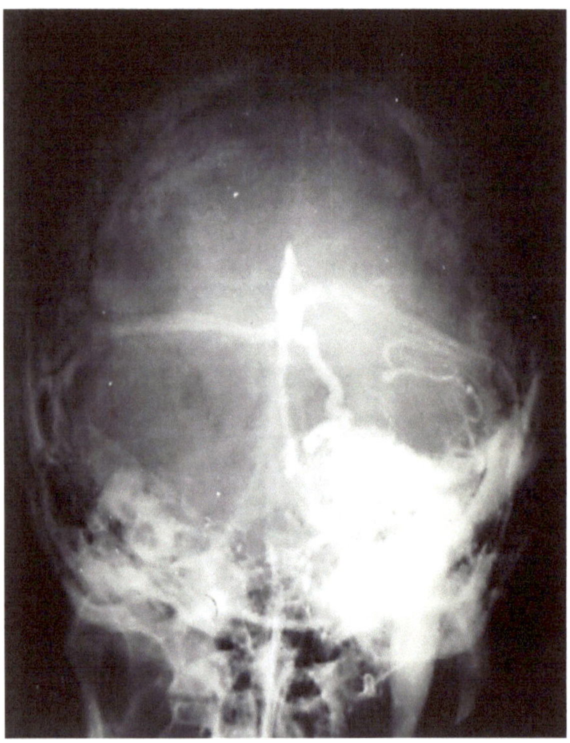

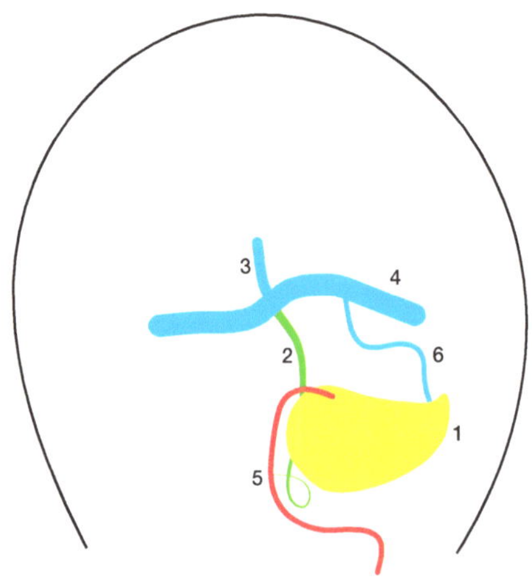

1 Angioma **2** Dors Dienceph V **3** GR Cereb V
4 Trans Sinus **5** Post Cereb A **6** Accessory Draining

Figure 8.26 Dorsal diencephalic arterio-venous malformation. Posterior cerebral artery feeder. Infra-tentorial angioma. Diencephalic vein drains into the great cerebral vein (AP) (Arterial).

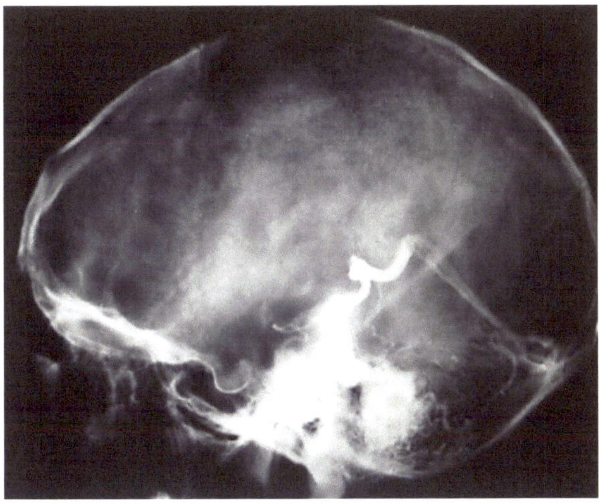

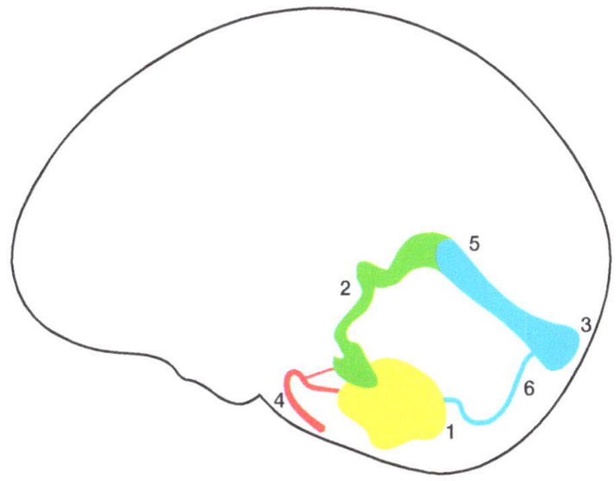

1 Angioma **2** Dors Dienceph V **3** Torcula
4 Baskar A **5** STR Sinus **6** Accessory Draining

Figure 8.27 Dorsal diencephalic arterio-venous malformation. Posterior cerebral artery feeder. Infra-tentorial angioma. Diencephalic vein drains into the great cerebral vein (AP) (Venous).

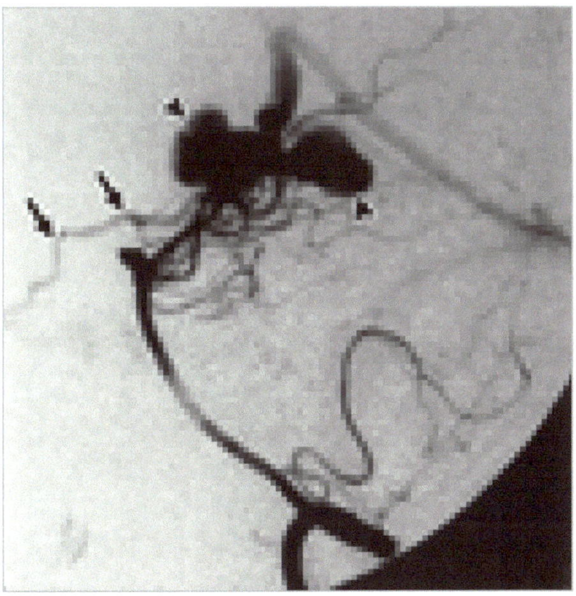

Figure 8.28 Posterior Cerebral Artery AVM Draining into internal cerebral vein (Geibpraser).[89]

Figure 8.44 shows an example of a dorsal diencephalic malformation where the venous drainage is directed laterally into the transverse sinus. This is exceptional, but can be explained on embryological terms. It was mentioned in the first section of the discussion that the segmental pia-arachnoidal veins drain primarily into the transverse sinus to be diverted medially subsequently into the internal cerebral vein with the development of the basal vein. Since the primary lateral drainage into the tentorial sinus is inefficient, it is not generally seen in the adult. The above example illustrates the persistence of the primary lateral drainage into the transverse sinus. Perhaps the development of the basal vein in this section of the brain was imperfect.

Occasionally, the basal vein itself drains laterally into the transverse sinus. After 80 mm, expansion of the dorsolateral walls of the brain is accompanied by the formation of the anastomotic veins of Labe and Trollard – transverse sinus, superior sagittal sinus, and middle cerebral veins. It is possible that the final drainage of the dorsal diencephalic vein may be shared by the superior sagittal sinus, thus obscuring the fundamental pattern of drainage. The exceptional pattern occurs when the mass of blood shunted is so large that the basal vein is unable to meet the requirements.

Summing up, the arteriovenous malformations related to the posterior cerebral artery drain through the dorsal diencephalic vein, and this may persist in the adult in three possible ways:

1. Through the tentorial sinus into the transverse sinus (the persisting primary feature)
2. Through the basal vein into the great cerebral vein (the most commonly seen pattern)
3. The vein of Labe and Trollard into the superior sagittal sinus (exceptional)

The Arterial Component: The Posterior Choroidal Artery

The posterior choroidal artery arises as a branch of the diencephalic artery posterior cerebral artery. This primary embryonic feature is retained in the adult.

Identification of the Angiomatous Malformation

The difficulties in recognising the choroidal branch from the other branches of the posterior cerebral artery, particularly in the presence of a large arterio-capillary tangle, is often responsible for including the former as 'abnormal arterial branches feeding the angioma'. Delman[61]

The Venous Elements of the Malformation

The dorsal diencephalic vein also crosses the posterior choroidal artery at approximately right angles, and an arteriovenous fistula between them is less possible.

Similarities of the Venous Pattern

As the posterior cerebral artery swings back approximately through a right angle to occupy the adult position, the posterior choroidal arteries are also carried with them to the same extent, and now occupy a more or less vertical position. The displacement of the dorsal diencephalic vein is similar, but as the segment of the vein involved is very short and deeply situated, the features are not often as dramatic as those of the posterior cerebral artery.

There were no cases in the present series where the posterior choroidal feeder could be recognised with certainty.

It is not uncommon to find where both posterior cerebral and posterior choroidal arteries appear to have been involved. For the above-mentioned reasons, the venous drainage is likely to be a common route, namely, the dorsal diencephalic vein.

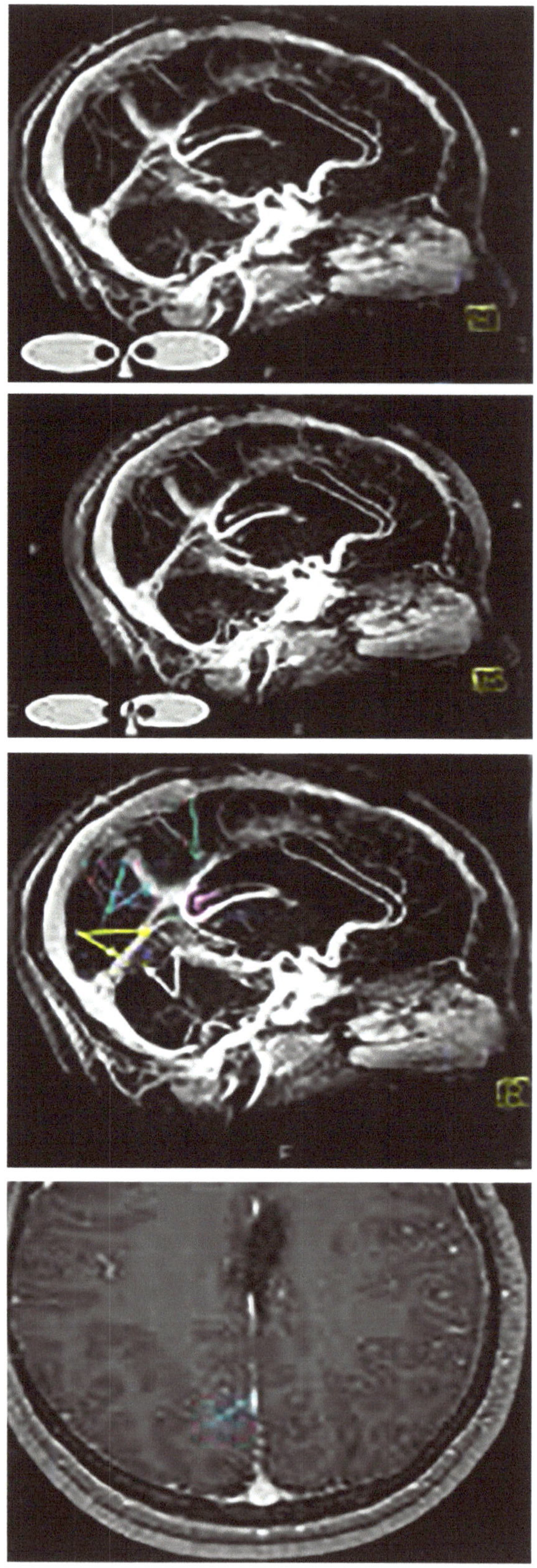

Figure 8.29 AVM nidus (black) draining into the false Galen (pink) and the Falxine sinuse (blue). The AVM is supplied via the posterior lateral choroidal arteries (Neurosurgery Focus).

Anterior Choroidal Artery: Ventral Diencephalic Vein

This section deals with the diencephalic malformations where the ventral diencephalic vein has persisted.

The Arterial Component

This artery arises from the internal carotid artery as its largest cranial division and reaches the choroid plexus through the diencephalon (see Figure 8.3 and Figure 8.4).

The Angiomatous Elements of the Malformation

The anterior choroidal artery is crossed by the ventral diencephalic vein at approximately right angles, and an arteriovenous fistula between these vessels can occur.

The Venous Elements of the Malformation

Like the dorsal diencephalic vein, a ventral diencephalic vein develops connections. The ventral diencephalic vein primarily drains laterally into the transverse sinus, but later definitive connections with the internal cerebral vein are established between the 60- and 80-mm stages.

Unlike in the case of the dorsal diencephalic vein, these connections occur in two different ways. The diencephalic vein makes a significant contribution to the formation of the basal cerebral vein, a pattern similar to that of the dorsal diencephalic vein. The second connection is unique to the ventral diencephalic vein. The massive choroid plexus drains ventro-laterally via the inferior choroidal vein into the ventral diencephalic vein (see Figure 8.3). This primary drainage of the choroid plexus is later replaced around the 80-mm stage by a medial drainage through the superior choroidal vein. This vein

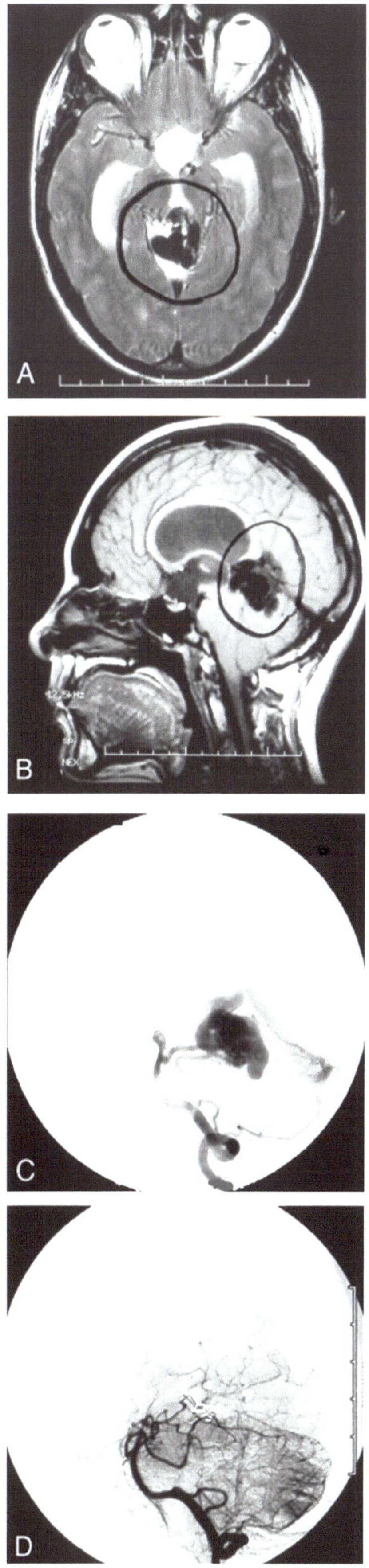

Figure 8.30 Posterior Chroidal Artery Malformation (Neurosurgery Focus).

continues as the primitive internal cerebral vein and, in the adult, is represented as a permanent tributary of the definitive internal cerebral vein. Thus, the primitive lateral drainage of the choroid plexus is completely annexed by the definitive medial drainage.

Regrouping of Cases According to Similarities of Venous Drainage

Although it is possible for the lateral drainage to persist in the extrauterine life, the medial drainage is likely to be more frequent. There are three possible routes by which this primary lateral drainage can be deviated medially:

1. Basal vein.
2. Drainage through the inferior choroidal vein and superior choroidal vein
3. Into the internal cerebral vein (This is a less likely occurrence, as it is very roundabout and inefficient.)

Therefore, when the changes in the tentorial sinus create a need for an alternate route, the blood flow is likely to be in the direction of least resistance, that is, into the basal vein.

Identification and Matching of Abnormal Vascular Channels with the Normal Embryonic Vascular Channels

The abnormal veins are, as a rule, directed upwards and medially into the great cerebral vein. Their course and direction resemble those of the ventral diencephalic vein. Although in the embryo the ventral and dorsal diencephalic veins appear very distinct, in the adult it is often difficult to distinguish the differences. This is due to the approximation of the anterior choroidal artery and posterior cerebral artery trunk in the adult. (Vidyasagar[337])

Regrouping of Adult Diencephalic Arteries with Reference to the Embryonic Region

The location of anterior choroidal artery in the adult is misleading. Its proximity to the anterior cerebral and middle cerebral artery is only a secondary feature. It is primarily the artery of the diencephalon, although part of its course is through the telencephalon.

The New Classification Based on the Embryological Site of Their Formation

The anterior choroidal artery malformation should, therefore, be grouped with posterior cerebral, posterior choroidal lesions, as they all belong to the diencephalon. The locations of these vessels are so far apart in the adult that a resort to embryology is necessary to appreciate the common pattern

Anterior choroidal AVM (Straus)

Figure 8.31 to Figure 8.38 illustrate the theoretical possibilities of the anatomical features of the ventral diencephalic malformation. The vascular channels marked Green represent the ventral diencephalic vein in these diagrams.

Hypothetical Illustration

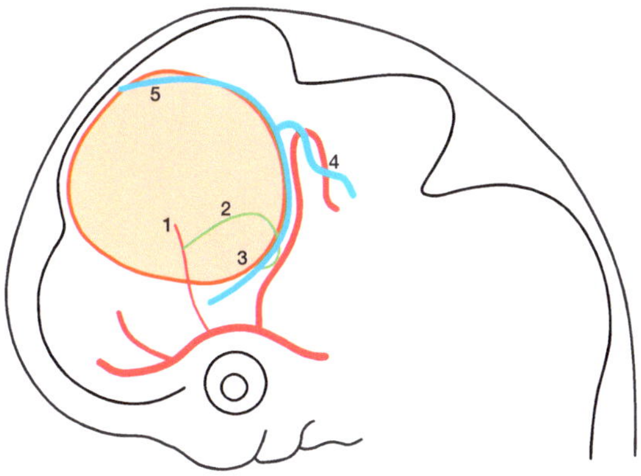

Figure 8.31 Diencephalic arterio-venous malformaion ventral diencephalic vein draining into the tentorial sinus at 20mm (Lateral).

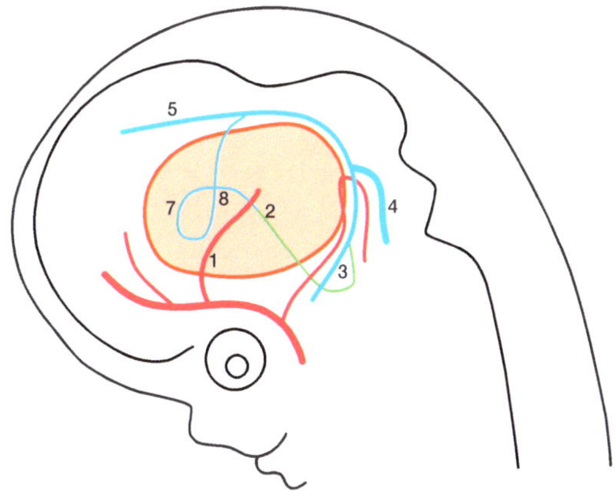

Figure 8.32 Ventral diencephalic vein draining into the tentorial sinus at 40mm (Lateral).

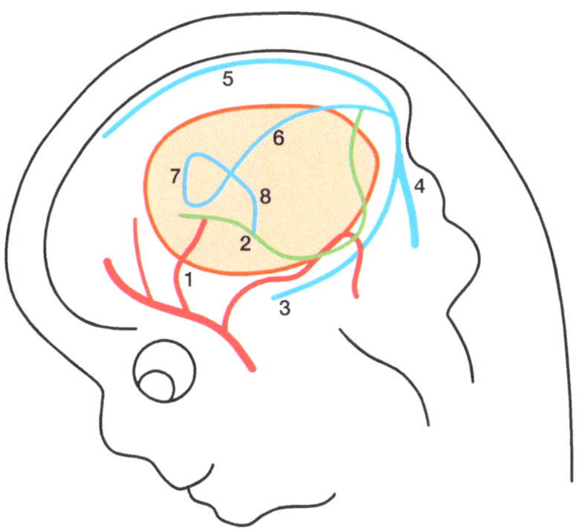

Figure 8.33 Ventral diencephalic vein draining into the tentorial sinus at 80mm (Lateral).

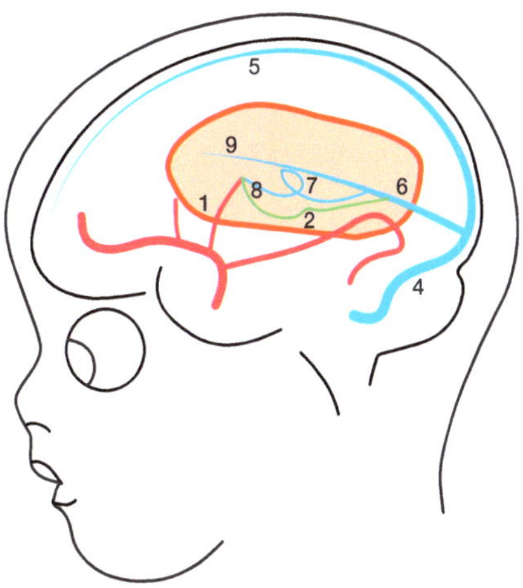

Figure 8.34 Ventral diencephalic vein draining into the sinus in the adult (Lateral).

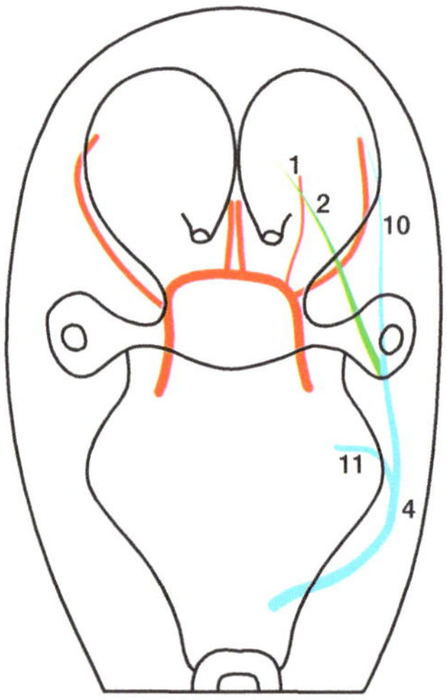

Figure 8.35 Ventral diencephalic vein draining into the tentorial sinus at 20mm (Basal).

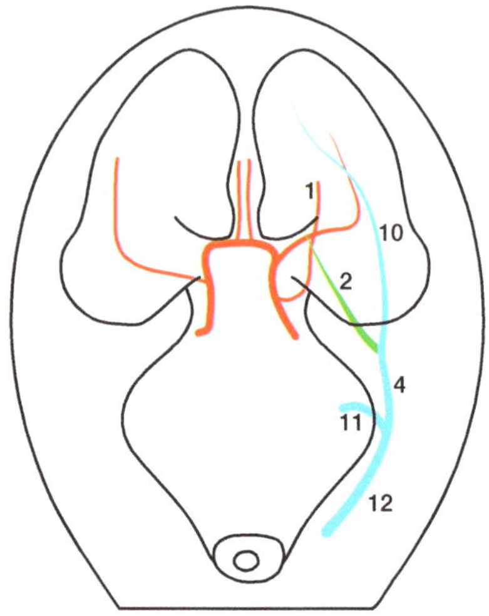

Figure 8.36 Ventral diencephalic vein draining into the tentorial sinus at 40mm (Basal).

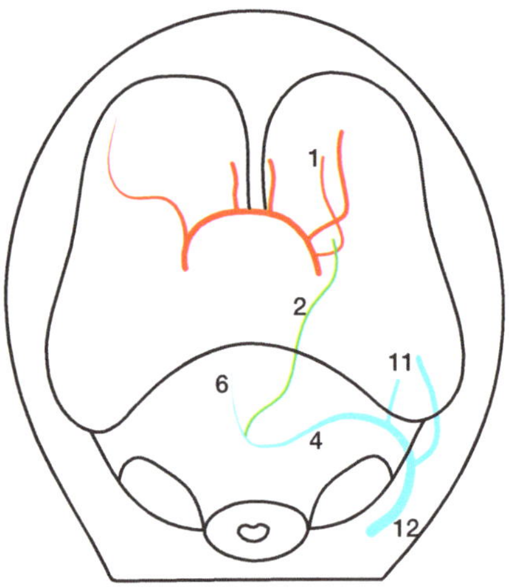

Figure 8.37 Ventral diencephalic vein draining into the tentorial sinus at 80mm (Basal).

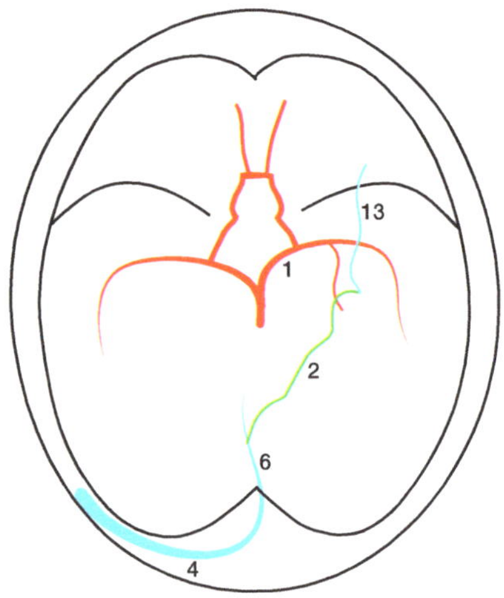

Figure 8.38 Ventral diencephalic vein draining into the tentorial sinus in the adult (Basal).

1 Ant Choroid A **2** Vent Dienceph V **3** Tent Sin **4** Trans Sin **5** Sup Sagitt Sin
6 Int Cerebral V **7** Sup Choroidal V **8** Inf Choroidal V **9** Inf Sagitt Sin
10 Marginal Sin **11** Pro-Otic Sin **12** Sigmoid Sin **13** Basal V

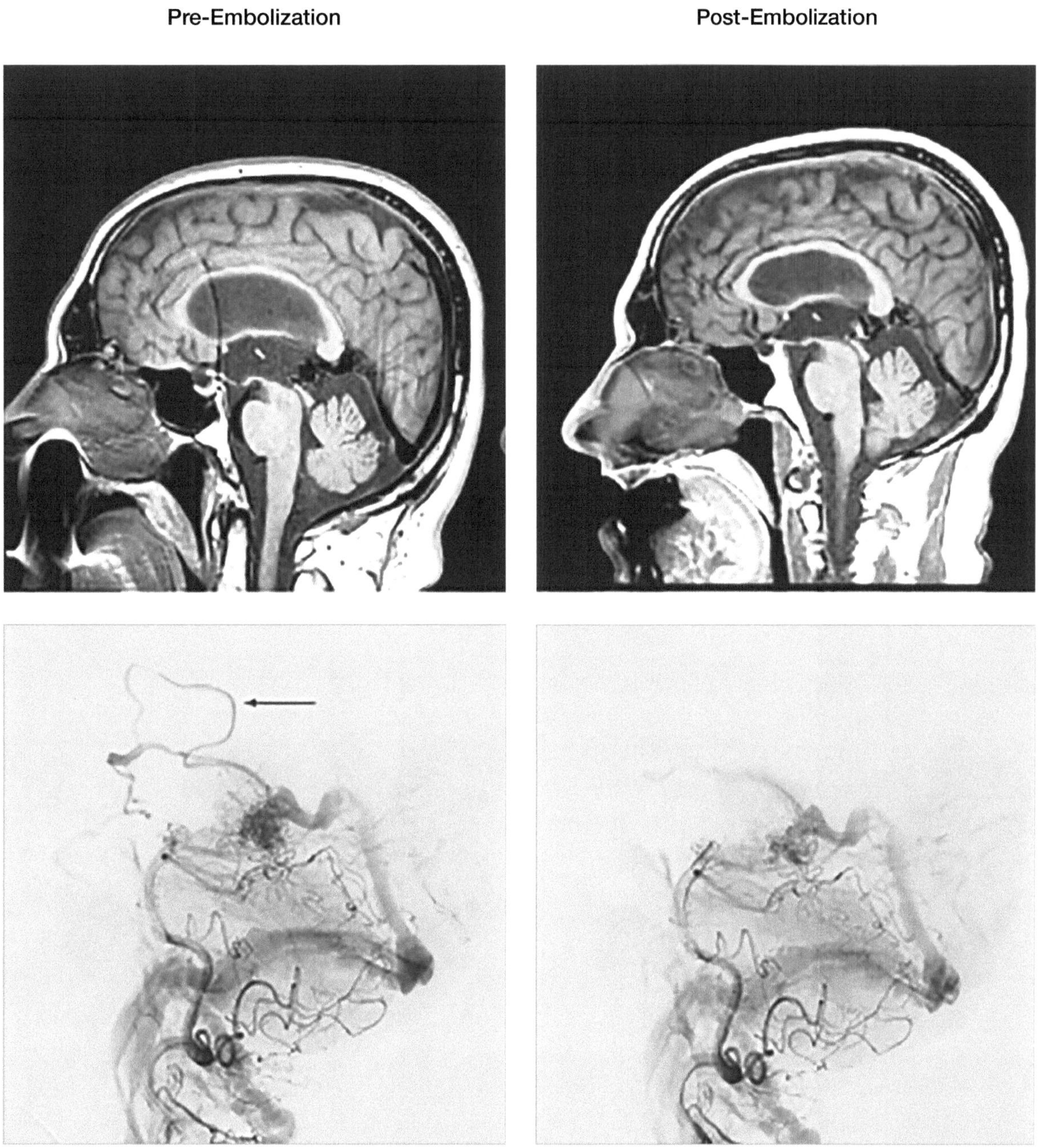

Figure 8.39 Anterior choroidal Artery – Ventral Diencephalic vein Malformations (Neurosurgery Focus).

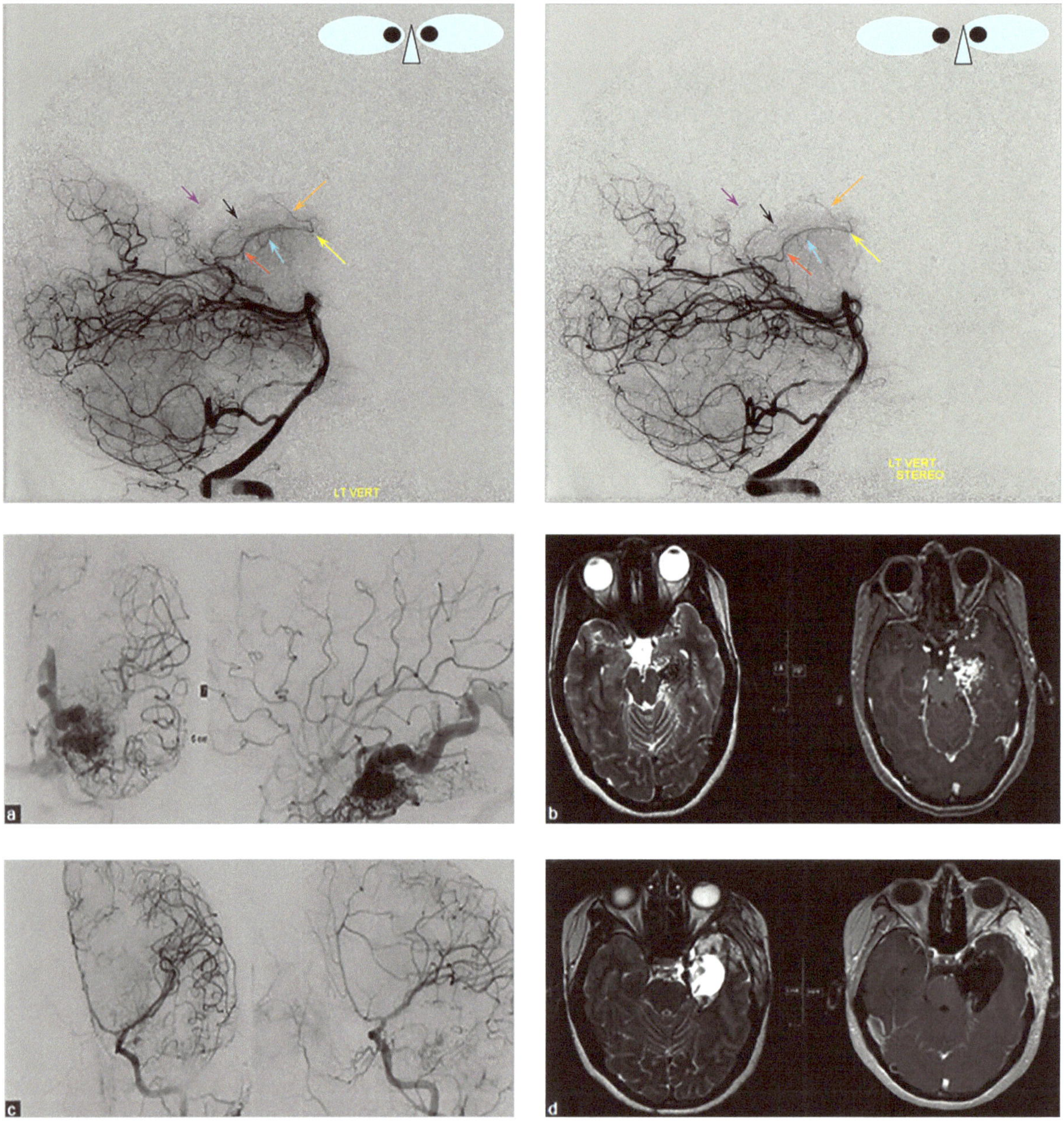

Figure 8.40 Anterior choroidal Artery – Ventral Diencephalic vein Malformations (Neurosurgery Focus).

Examples

Figure 8.41 to Figure 8.42 illustrate an example where the malformation has been used by the anterior choroidal artery. The venous channel is directed backwards and medially into the straight sinus. The course and direction of this vessel are easily comparable to those seen in Figure 8.34.

Figure 8.43 is a reproduction from the work of Yasargil (1971)[354]. The anterior choroidal malformation here is draining laterally into the transverse sinus. As under section 1, the lateral drainage here is an infrequent phenomenon, but when it occurs, the vessel would be coursing downwards, laterally, and backwards.

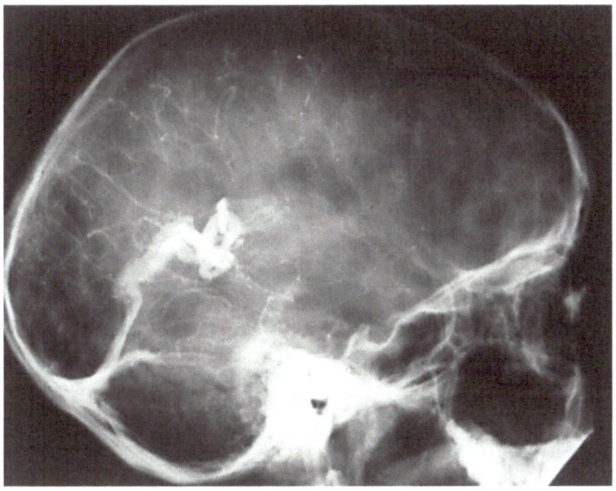

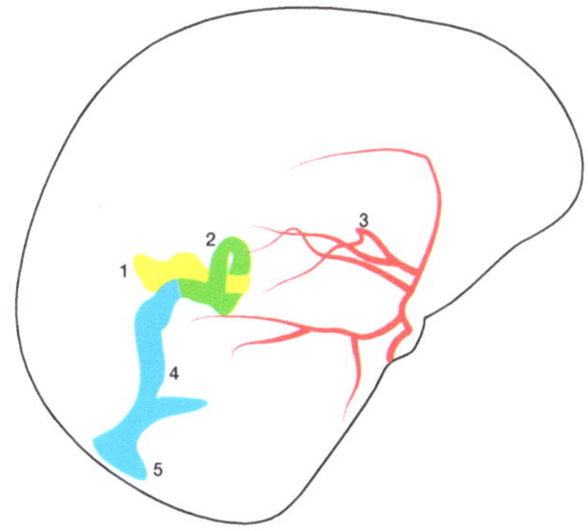

1 Angioma **2** Vent Dienceph V **3** Ant Choroid A **4** STR Sinus **5** Torcula

Figure 8.41 Diencephalic arterio-venous malformation. Anterior choroidal artery feeder. Ventral diencephalic vein draining into the great cerebral vein (Lateral) (Venous).

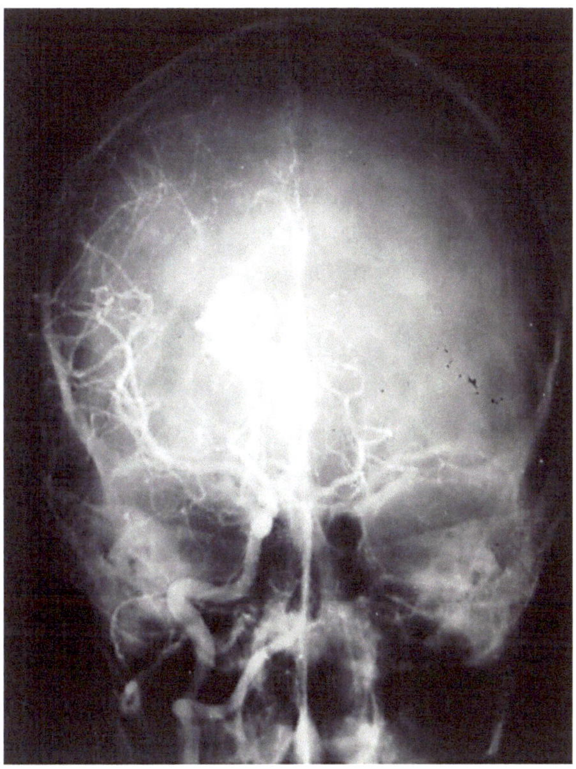

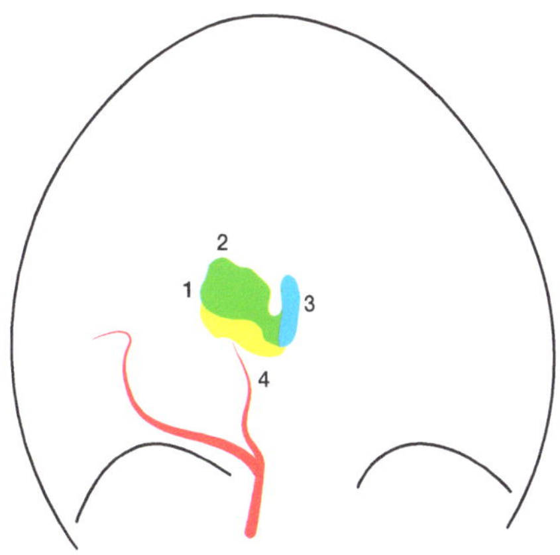

1 Vent Dienceph V **2** Mid Cereb A **3** GR Cereb Vein **4** Ant Choroid A

Figure 8.42 Diencephalic arterio-venous malformation. Anterior choroidal artery feeder. Vantral diencephalic vein draining into the great cerebral vein (AP).

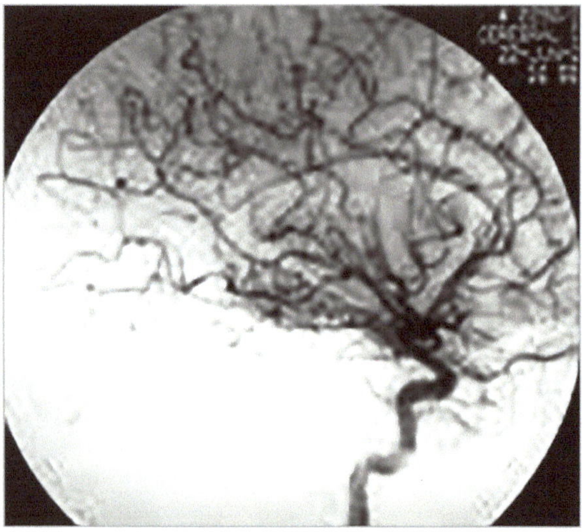

Figure 8.43 Cerebral angiography showing the artersovenous malformation supplied by the anterior choroidal artery.

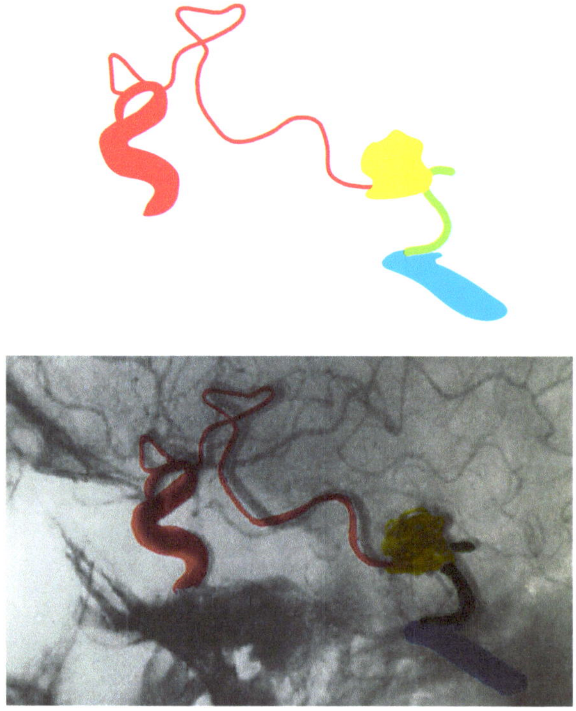

Figure 8.44 Diencephalic arterio-venous malformation. Dorsal diencephalic vein drains laterally into the transverse sinus.

Choroid Plexus

When an angioma is situated in the convexity of the choroid plexus, it is often thought that this tangle of vessels represents a segment of the choroid plexus. This concept is based on the idea that the choroid plexus contains numerous persisting embryonic fistulae (O'Brien and Schechter[223&224]), which are made obvious by an excess flow. If such a drainage through the meshes of choroid plexus does occur, then it should be possible to see the anterior choroid plexus involved, but such extensive inclusion of choroid plexuses is seldom seen. On the contrary, it is often possible to come across malformations in this region without an angioma.

These facts substantiate the concept that the arteriovenous fistula occurre between definite arteries and veins, and the angiomas do not represent persisting embryonic fistula.

Thus, it can be summed up that a diencephalic malformation is produced by a posterior cerebral, posterior choroidal, and the anterior choroidal arteries. The abnormal vessels seen in these malformations represent dorsal and ventral diencephalic veins. The drainage of the shunted blood is primarily into the transverse sinus and is later diverted medially into the great cerebral vein with the formation of the basal vein. The medial drainage being in keeping with the normal developmental pattern is seen more frequently. The presence and location of the arterio-capillary tangle are very variable and do not follow any predictable pattern. They are related to the choroid plexus. The presence of the latter is only coincidental.

9

Telencephalic Abnormalities

The cerebral hemispheres are the major derivatives of telencephalon. The anterior and middle cerebral arteries supply this part of the brain. Arteriovenous malformations occur in three distinct sites: (a) in the midline,(b) in the sylvian fissure, and (c) over the convexity of the cerebral hemisphere. Primitive segmental embryonic veins are closely associated with the corresponding primitive arteries in these areas. The anatomical features of arteriovenous malformations in these areas have distinct features.

The development of the telencephalon is the most complex of all segments of the primitive brain. The segmental pattern is completely overshadowed by the developmental process (see Figure 8.1 and Figure 8.2). Correspondingly, the vascular system has no features easily attributable to the segmental pattern, but on closer examination it is possible to appreciate the primary scheme, and the anatomical aspects of the malformations are predictable.

For the purpose of clarity, these lesions are dealt with separately in three sections, namely,

1. Surface of Telencephalon
2. Sylvian Malformations
3. Deep Telencephalic Malformations

Surface of Telencephalon

The Arterial Component of the Malformation

This section deals with the arteriovenous malformations situated on the cortical surface of the brain. This consists of the frontal, temporal, parietal, and occipital cortices of the adult. The anterior cerebral and middle cerebral arteries supply principally this part of the brain. The medial surface is primarily the territory of the anterior cerebral, and the lateral surface that of the middle cerebral.

The Angiomatous Elements of the Malformation

The terminal branches of the anterior middle cerebral arteries are closely associated with the tributaries of the superior sagittal sinus. In a situation like this, an arteriovenous fistula between these vessels is easily possible. The fistula so produced could be situated anywhere between the frontal and occipital poles. Padget (1956), however, contended that a primary arteriovenous fistula in such a shifting and plexiform marginal sinus is not likely. It is difficult to accept this concept entirely until a more satisfactory explanation is available to account for the frequent occurrence of the arteriovenous lesions in this area.

The Venous Elements

The superior sagittal sinus constitutes the principal outlet for the veins over the surface. The development of the sinus and its tributaries begins around 40-mm stage. This period corresponds to the time when the pial arteries and veins are crossing each other at right angles in other areas of the brain. Because of the numerous vessels involved in these plexuses, the possibilities of a fistula are very high.

Regrouping of Cases According to Similarity of Venous Pattern

The abnormal venous channels are directed backwards and superiorly towards the superior sagittal sinus. They are situated either on the lateral or on the medial surface of the cerebral cortex, depending upon the source of the arterial feeder.

Identification and Matching of the Abnormal Venous Channels with the Normal Embryonic Venous Channels

The venous channels extending between the fistula and the superior sagittal sinus are generally directed backwards and medially. They, as a rule, end in the superior sagittal sinus. Occasionally, venous channels could be seen extending to the transverse sinus by way of the anastomotic veins of Labe and Trollard.

Regrouping of the Arteries According to Their Site of Origin in the Embryo

Both anterior and middle cerebral arteries belong to the telencephalon, and the arteriovenous malformations arising from them have similar features. The entire cerebral cortex is formed by the telencephalon, and the anatomy of the arteriovenous malformations is identical.

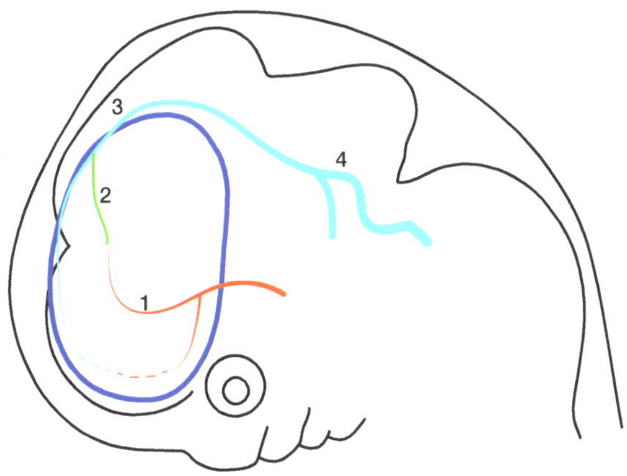

Figure 9.1 Vein on the surface of the telencephalon draining into the superior sagittal sinus at 20mm (Lateral).

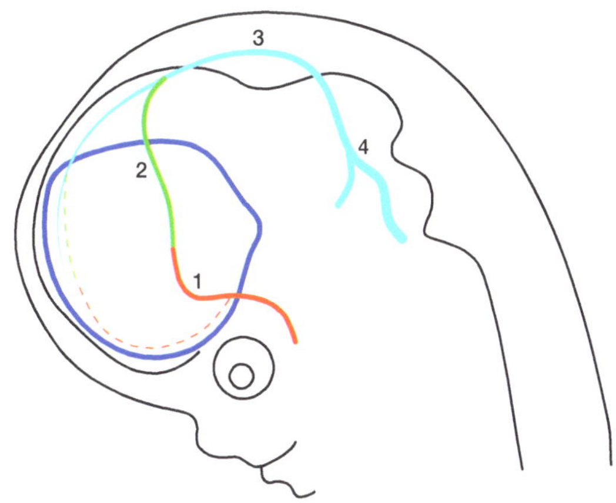

Figure 9.2 Vein on the surface of the telencephalon draining into the superior sagittal at 40mm (Lateral).

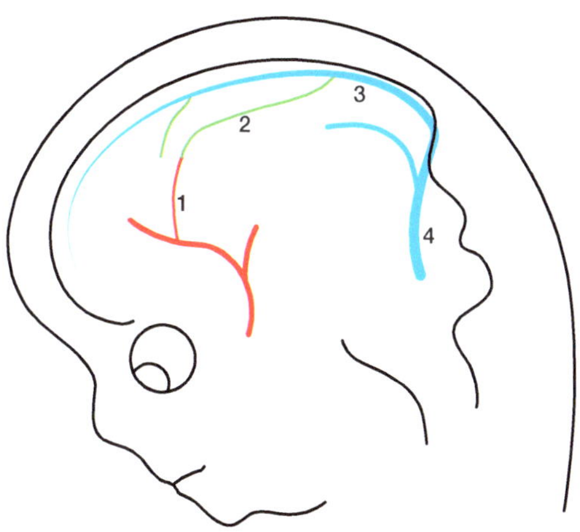

Figure 9.3 Telencephalic vein draining into the superor sagittial sinus at 80mm (Lateral).

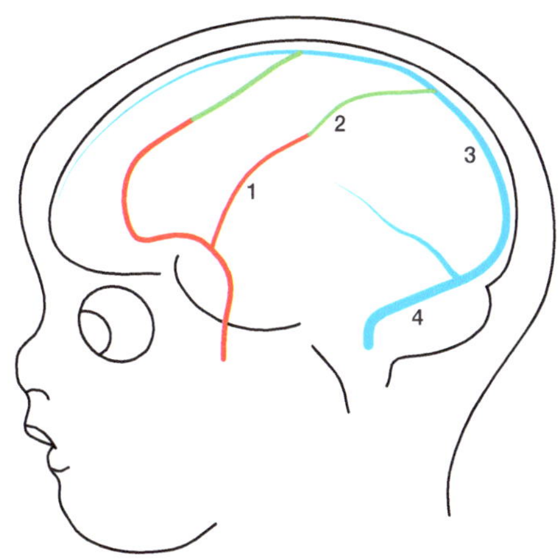

Figure 9.4 Telencephalic vein draining into the superor sagittal sinus in the adult (Lateral).

1 Sup Sagitt Sin **2** Tent Sin **3** Telenceph V **4** Mid Cer A
5 Trans Sin **6** Int Car A **7** Int Cer V **8** Ant Cer A
9 Sigmoid Sin **10** Margin Sin **11** Pro-Otic Sin **12** Sup Mid Cer V

Regrouping of the Cases with Reference to the Embryonic Regions

Malformations in this area have always been described with reference to the site in terms of adult anatomy, namely, the temporal, the frontal, the parietal, and the occipital. It has been mentioned earlier how these regions of the brain have a common developmental origin (telencephalon). Therefore, it becomes necessary to classify them all as a single entity. Their anatomical features are, in fact, similar.

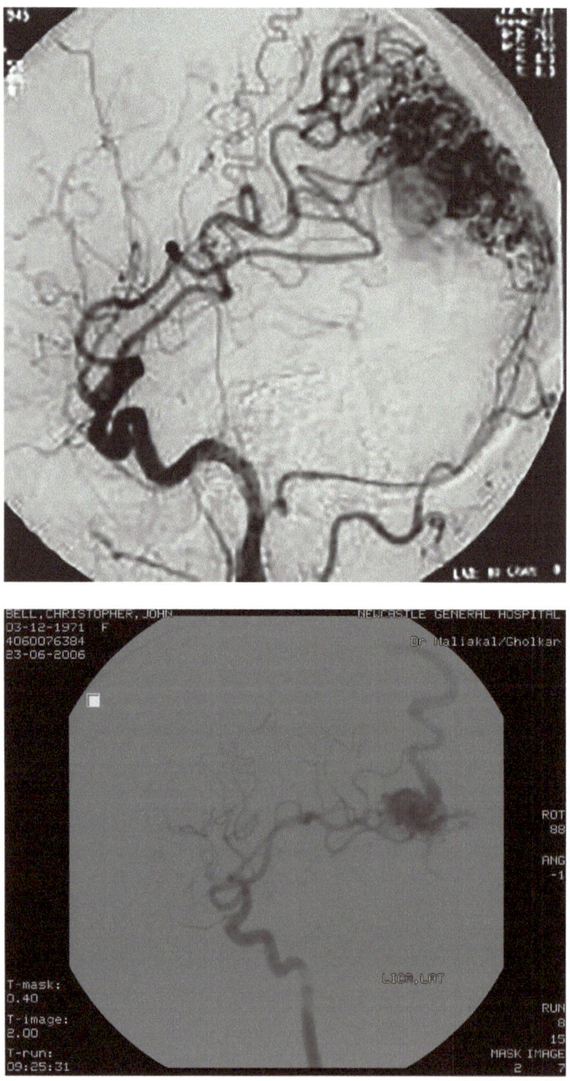

Figure 9.5 Mid Cereb A AVM draining into SSS (Ogilvy).[226]

Hypothetical Illustrations

Figure 9.1 to Figure 9.4 show diagrammatically the theoretical possibilities of the malformations. It is clear from these diagrams how a lesion situated in the frontal region in the earlier part of the development migrates to the parietal or occipital area (Vidyasagar[338]).

Examples

Fig 9.5 and 9.6 show examples of the malformations situated in various areas of the cortex. In spite of this apparent variation, they appear to have common features. The drainage of the veins has always been into the superior sagittal sinus.

Sylvian Malformations

The Arterial Component of the Malformation

The lesions situated in the region of the sylvian fissure arise mainly from the middle cerebral arteries. Since the branches arising in this segment of the middle cerebral artery are very close to its point of origin, the size of the fistulae tends to be large.

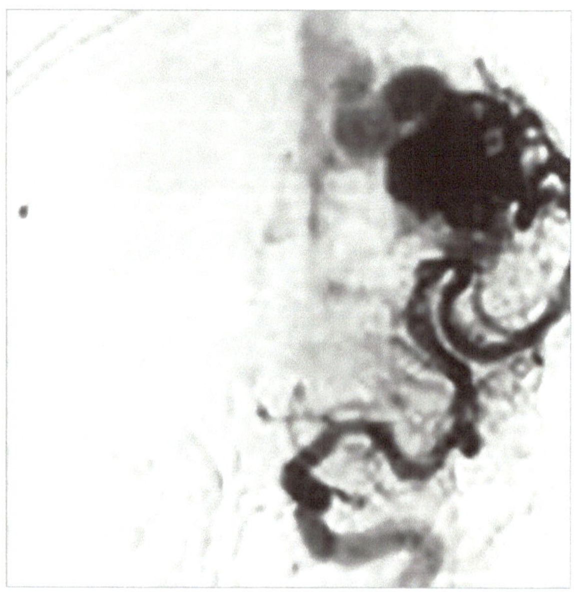

Figure 9.6 Mid Cereb A feeder drainage into SSS (Ogilvy).[226]

The Angiomatous Elements of the Malformation

Although both superficial and deep middle cerebral veins are situated in the sylvian fissure, the deep veins are related closely to the middle cerebral arteries. Therefore, the arteriovenous fistula occurs primarily between the middle cerebral artery and the deep middle cerebral veins. The angioma tends to be confined to the sylvian area.

The Venous Elements

The pattern of venous drainage tends to be very variable in these lesions. There are generally as follows:

1. Laterally, downwards, and posteriorly into the transverse sinus
2. Medially, posteriorly into the internal cerebral vein
3. Superficially into the superior sagittal sinus

There may be, in addition, secondary connections between these channels.

Regrouping of the Cases According to the Similarity of the Venous Pattern

The sylvian malformations can be grouped into three types, depending upon the manner in which the venous drainage occurs. The venous drainage may be into the transverse sinus, into the cerebral vein, or into the superior sagittal sinus. In addition, any combination of these three variations can also occur.

Identification and Matching of the Abnormal Venous Channels with the Normal Embryonic Venous Channels

All the three venous channels mentioned above can be recognised in the embryo at various stages. The channel draining laterally and backwards into the transverse sinus has a course and direction similar to those of the primitive tentorial sinus. The channel draining medially into the internal cerebral vein represents the basal vein and whilst that draining into the superior sagittal sinus represents the tributaries of the primitive marginal sinus situated on the convexity of the hemisphere.

Regrouping of the Arteries According to Their Site of Origin in the Embryo

Both anterior and middle cerebral arteries belong to the telencephalon, and the arteriovenous malformations arising from them have similar features. The entire cerebral cortex is formed by the telencephalon, and the anatomy of the arteriovenous malformations is identical.

Regrouping of the Cases with Reference to the Embryonic Regions

Malformations in this area have always been described with reference to the site in terms of adult anatomy, namely, the temporal, the frontal, the parietal, and the occipital. It has been mentioned earlier how these variations arise and the brain has a common developmental origin. Therefore, it becomes necessary to classify them all as a single entity. Their anatomical features are, in fact, similar.

Hypothetical Illustrations

Figures 9.8-9.15 indicate the hypothetical configuration of the vascular channels in these malformations. It will be noted that the vessels marked Green represent the persistent telencephalic vein. Not all the variations mentioned earlier have been included in the diagram, to preserve the clarity, but they have been shown separately in Figure 9.7 and Figure 9.14.

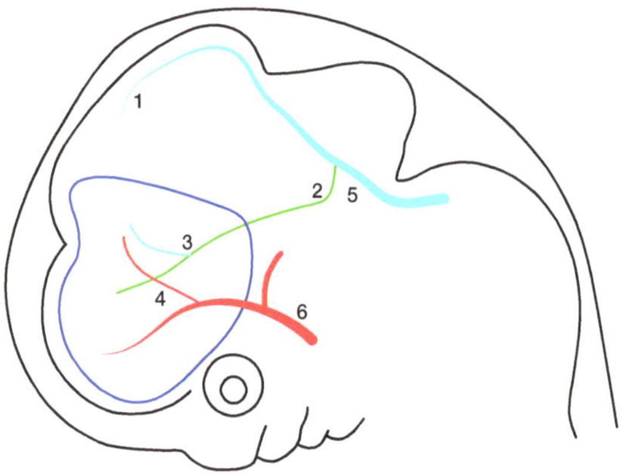

Figure 9.7 The Telencephalic vein draining into the Transverse Sinus at 20mm (Lateral).

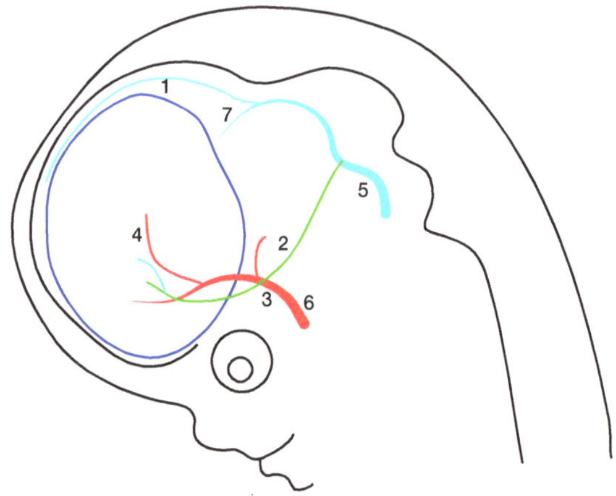

Figure 9.8 The Telencephalic vein draining into the Transverse Sinus at 40mm (Lateral).

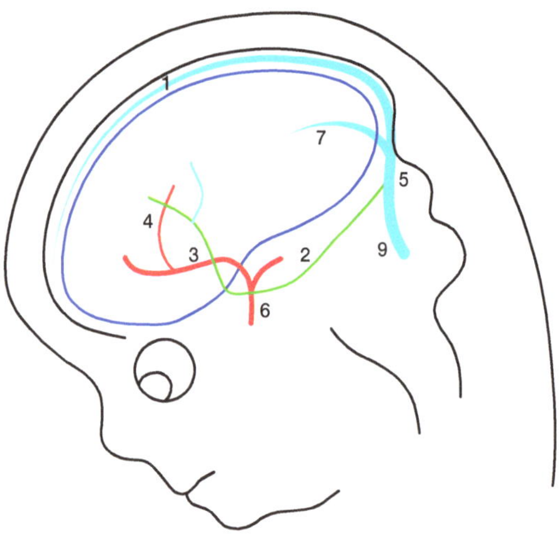

Figure 9.9 The Telencephalic vein draining into the Transverse Sinus at 80mm (Lateral).

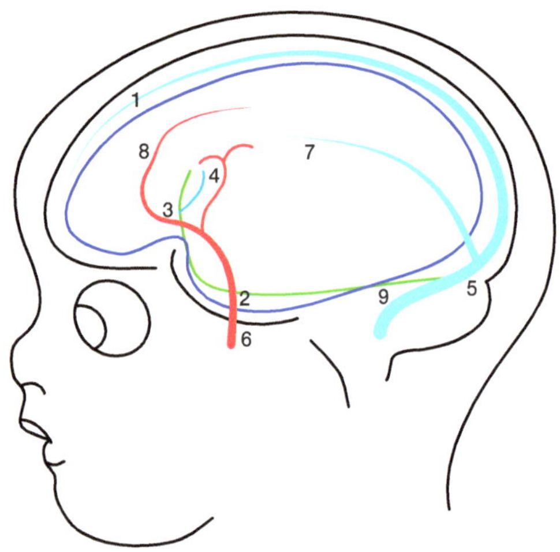

Figure 9.10 The Telencephalic vein draining into the Transverse Sinus in the adult (Lateral).

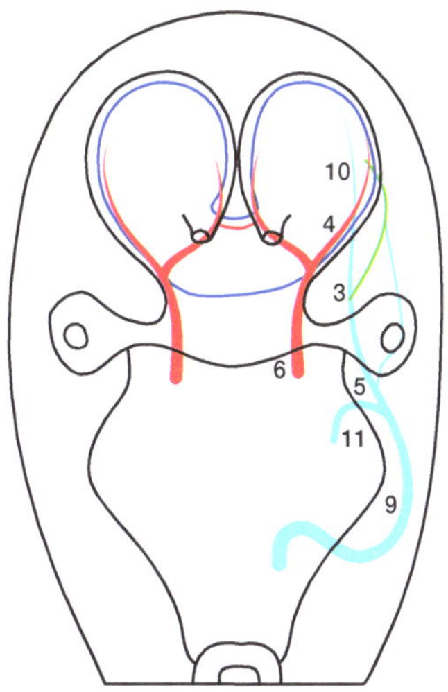

Figure 9.11 The telencephalic vein draining into the Transverse Sinus at 20mm (Basal).

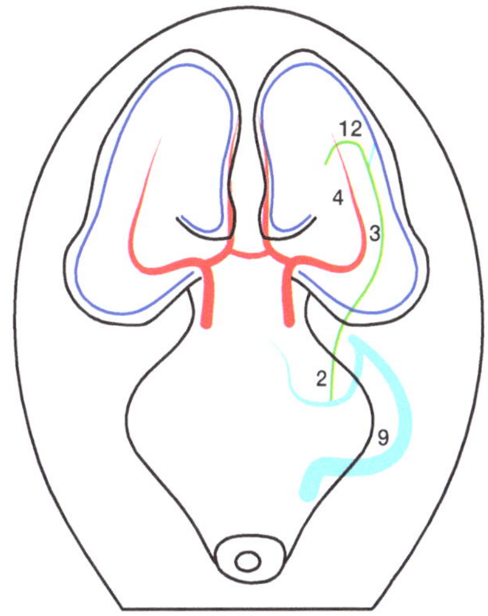

Figure 9.12 The Telencephalic vein draining into the Transverse Sinus at 40mm (Basal).

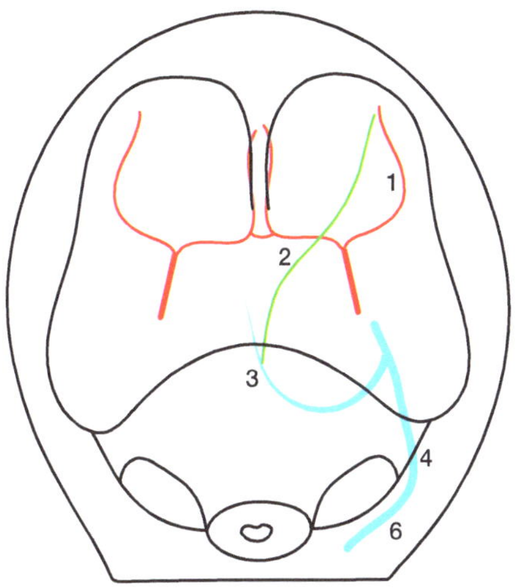

Figure 9.13 The Telencephalic vein draining into the Transverse Sinus at 80mm (Basal).

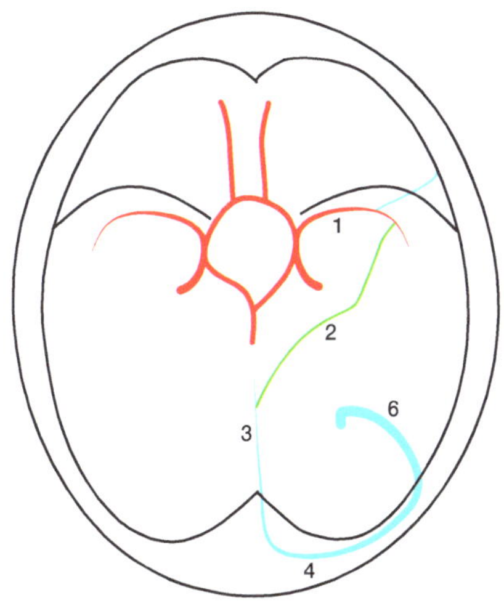

Figure 9.14 The Telencephalic vein draining into the Transverse Sinus in the adult (Basal).

1 Sup Sagitt Sin **2** Tent Sin **3** Telenceph V **4** Mid Cer A
5 Trans Sin **6** Int Car A **7** Int Cer V **8** Ant Cer A
9 Sigmoid Sin **10** Margin Sin **11** Pro-Otic Sin **12** Sup Mid Cer V

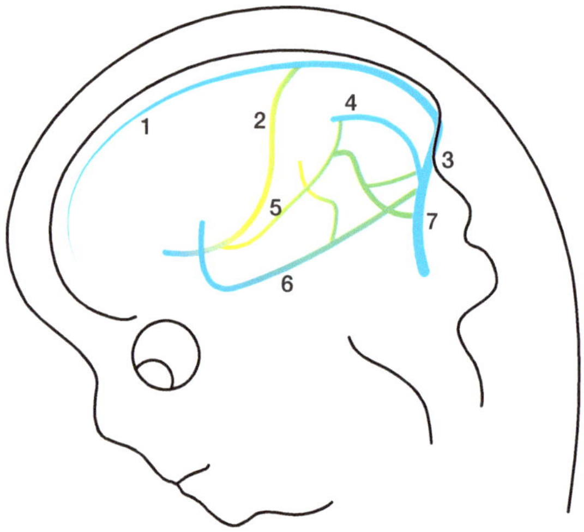

Figure 9.15 Variations in the draining of telencephalic arterio-venous malformation in the region of the sylvian fissure (Lateral).

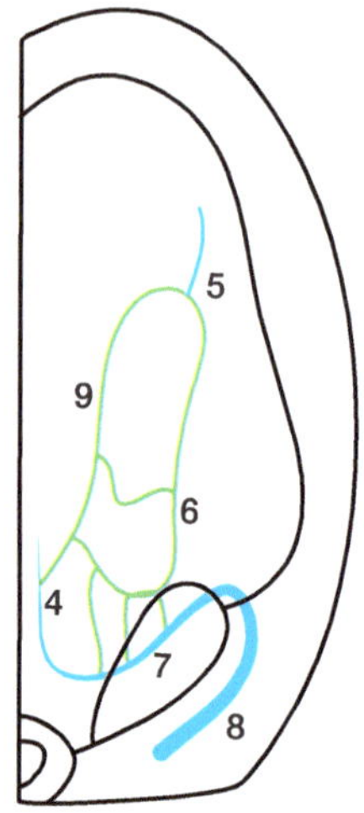

Figure 9.16 Variations in the draining of the telencephalic arterio-venous malformations in the region of the sylvian fissure (Basal).

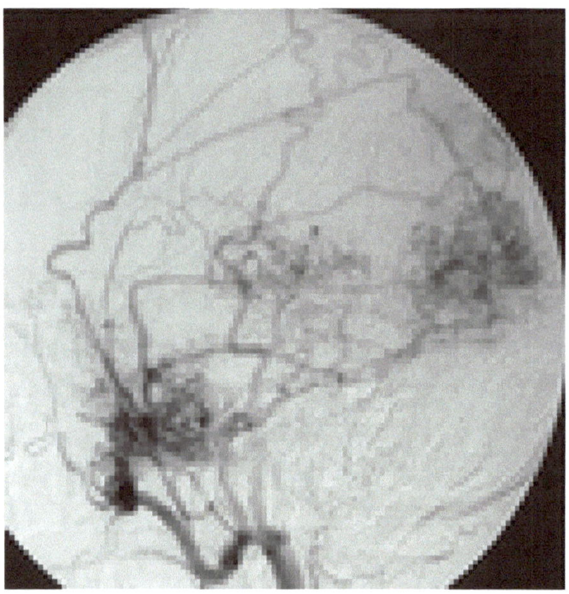

Figure 9.17 Sylvian AVM drainage into Sup Sagital Sinus (Radiopedia).

Examples

Figure 9.18 show examples of a sylvian arterio-venous malformation. The arterial contribution from the middle cerebral artery is clearly seen. The venous drainage is into the great cerebral vein. The venous channels marked Green represent the persisting telencephalic vein and parts of the primitive basal vein draining into the great cerebral vein. There is also some reflux filling into the tentorial sinus, which has preserved its embryonic nature to a certain extent. The explanation for the persistence of embryonic characters of the channels when there is retrograde filling has been mentioned earlier.

Figure 9.18 –Figure 9.19 show examples of sylvian malformations where the venous drainage is into the transverse sinus. The persistent embryonic tentorial sinus can be seen coursing laterally and downwards to reach the transverse sinus. In this example there is no distinction between the telencephalic vein and the tentorial sinus. This is because the cranial end of the tentorial sinus receives the telencephalic vein, and therefore, it appears as if the tentorial sinus and the telencephalic vein appear as a single channel. There is a second embryonic channel situated more posteriorly, which also drains into the transverse sinus. The course and direction of this vein appear to be comparable to those of the ventral diencephalic vein. The involvement of the diencephalic vein in a telencephalic malformation seems out of pattern. Although the venous drainage of the primitive brain is segmental, there are potential channels existing between them. The basal vein was one such commonly seen. But the most common connections, which as a rule are atritic, can be

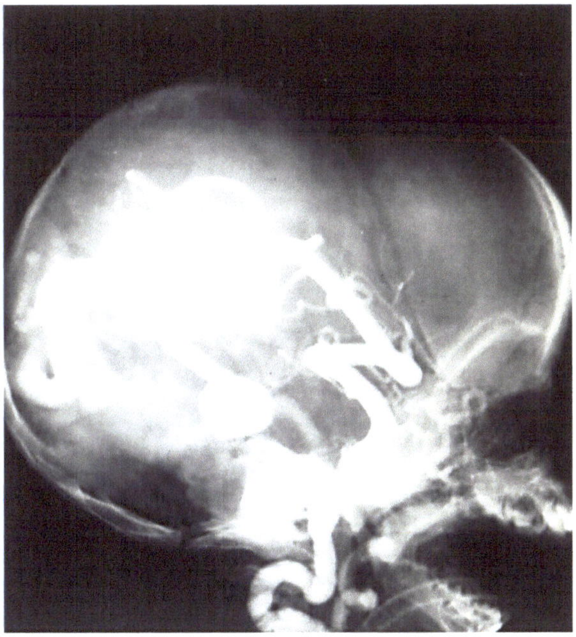

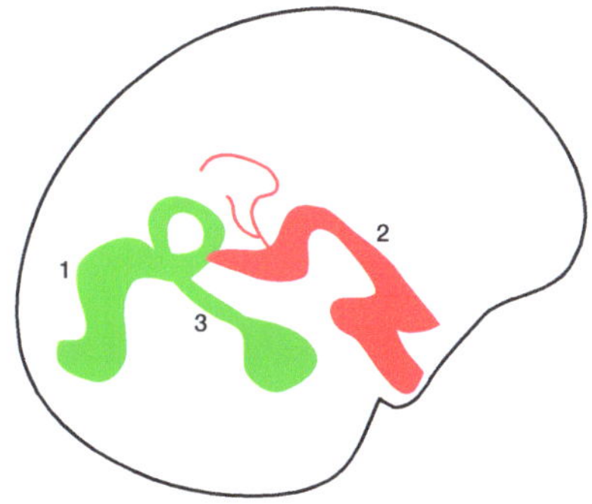

1 STR Sinus **2** Mid Cereb A
3 Retrograde Filling of Telenceph V and Tentorial Sinus

Figure 9.18 Telencephalic arterio-venous malformation middle cerebral artery feeder. Telencephalic vein draining into the great cerebral vein (Lateral).

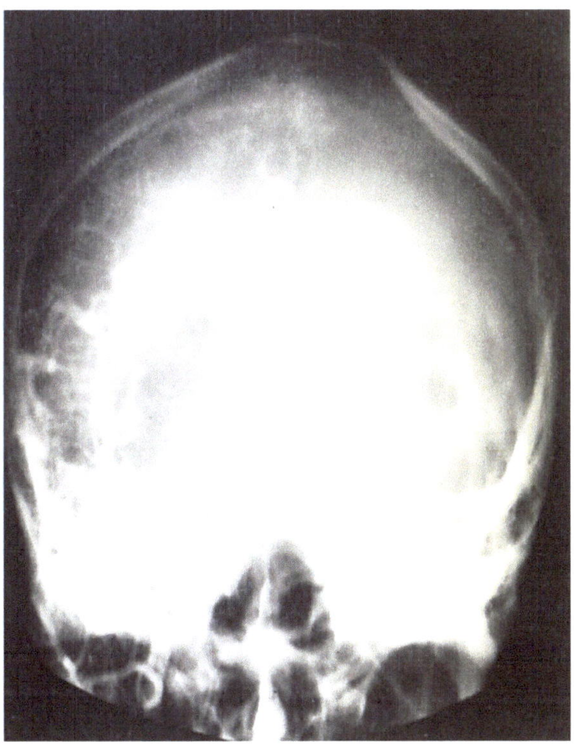

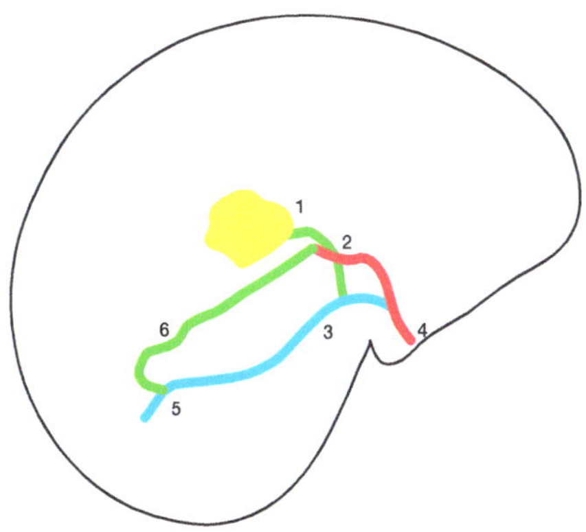

1 Angioma **2** Mid Cereb A **3** Tent Sinus
4 Int Cer V **5** Trans Sinus **6** Vent Dienceph V

Figure 9.19 Telencephalic Arterio-Venous malformation middle cerebral artery feeder. Lateral draining into the transverse sinus (Lateral).

seen in the earlier stages of the development. When an arteriovenous fistula occurs in one of the segmental veins, and if the venous outflow is enormous, the adjoining channels are naturally made use of. In this example the arterial feeder is from a principal branch of the middle cerebral artery. The quantity of blood flow in such a fistula is not surprisingly large. It is very likely that the telencephalic vein, being unable to deal with all the blood shunted by the adjoining diencephalic vein, was used as an accessory drainage. The atritic process has not occurred in the latter.

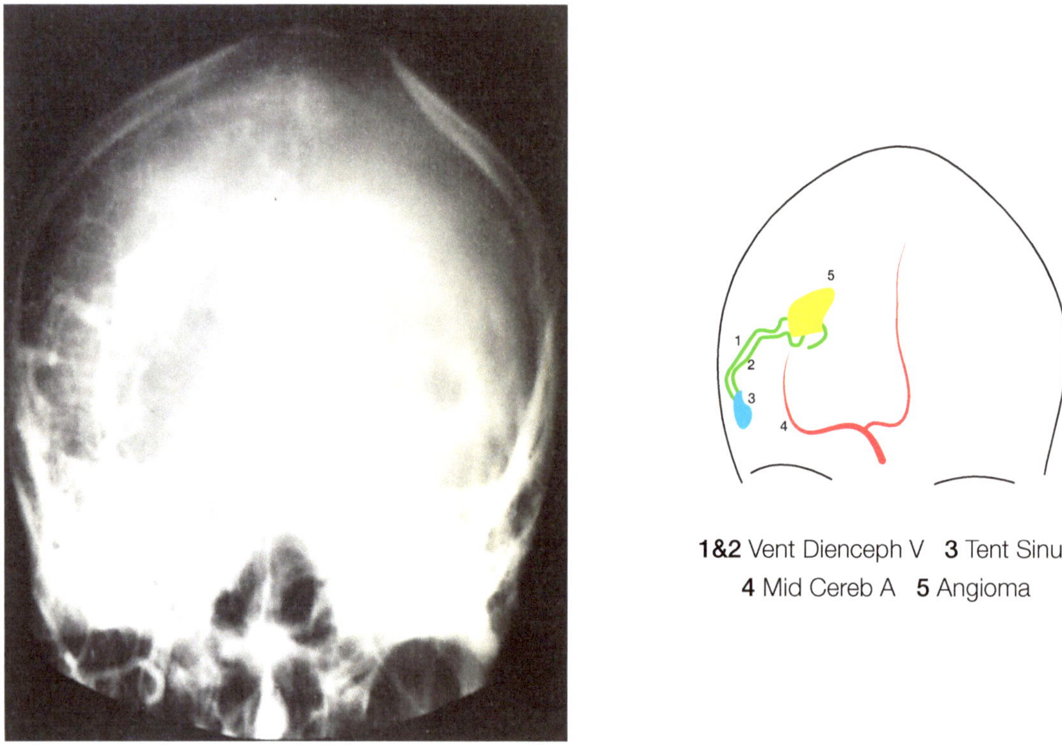

Figure 9.20 Telencephalic arterio-venous malformation middle cerebral artery feeder. Lateral drainage into the transverse sinuus (AP).

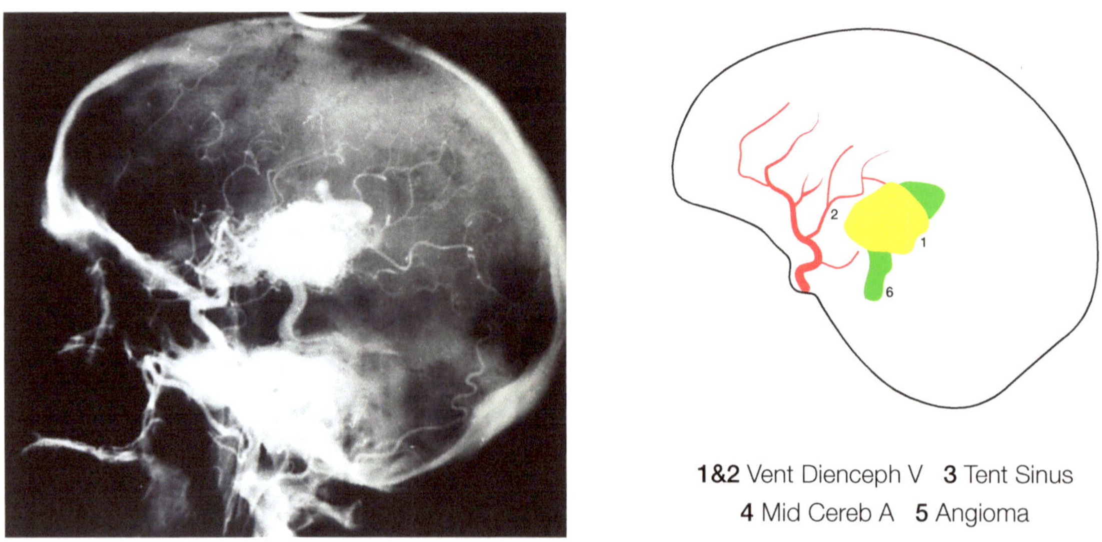

Figure 9.21 Telencephalic arterio-veous malformation middle cerebral artery feeder (Lateral).

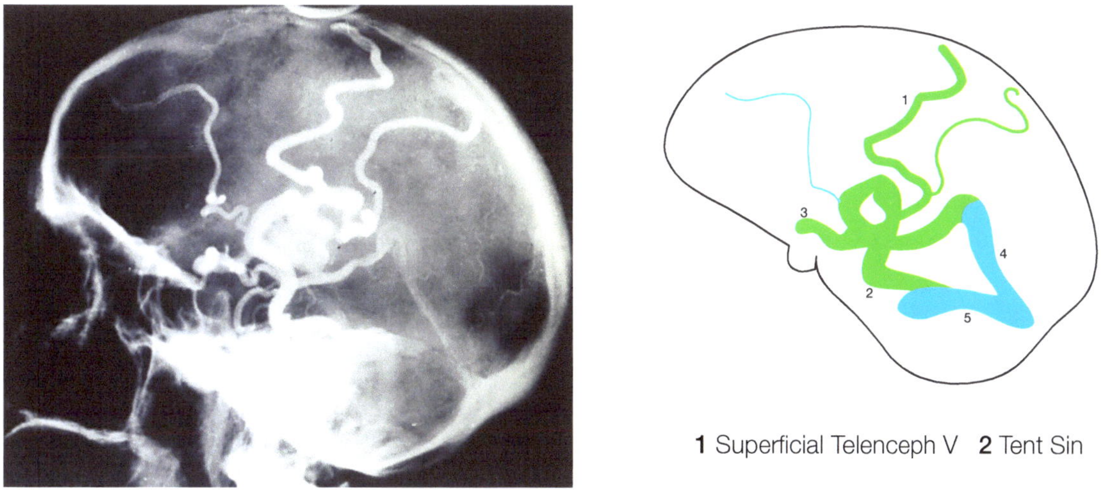

Figure 9.22 Telencephalic arterio-venous malformation venous drainage into transverse, superior sagittal and straight sinuses (Lateral).

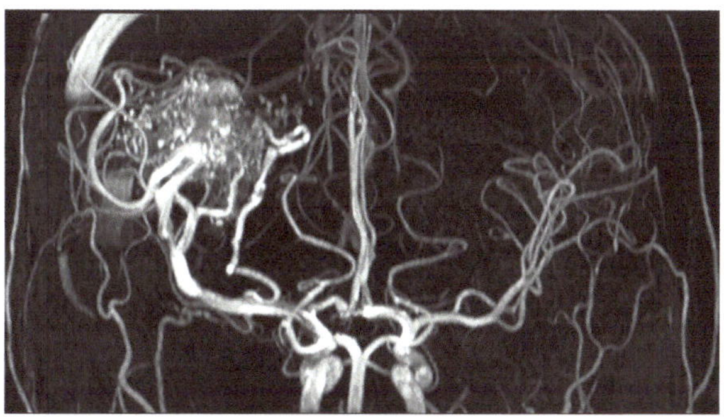

Figure 9.23 Sylvian AVM draining laterally (Geibpraser).[89]

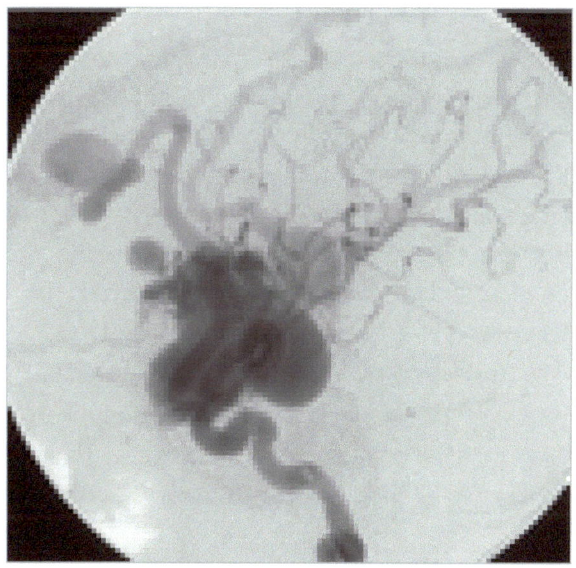

Figure 9.24 Sylvian AVM draining into Superior Sagital Sinus (Geibpraser).[89]

Figure 9.22 show another example of a sylvian arteriovenous malformation. The arterio-capillary tangle is situated in the sylvian area. The venous drainage has occurred through all the three possible routes, namely, the tentorial sinus, the basal vein, and the superior sagittal sinus. The size of the fistula is responsible for the persistence of all the three channels. It must be recognised that the tentorial sinus is the primary route of exit. The relationship between the arterial feeders, the size of the fistula, and the capacity of the venous channels is discussed in the appendix. The three examples sited in this section are basically similar. The variations seem to be in the pattern of the venous drainage. There are a number of variations possible on this basic pattern, but they follow the same principle (see Figure 9.22).

The Deep Telencephalic Malformations

The Arterial Component of the Malformations

The medial striate and primitive ophthalmic branches of the anterior cerebral artery constitute the arterial elements of the malformation.

The Angiomatous Elements of the Malformation

As in the case of the sylvian malformations, the arterio-capillary tangle is often situated in the region of the basal ganglia. Complete absence of the angioma is also a frequent feature of this group of lesions.

The Venous Elements

The inferior striate tributaries of the deep telencephalic pial veins cross the medial striate arteries at approximately right angles. The complexity of the development of the telencephalon obscures the segmental pattern. The inferior striate vein drains through the telencephalic veins into the tentorial and transverse sinuses respectively. The formation of the basal vein can divert the blood flow medially into the great cerebral vein.

Regrouping of the Cases According to the Similarity of the Venous Pattern

The abnormal venous channels have a very distinct appearance in this region. They are directed backwards and medially and reach the internal cerebral vein near its anterior end.

Identification and Matching of the Abnormal Venous Channels with the Normal Embryonic Venous Channels

The venous channels involved in these lesions are usually directed backwards and medially into the great cerebral vein, and they represent segments of the primitive basal vein. It was mentioned earlier that the drainage primarily is into the tentorial and transverse sinuses. It is extremely rare to see this persisting into the adult life. The drainage from the inferior striate vein via the deep middle cerebral, superficially middle cerebral, the tentorial sinus, and finally into the transverse sinus is a very devious and inefficient route to persist. The basal vein seems to be the naturally preferred route. As the fistula occurs close to the origin of the anterior cerebellar artery, the quantity of blood flowing across is very likely to be enormous, and nothing short of the most efficient route is practicable. The capacity of the internal cerebral vein is nearly unlimited.

Aneurysm of the Vein of Galen

The inferior striate vein, not infrequently, has a connection with the great cerebral vein, in addition to the basal vein already mentioned. The inferior striate vein courses through the caudate closely related to the caudate tributaries of the terminal vein. An anastomosis between these can occur. The primitive internal cerebral vein is mainly extracerebral until after the 80-mm stage and receives only one intracerebral tributary (in the region of the intraventricular foramena), namely, the terminal vein. Therefore, the shunted blood will find its way thus into the primitive internal cerebral vein. Since the latter is mainly extracerebral, there is scope for unlimited expansion as there are no restrictions from the surrounding tissues. (Agee[2&3], Amachar[7], Askenasy[48], Bedford[81], Boldrey[84], Claireux[46], Cohen[41], French[69], Gagnon[70], Gibbs[92], Gold[97], Gomez[101], Hirano[123], Hochsetter[124], Litvak[167], Lumsden[176], Poppen[253], Rosenberg[276], Thomson[325], Weir[346]).

Since the terminal vein marks the beginning of the intracerebral vein, location of the drainage is likely to be at the anterior end of the latter. Since the medial striate artery is one of the earliest branches of the main trunk, and since the capacity for venous system to expand is unlimited, the degree of shunting is proportionately very high, compared with the other types in this group. (See the chapter on the Hemodynamics properties of arteriovenous shunting.)

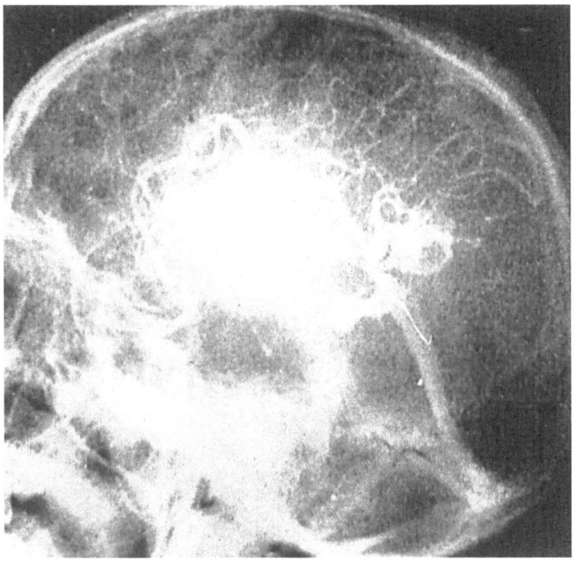

Figure 9.25 Telencephalic arterio-venous malformation. Arterior cerebral artery feeder. Telencephalic vein draining into the great cerebral vein (Lateral).

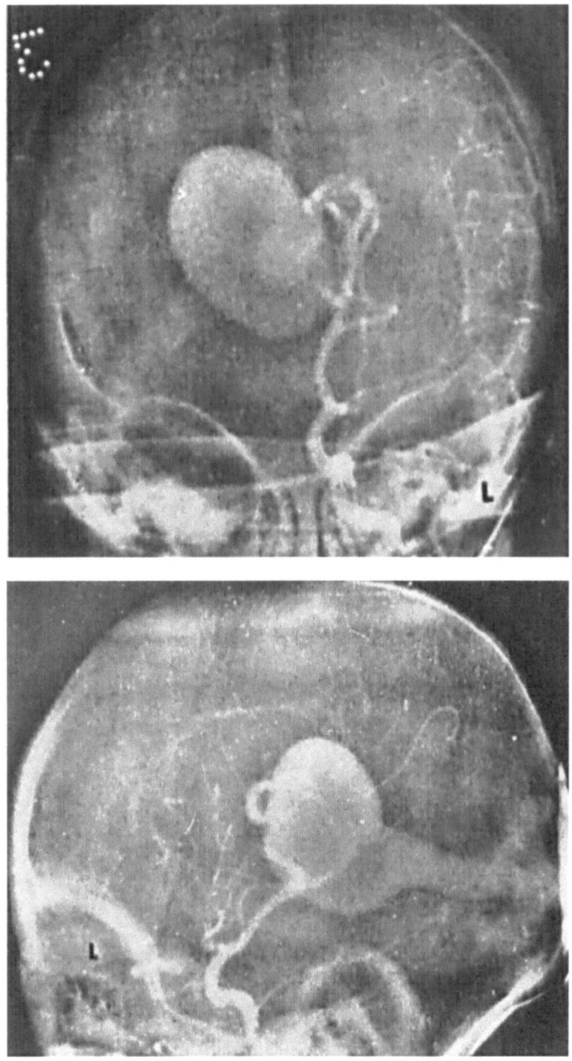

Figure 9.26 Telencephalic arterio-venous malformation. Anterior cerebral artery feeder. Telencephalic vein draining into the great cerebral vein.

The examples of aneurysm of the vein of Galen described in the literature belong to the category of arteriovenous malformations. The dilatation of the vein is so obvious, the importance of the arterial feeder is generally overlooked.

Figure 9.28 also shows an arteriovenous fistula produced by the anterior cerebral artery and very dilated internal cerebral vein. Although at first sight this example appears to be similar to the ones cited earlier (Figure 9.25-Figure 9.27), there are certain variations. The anterior cerebral artery here enters the internal cerebral vein at its anterior end. This is not just a variation of the earlier examples. The involvement of the terminal vein in the malformation is responsible for the production of this pattern. Many of the cases published in the literature in the category of aneurysm of the vein of Galen have this feature (Wolf[350&351]).

Sometimes the inferior striate vein joins the superior striate vein, and this, in turn, joins the anterior terminal vein. Since this anastomosis occurs in post-natal life, it is unlikely to play a significant role in the present context.

Summing up, the arterial components of the telencephalic arteriovenous malformations arise from the anterior cerebral and middle cerebral arteries. The complexity of the developmental process in this region obscures the fundamental segmental pattern. There are three regions where the primitive pial vessels cross at right angles; they are as follows:

1. Over the convexity of the cerebral hemisphere
2. In the sylvian territory
3. In the region of the basal ganglia

The malformations over the surface drain into the superior sagittal sinus. The sylvian and deep telencephalic malformations drain primarily into the tentorial sinus, and this is often replaced by a medial drainage into the internal cerebral vein through the tributaries of the basal vein.

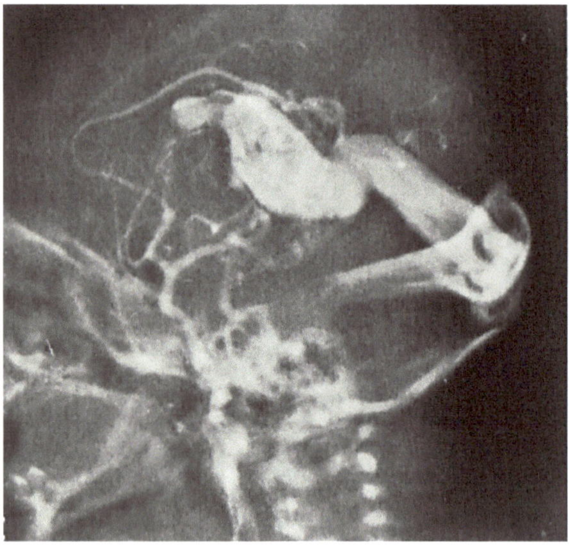

Figure 9.27 Telencephalic arterio-venous malformation. Anterior cerebral artery feeder. Telencephalic vein draining into the great cerebral vein (Lateral).

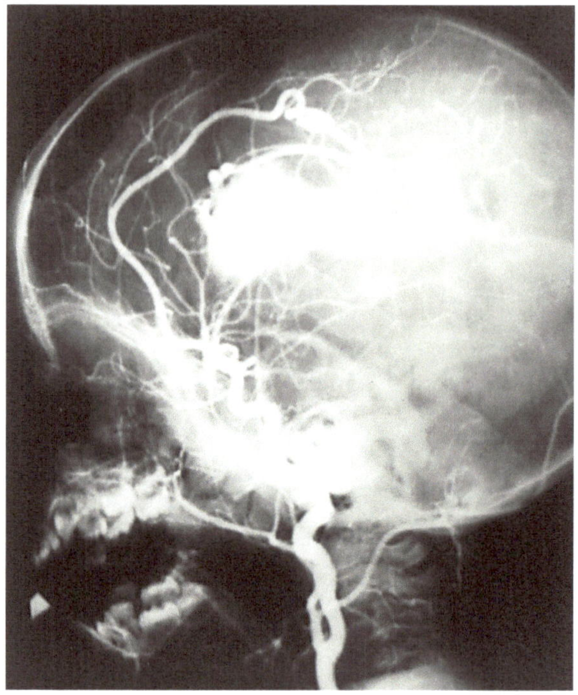

Figure 9.28 Vein of Galen Malformation.

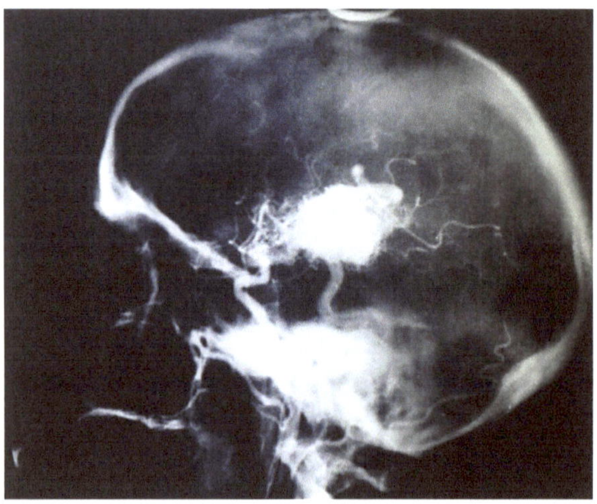

Figure 9.29 MCA Feeder Sylvian Malformation. Shift the end of this section along ith other pictures.

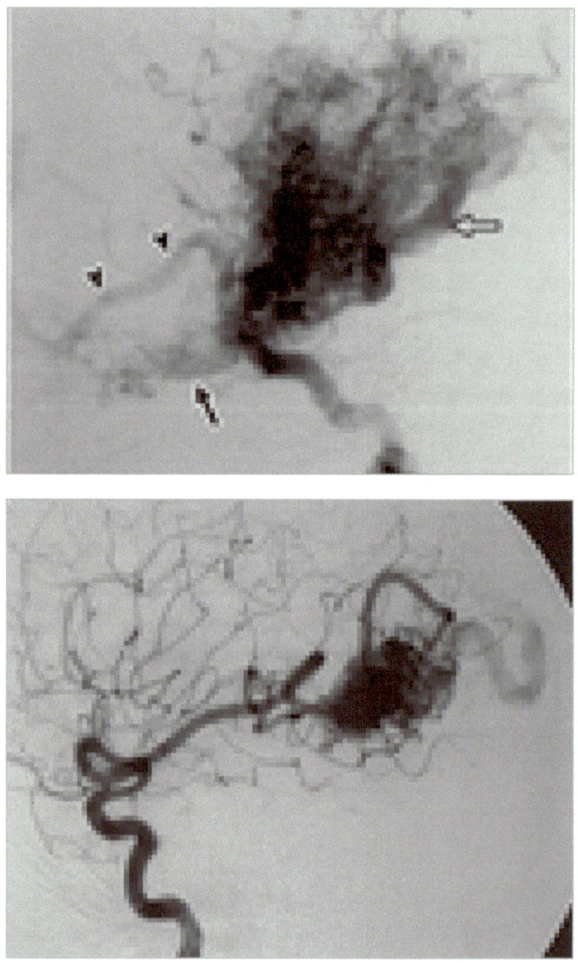

Figure 9.30 Sylvian AVM draining laterally. (Geibpraser)[74] Locate above as no indicates.

10

Dural Arteriovenous Malformations

The anatomy of dural arteriovenous malformations is often difficult to understand. The dural lesions have features common with those of internal carotid arterial feeders, since they have a common origin during the early stages of development. The vascular malformations of the scalp are from the external carotid feeders and have a different pattern.

The arteriovenous malformations of the coverings of the brain (the dura) have the same general pattern as those of the intracerebral lesions (Vidyasagar[334&335]).

The Arterial Component

The middle meningeal artery is the principal dural artery from which the arteriovenous malformations arise frequently. The less-frequent arterial source includes the ophthalmic artery, the tentorial artery, and the meningo-hypophyseal artery. The occipital artery is frequently seen to be involved in the dural malformations, but its role is secondary, and this is explained later in this chapter (Stattin[311], Wilson[349], Amico[8], Nakumara[207], Nomura[214]).

The Angioma

The location of the angioma is very variable and has no predictable feature. In a majority of cases no angioma is seen.

As an exception, the dural malformation in the region of the cavernous sinus frequently contains an angioma.

The Venous Elements

The venous drainage of the dura is either into the superior sagittal sinus or into the transverse sinus. The veins draining into the superior sagittal sinus course upwards and medially, whilst those draining into the transverse sinus course laterally and downwards (Balo[14]).

Regrouping of Cases According to the Similarity of Venous Pattern

There are, therefore, two principal types of dural lesion:

1. Venous drainage through the tributaries of the middle meningeal sinus into the superior sagittal sinus over the convexity of the developing brain.
2. Less frequently in a certain group of cases, the venous drainage occurs laterally into the junction between the transverse and sigmoid sinuses.

Matching of the Abnormal Vascular Channels with the Normal Embryonic Venous Channels

Middle Meningeal Sinus

The venous drainage from the meninges reaches the pro-otic sinus (40 mm) by a lateral tributary, the middle meningeal sinus. The pro-otic sinus, by a process of secondary anastomosis, reaches the junction between the transverse and sigmoid sinuses (superior petrosal sinus). Subsequent development of the external jugular vein and cavernous sinus, as an alternate route, diverts the flow partly away from the transverse and sigmoid sinuses.

Superior Sagittal Sinus

This sinus shares the drainage of the dura with the transverse sinus. The middle meningeal sinus drains partly into the superior sagittal sinus over the convexity of the developing brain. These are retained in the post-natal period as diverticula of the superior sagittal sinus (see Figure 10.1).

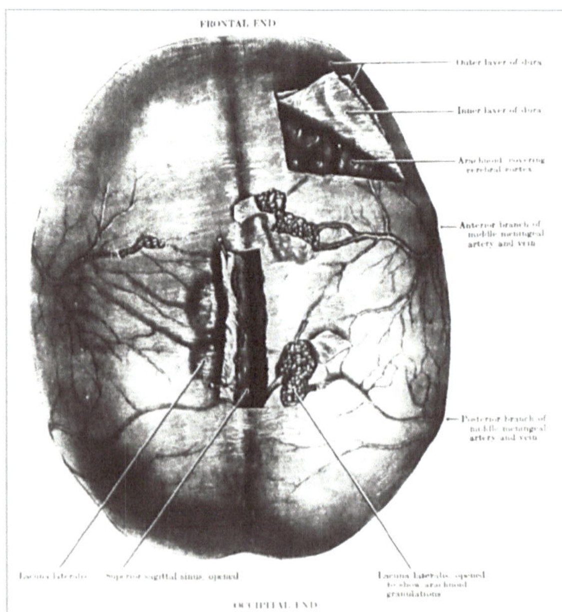

Figure 10.1 Middle meningeal vein draining into the superior sagittal sinus via the lateral lacunae (Grant).[102]

Cavernous Sinus

It was mentioned earlier that the involvement of the cavernous sinus through the inferior petrosal sinus is not common, as these venous connections are established only in the post-natal period. In certain instances, the primitive cavernous sinus can play a primary role in the dural malformations. The cavernous sinus in the early period of development is in the form of venous sinusoids and closely related to the meningio-hypophyseal trunk. An arteriovenous fistula in this situation is possible.

Regrouping of the Malformations with Reference to the Embryological Location of the Adult Cerebral Arteries

The middle meningeal artery in the adult arises from the external carotid artery. Therefore, it has been a common practice to group the malformations related to this artery with the scalp malformations. See classification – Newton and Cronqvist. The reader is referred to the reference list and not to the chapter in the book. The middle meningeal artery primarily is a branch of the internal carotid artery (Elkin[75&76], Fincher[79] Hassler[117]. The following developmental changes occur. The primitive stapedial artery arising from the internal carotid artery consists of two principal branches, namely, the supraorbital and the maxillo-mandibular. Around the 20-mm stage, an anastomosis between the maxillo-mandibular artery and the internal maxillary artery (branch of the external carotid artery) occurs. Thus the origin of the middle meningeal artery is secondarily shifted to the external carotid system (see Figure 10.2 and Figure 10.3). The supraorbital division now represents the segment of the middle meningeal artery within the dural coverings of the brain.

A similar anastomosis also occurs between the divisions of the external and internal carotid

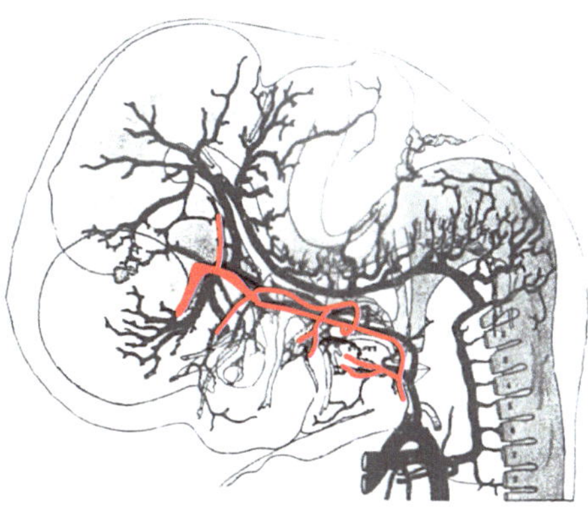

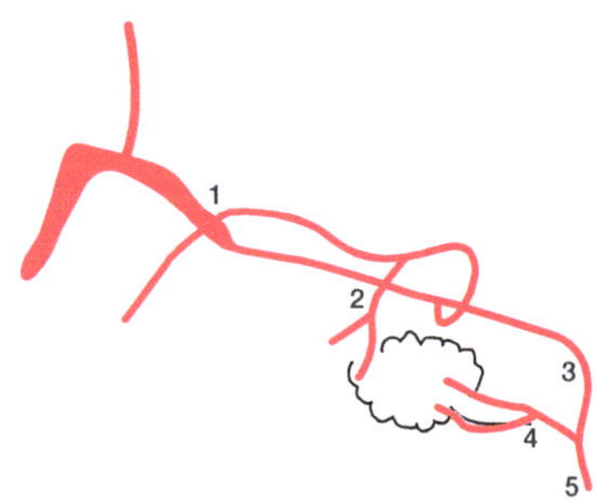

1 Supraord Div of Staped A **2** Max-Mand Div of Staped **3** Int Carot A **4** Ext Carot A **5** Comm Carot A

Figure 10.2 Middle meningeal artery arising from the internal carotid artery (Stapedial Artery).

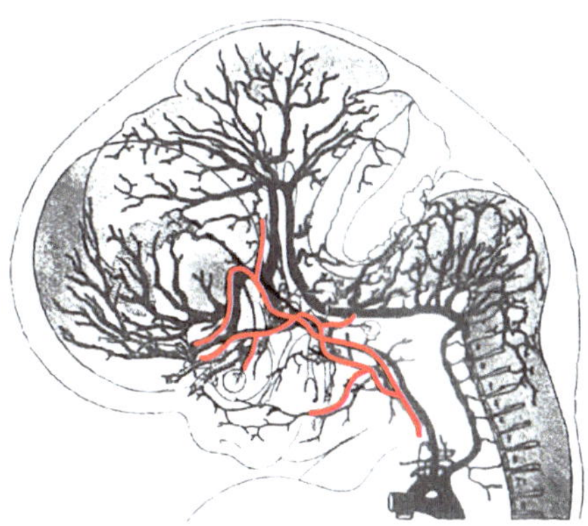

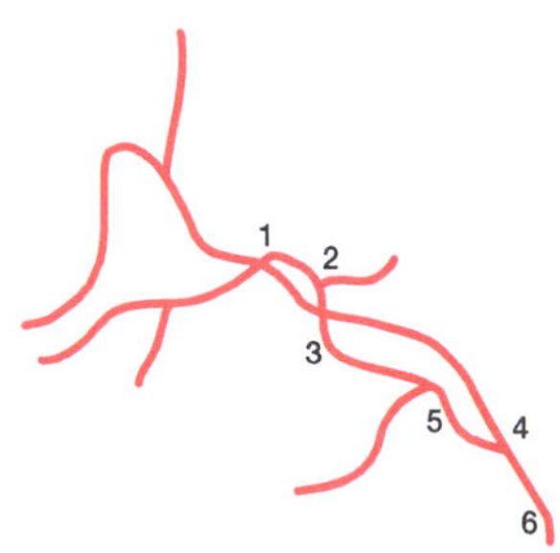

1 Mid Mening A **2** Stem of Staped A **3** Int Max A **4** Ext Max A & Int Carot A **5** Ext Carot A **6** Comm Carot A

Figure 10.3 Middle mentingeal artery arising from the external carotid artery.

arteries in the region of the orbit. The stapedial artery (the definitive middle meningeal artery) gives rise to supraorbital branches, in the process forming a part of the vascular ring around the optic nerve. The remaining part of this ring is completed by the branches of the ophthalmic artery. Between the 20–40-mm stage, a secondary anastomosis develops between the supraorbital branches of the middle meningeal artery and the stem of the lacunal branch of the ophthalmic artery. This disappears in the latter stages so that the supraorbital branches of the middle meningeal artery are incorporated in the ophthalmic artery (see Figure 10.4, Figure 10.5 and 10.6). The persistence of this embryonic connection can sometimes be seen in the adult near the lateral end of the sylvian fissure. (Kosnik[151], Nizzoli[213], Pakarinen[236] Vidyasagar[340]).

It was mentioned earlier that the occipital artery is frequently seen hypertrophied in the dural malformations. Like the middle meningeal artery, the origin of the occipital artery from the external carotid artery is a secondary phenomenon. It is a branch of the internal carotid artery primarily (Adams[1] Fadhli[78], Schnurer[292] (see Figure 10.6).

The Classification Based on the Embryological Site of the Malformation

Newton and Cronqvist[209] classified the arteriovenous malformations into pial, mixed, and the dural. This classification is based on the concept that

1. the dural arteries are different from the pial arteries.
2. some dural arteriovenous malformations receive arterial feeders from both external and internal carotid systems.

The dural vascular system is closely related to that of the pial and is different from the external carotid system. The post-natal configuration is a secondary development. It is often recorded that the venous systems of the skull and the dura are interconnected and later separated by the membranous skull, except in the region of the emissary veins. This is an error (Takahashi[321] Takekawa[322] Urdanibia[329] Van Der Eecken[330].

Except in the region of the emissary veins, the two systems are primarily separate. The purely extradural arteriovenous malformations are related to scalp arteries and external jugular

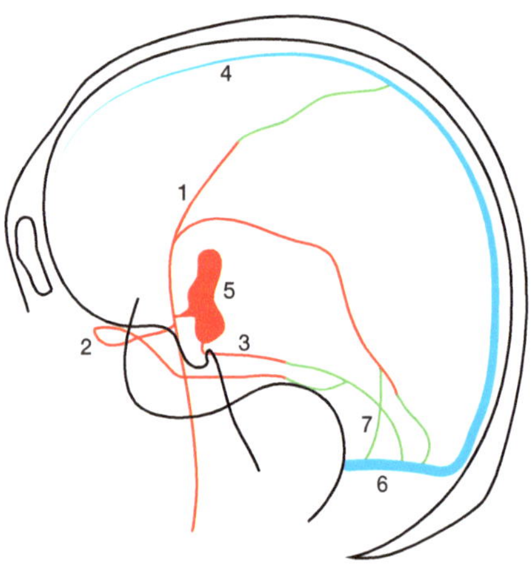

Figure 10.4 Theoretically possible variations in the drainage of dural arterio-venous malformations (Lateral).

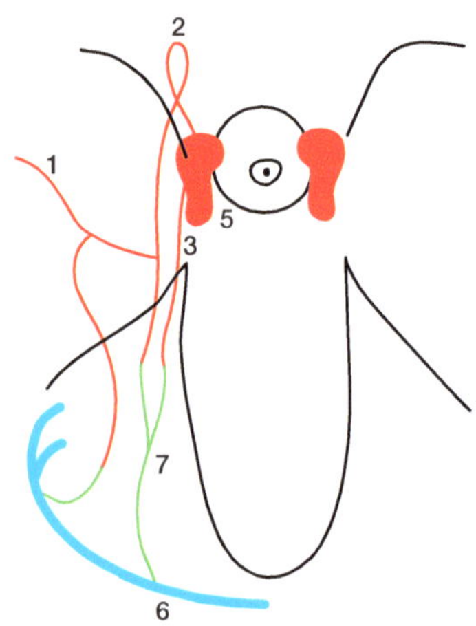

Figure 10.5 Theoretically possible variations in the drainage of dural arterio-venous malformations (Basal).

1 Mid Mening A **2** Ophthalmic A **3** Tentorial A **4** Sup Sagitt Sin
5 Int Carotid A **6** Trans Sin **7** Mid Mening Sin

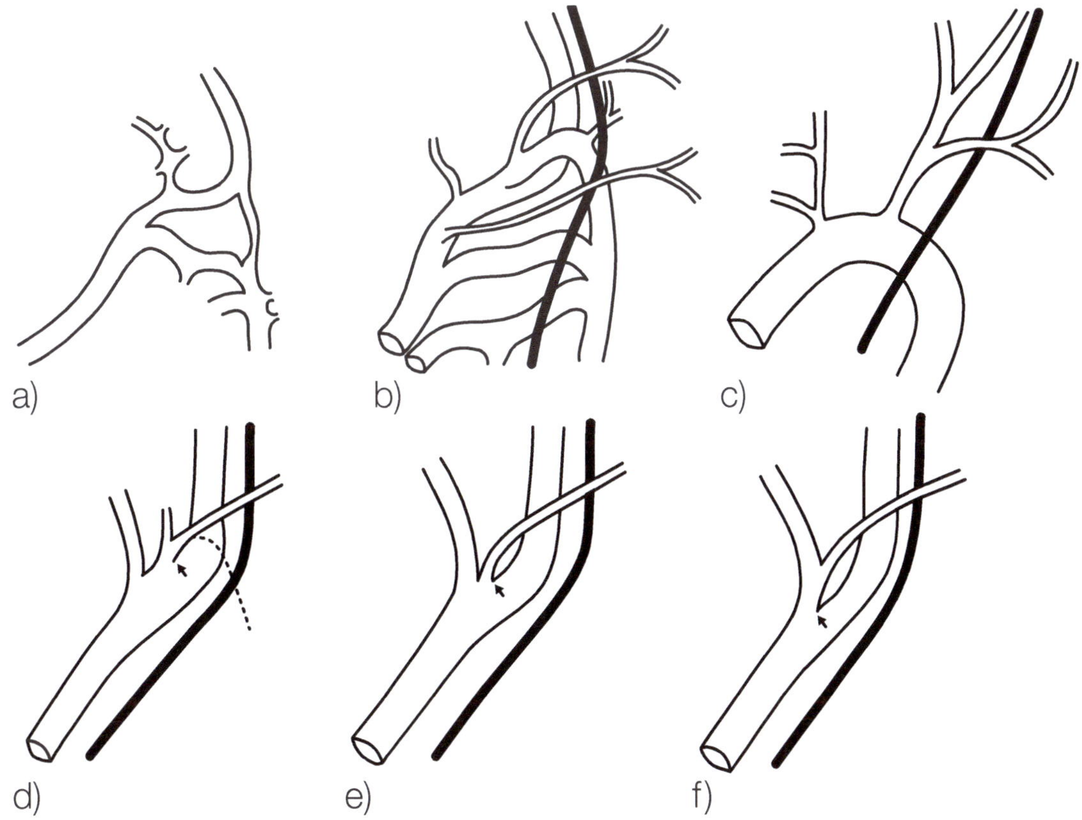

Figure 10.6 Secondary migration of the occipital artery from the internal carotid to the external carotid system.

veins. They have no direct communications with the dural vessels. The scalp is developed very late and is vascularised after the 80-mm stage. By this time, the cerebral and dural vessels are well advanced in development and are less likely to be involved in these malformations.

Possible Anatomical Configurations of Dural Arteriovenous Malformation

Like the pia-arachnoidal vessels, the dural arteries and veins also cross each other at approximately right angles. The venous tributaries are interposed between the branches of the artery and the bone. Occurrence of an arteriovenous fistula in this situation is just as easily possible here as elsewhere. Since the meningeal arteries arise primarily from the internal carotid artery, the venous anatomy of the malformation has the basic features similar to that of the cerebral lesions. The drainage is laterally into the transverse sinus and superiorly into the superior sagittal sinus Robinson[274]. Since the middle meningeal sinus drains into the transverse sinus directly (pro-otic sinus), the developmental changes in the tentorial sinus do not affect the lateral drainage. Therefore, the primary drainage into the transverse sinus persists in the adult. It is very rare to see the drainage into the great cerebral vein.

Examples

Middle Meningeal Artery – Transverse Sinus

Markham[190] reported an arteriovenous fistula between the middle meningeal artery and the greater petrosal sinuses. 'The middle meningeal artery was noted to be somewhat larger in diameter than usual. Also demonstrated was a fistulous communication between the proximal portion of the right middle meningeal artery and the greater petrosal sinus. The venogram revealed some dye remaining in the sinus, and some could be traced without difficulty into the jugular bulb.' (Reproduction of the actual figure was not possible because of technical difficulties).

Superior Sagittal Sinus

Figure 10.7 and Figure 10.8 (lateral) show an arteriovenous fistula produced by the middle meningeal artery. The venous drainage is into the superior sagittal sinus near the torcula. The point of entry into the superior sagittal sinus near its torcula end appears to be a fairly frequent pattern. The caudal migration of the torcula and the cerebral hemisphere produced a corresponding backward swing of the superior sagittal sinus. It is possible that this process is responsible for the location of the drainage seen in the above examples.

Primary drainage into the torcula region directly is unusual. A secondary (perhaps post-natal) anastomosis may divert the blood via the occipital veins into the torcula area.

Meningio-Hypophyseal Artery

In the example cited by Newton and Hoyt[211], the fistula has occurred within the venous meshes of the cavernous sinus and the meningeal branch of the meningio-hypophyseal trunk.

Figure 10.12 shows a further variation of the above example. Here the fistula has occurred outside the region of the cavernous sinus. The tentorial sinus is closely related to the tentorial branch of the meningio-hypophyseal trunk. So if a fistula occurs in this area, the venous drainage is naturally into the tentorial sinus. Since the outcome of such a lesion depends upon the fate of the tentorial sinus, the final drainage is very likely to be into the great cerebral vein. See Figure 10.9 and Figure 10.12. Hanford[116]

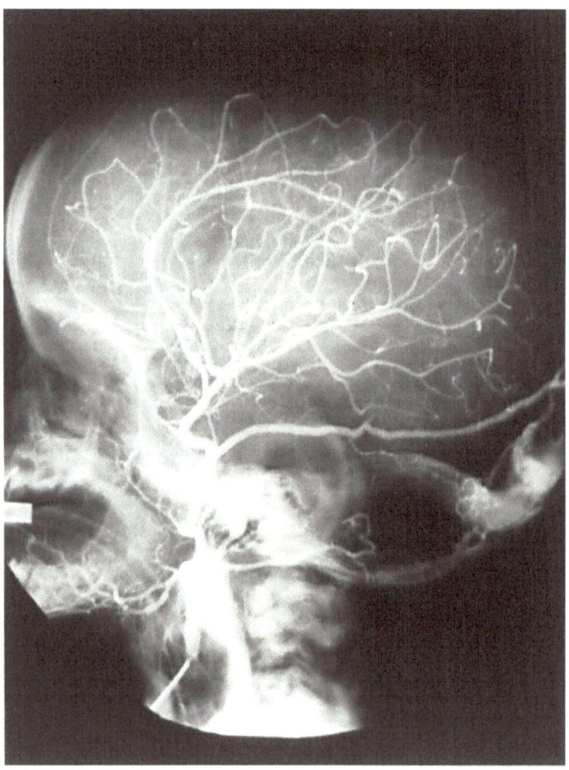

Figure 10.7 Venous drainage into SSS - Torcula junction

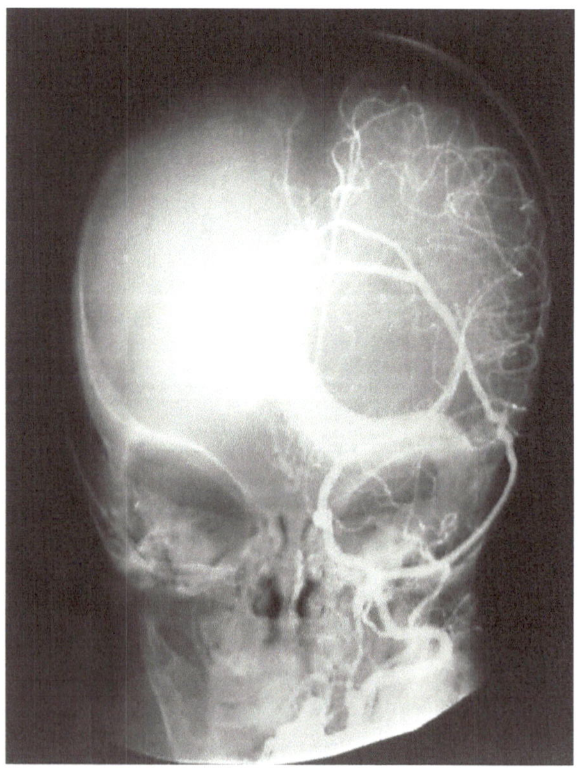

Figure 10.8 Venous drainage into SSS - Torcula junction

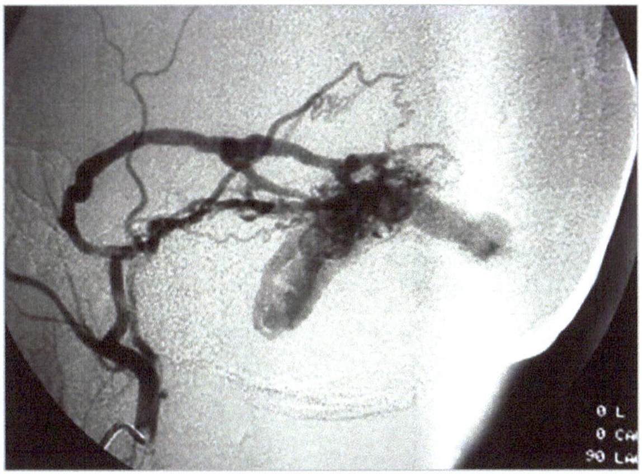

Figure 10.9 Dural arterio-venous malformation. Venous draining into the tentorial sinus (Lateral).

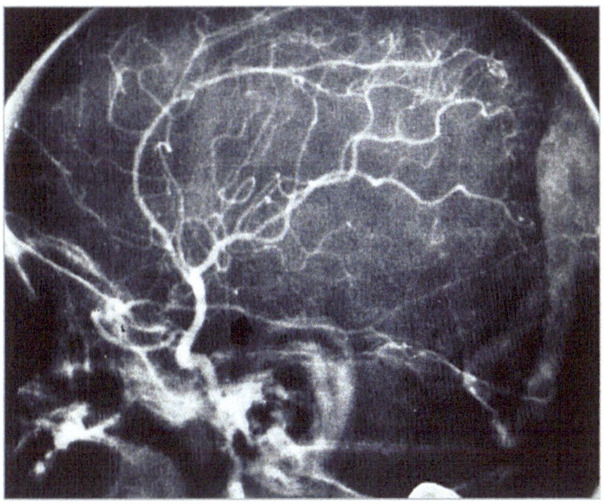

Figure 10.10 Dural Arterio-Venous Malformation. Ophthalmic artery feeder. Venous drainage into the transverse sinus (Lateral).

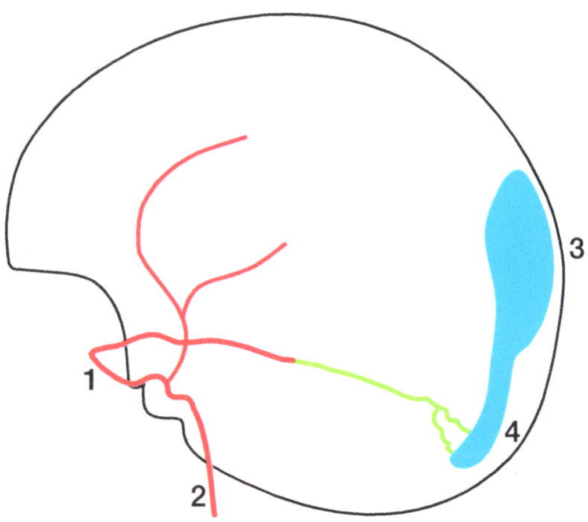

Figure 10.11 Colour tracing of Figure 10.10.

1 Ophthalmic A **2** Int Carot A **3** Torcula **4** Transv Sin

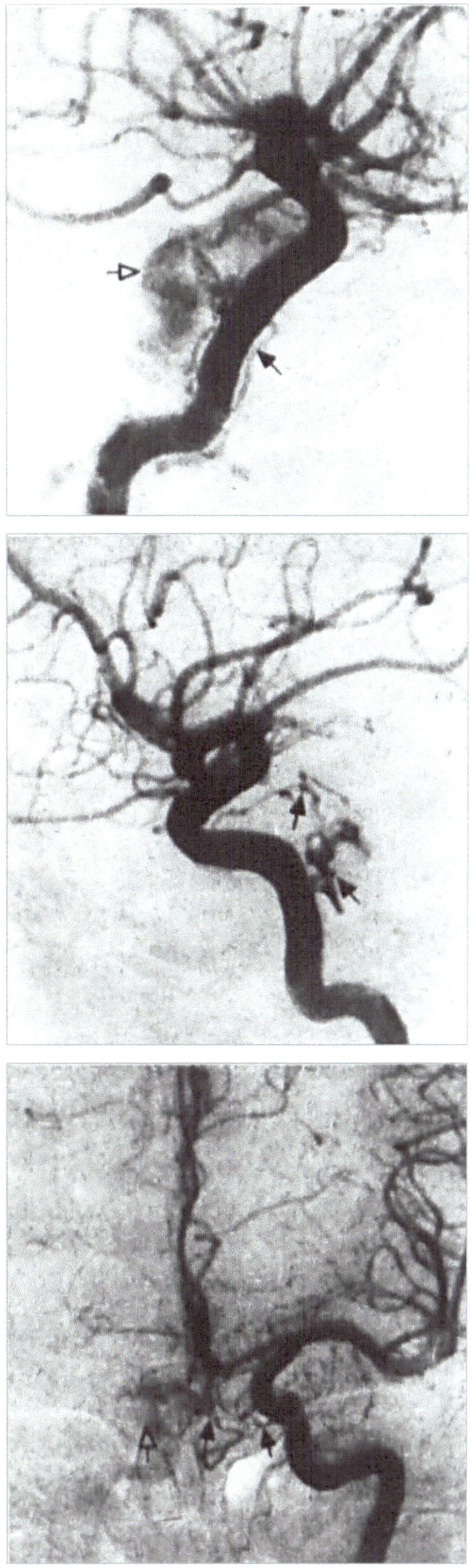

Figure 10.12 Dural arterio-venous malformation meningio-hypophyseal artery feeder.

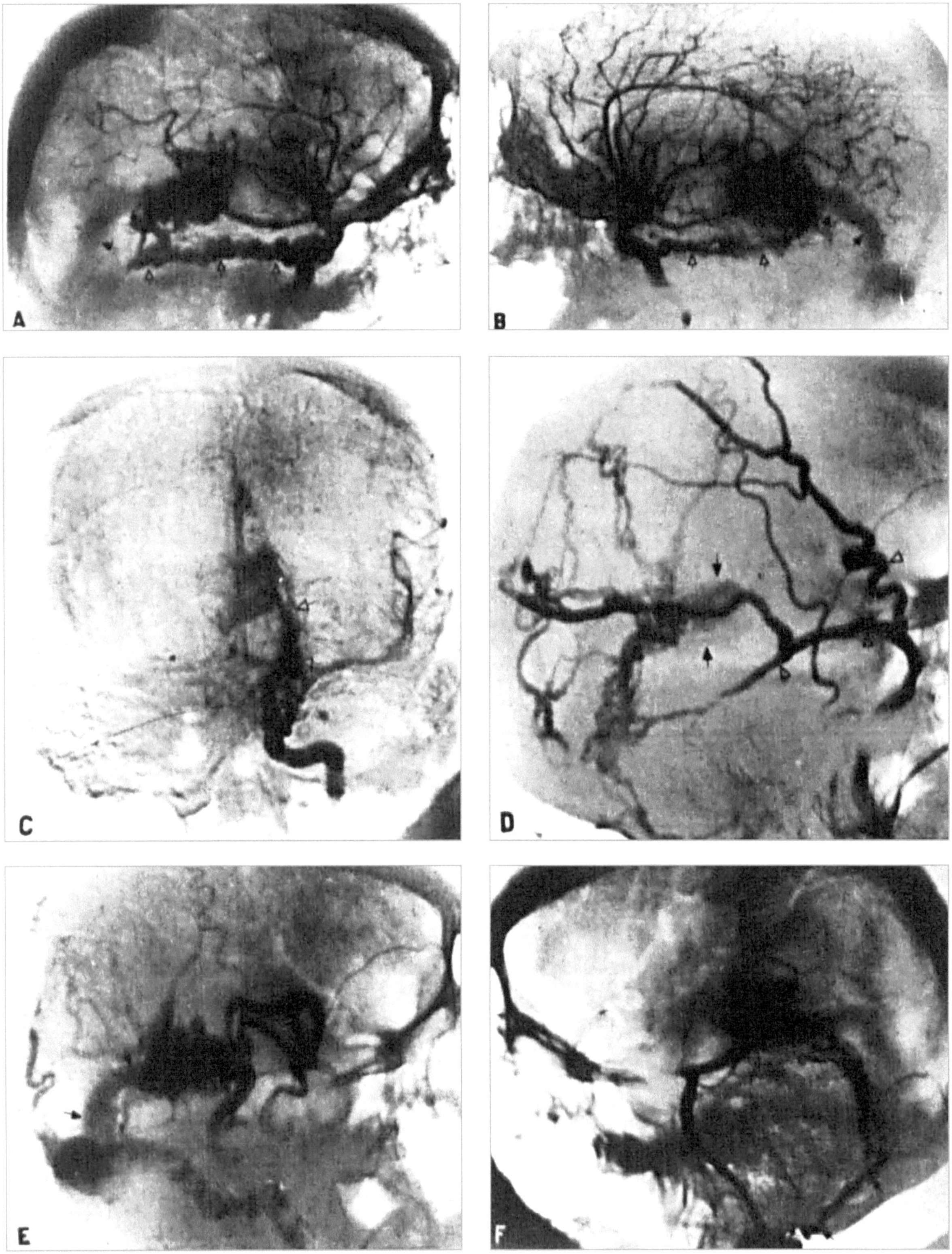

Figure 10.13 Dural arterio-venous malformation. Tentorial artery feeder. Yasargil[354]

Some Less-Frequent Patterns

Figures 10.10 & 10.11 are examples cited by Pool[250-252] and show the arterial component arising from the ophthalmic artery, a dilated and tortuous vessel that extends to the sigmoid sinus. This segment of the vessel represents the middle meningeal sinus leading to the sigmoid sinus. The segment of the artery extending from the ophthalmic artery to this vessel perhaps represents the persisting embryonic connection.

It is possible in this case that the connection between the ophthalmic and middle meningeal arteries (which would normally have disappeared) has been retained as a supplementary channel, in an attempt to reduce the arteriovenous gradient.

Vein of Galen

It is exceptional for the dural vein to drain into the vein of Galen. But potential channels exist via the inferior cerebral vein and tributaries of tentorial sinus (see Figure 10.13).

In a series of sixteen dural arteriovenous malformations, Newton, Weidner, and Greitz[212] attributed vein of Galen involvement in three cases. The feeding arteries were as follows:

1. Tentorial artery (Figure 10.13A & 10.13B)
2. Posterior branch of the middle meningeal artery (Figure 10.13C & 10.13D)
3. Vertebral artery (Figure 10.13E & 10.13F)

Example 2 is a rare feature and has probably occurred through the potential connection mentioned earlier.

But in example 3, in addition to the meningeal branch of the vertebral artery, the posterior cerebral artery is hypertrophied and appears to be the principal contributor. The vertebral artery involvement is not very convincing and is probably of secondary importance. (Vein of Galen drainage in relation to the posterior cerebral artery lesion is, as described earlier, a very common feature.)

Occipital Artery

Newton and Greitz[209] reported a series of five cases of dural arteriovenous malformations. In each of these cases a prominent occipital artery and transverse sinus were seen in the angiograms. These findings were interpreted as to show communications between the occipital artery and the transverse sinus, indicating a congenital arteriovenous communication between the external carotid artery and the emissary veins at the base of the skull.

But certain important aspects appear to have been overlooked in this reasoning. In each of these cases cited, a prominent middle meningeal artery was also seen reaching the region of the transverse sinus.

Hypertrophy of the occipital artery with or without the opacification of a middle meningeal contribution seen in angiograms is not in itself a conclusive evidence of the role played by the occipital artery.

In all the instances cited in the literature where ligation of the occipital artery was carried out based on the reasoning that it was the prime feeder, the arteriovenous malformations either persisted or recurred soon after (Newton, Weidner, and Greitz[212]. In one case, it in fact appeared, having been absent during the earlier operative measures. Enlargement of the meningeal arteries are secondary effects of the primary lesion.

Kosnik, Hunt, and Miller[151] again reported two cases of dural arteriovenous malformations with prominent occipital arteries. In one the occipital artery appeared to drain into the sigmoid sinus. Following external carotid ligation, the symptoms recurred, although there was some initial improvement. The dilated vertebral artery was ligated at the second operation, with no symptomatic improvement. At the third exploration, 'dural arteries were ligated and sigmoid sinus partially blocked', followed by permanent recovery.

In the second case, external carotid artery branches drained into an arteriovenous malformation in the region of the torcula with reflux filling of the superior sagittal sinuses. Bilateral external carotid ligation produced only temporary improvement in symptoms. At the second operation an enlarged branch from the vertebral artery draining into the lateral sinus was ligated. Again the symptoms were relieved for nine months. The third angiograph showed a 'fistula' in the tentorium fed by the left and right occipital arteries leading to the posterior part of the superior sagittal sinus with a measured contribution from both tentorial arteries. Torcula, falx, and adjacent tentorium were excised, and superior sagittal sinus, right lateral sinus and sinus rectus up to the junction of the vein of Galen with inferior sagittal sinus were ligated, followed by recovery from symptoms. In both these cases, ligation of the prominent occipital and vertebral arteries only improved the symptoms, sometimes temporarily, and permanent recovery was possible only when the main fistula was obliterated.

The temporary improvement in the symptoms was perhaps due to reduction of the blood flow through the fistula via the collaterals. Symptoms recurred once a fresh collateral circulation was re-formed. These collaterals included meningeal branches of the vertebral and occipital arteries, which, in fact, occurred following the external carotid ligation. In fact, the ligation of the external carotid reduced the blood to the fistula, and collateral channels were opened. The same effect could be seen if the fistula is too large and a middle meningeal artery is unable to meet the demand. The effects of ligating collateral feeders and an inequilibrium between the supply and demand of the fistula are the same.

A similar explanation is possible where there is a temporary improvement following ligation of 'multiple feeders' of the malformation. The arterialised veins collapse and the angioma shrivels up. If the process has included the obliteration of the shunt, the results of such a procedure are likely to be permanent. If not, after a period, 'fresh feeding arteries and angioma' develop at the same or different sites(Maroum[191]).

Ramamurthi and Balasubramanian[262] reported a case where the malformation was fed by both middle meningeal and occipital arteries. Ligation of both the vessels cured the symptoms completely (18 months' follow-up). This is an unusual response, and it is likely that there were no other potential feeders shunting into the fistula.

This example was classified by the authors as 'arteriovenous malformations with a purely external carotid contribution'. It was mentioned at the beginning of this chapter how the middle meningeal artery secondarily shifts from the internal carotid to the external carotid artery.

By a similar process, the occipital artery is also shifted from the internal carotid to the external carotid circulation.

Adams[1] wrote on the possible homologies of the occipital artery in mammals and certain anomalies of the subclavian and carotid arteries (see Figure 10.5).

Although the occipital artery has many features similar to the middle meningeal artery with regard to its origin, dural arteriovenous malformations produced exclusively by the former appear to be rare. There is, so far, no evidence of such an example reported in the literature. (Dilated occipital artery in conjunction with middle meningeal artery or other arteries have to be excluded here). This is perhaps attributable to the fact that the venous elements in this region of the occipital artery are mainly related to the external jugular system and, therefore, appear very late. It is possible that by the time the vein appears, the formation of the artery is too far advanced to have endothelial defects still persisting, to produce a shunt.

11

Multiple Arteriovenous Malformations

The segmental anatomy is retained even in arteriovenous malformations extending across vast areas of the adult brain, with multiple arterial feeders. The common pattern in such complex lesions is described. Possibility of multiple defects in different segments of the brain is discussed.

In some instances more than one arterial feeder is seen to be involved in the malformation. They are generally described as 'a few of the many embryonic vascular shunts persisting in the post-natal life'. Even here, the pattern is not as complex as it may seem in the first instance. Some basic principles as seen in the solitary feeders are also applicable here (Mulvihill[204]). The arteriovenous shunts are produced between the individual vascular channels; the defect occurs at more than one point.

The Arterial Component

This can be classified into two types:

1. The feeding artery belonging to the same embryonic segment
2. The feeding arteries belonging to the different embryonic segments

When the feeding arteries belong to the same embryonic segment, the pattern is likely to be very similar to that of the individual lesion.

The diencephalic area is where these lesions are likely to occur most frequently. This is not surprising since this segment consists of the maximum number of arteries (three) (Figure 11.1).

The Angioma

When an angioma is present in these multiple feeders, the general appearances suggest that both the arteries are involved in a common lesion, but this is misleading. Each lesion is separately produced, and the overlap of their territories is only apparent.

Figure 11.2 show an example where a clear distinction between the areas involving the anterior cerebral and middle cerebral artery lesions can be made. Such definite demarcation perhaps exists in all these multiple lesions.

The Venous Elements

The pattern of venous drainage is more complex in this type of malformation. When the feeders arise from the same embryonic segment, the mode of drainage common to that segment is usually seen. In the example cited in Figure 11.2 both the posterior cerebral and anterior choroidal arteries belong to the diencephalon. The venous drainage into the great cerebral vein through the diencephalic veins has occurred. When the feeders belong to different embryonic segments, the pattern of final venous drainage is not predictable.

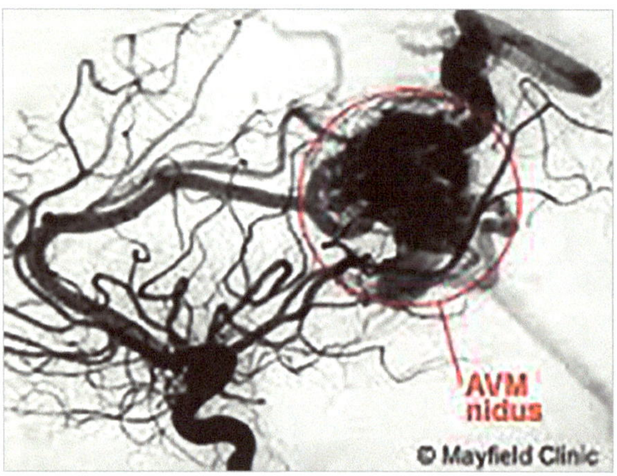

Figure 11.1 Multiple arterial feeders (Mayfield Clinic).

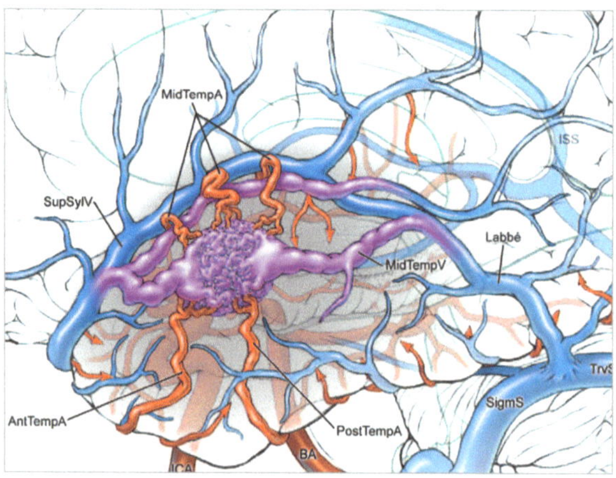

Figure 11.2 Multiple Arterial Feeders (Radiopedia).

12

Vein of Galen Malformations

Arteriovenous fistulae between the embryonic vessels situated in the midline are often associated with aneurismal dilatation of the great cerebral vein. These fistulae occur in the telencephalic, diencephalic, and mesencephalic segments of the primitive brain. The evolution of these malformations is described.

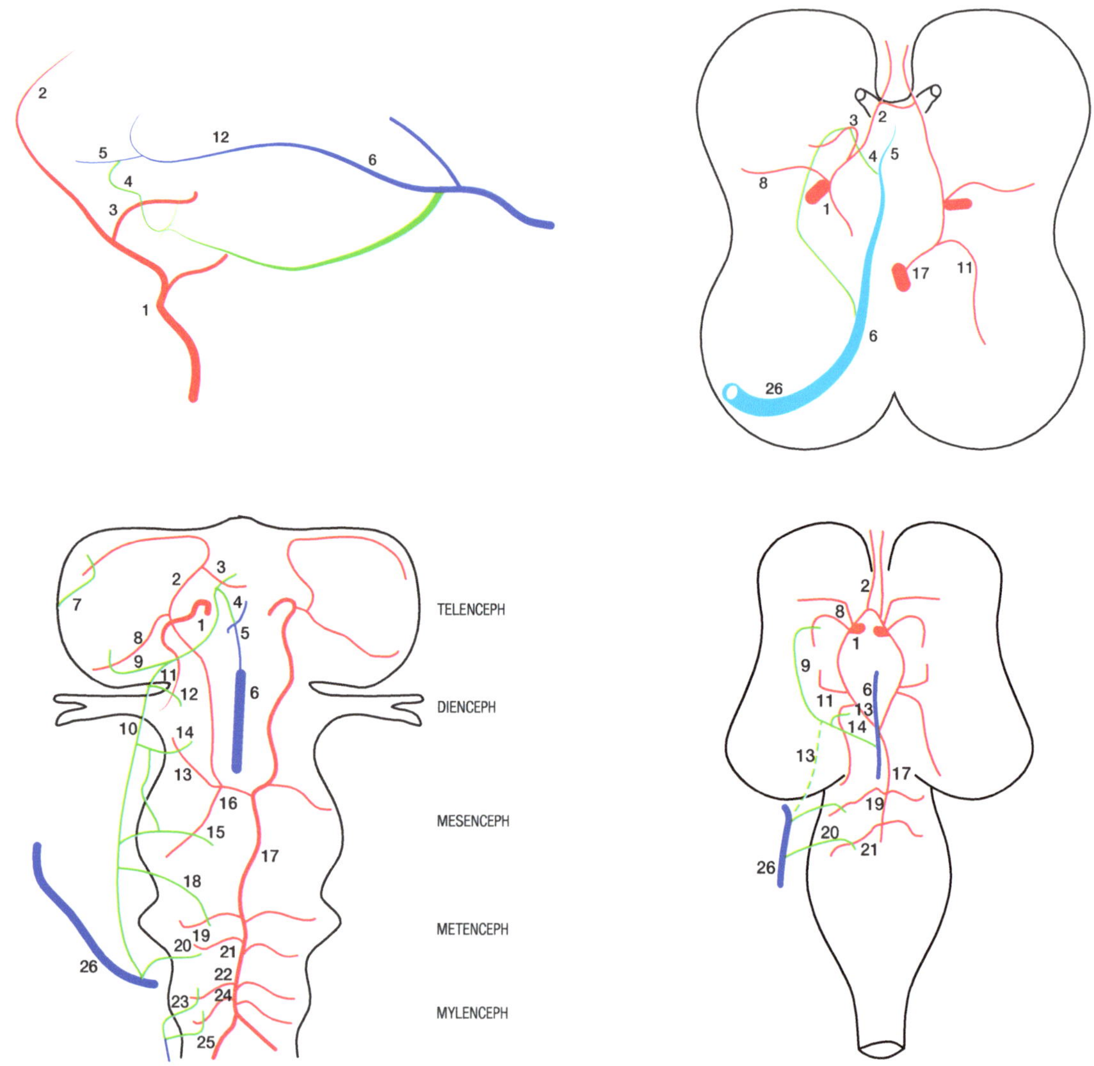

1 Int C A **2** Ant C A **3** Medical Striate A **4** Ant Striate V **5** Terminal Vein **6** Int Cereb V **7** Sup Telenceph V **8** Mid C A **9** Deep Telenceph V **10** Basal Vein **11** Ant Choridal V **12** Dors Dienceph V **13** Post Ch A **14** Vent Dienceph V **15** Vent Mesenceph V **16** Mesenceph A **17** Basilar A **18** Dors Metenceph V **19** Dors Metenceph A **20** Vent Metenceph V **21** Vent Metenceph A **22** Dors Mylenceph A **23** Dors Mylenceph V **24** Vent Mylenceph A **25** Vent Mylenceph V **26** Trans-Sigmoid Sin

Figure 12.1 Vein of Galen AVM variations (Diagramatic).

In the region of the telencephalon the segmental pial vessels are represented by the medial striate artery and the inferior striate vein. These cross each other at right angles.

If an arteriovenous fistula occurs between medial striate artery and the inferior striate vein the direction of flow of blood would be inferior striate vein, deep telencephalic vein, superficial telencephalic veins, tentorial sinus, and finally into the transverse sinus.

Between 60–80-mm stage, there is a backward swing of the developing brain. This stretches the tentorial sinus, reducing the size of the lumen. The shunt now changes into more medially situated, more direct channel – the basal vein – and drains into the great cerebral vein.

Sometimes in the embryo the inferior striate vein anastomoses with the caudate tributaries of the terminal vein. On such occasion the shunt is directed into the anterior end of the internal cerebral vein via the terminal vein.

In this angiogram the feeding artery entering the dilated internal cerebral vein can be clearly seen.

An arteriovenous fistula between the medial striate artery and inferior striate veins can either shunt along the basal vein into the great cerebral vein, or along the terminal vein into the internal cerebral vein. The latter usually dilates more as it is mainly extracerebral till 80-mm stage. It has no restraints of the surrounding brain. Many examples of the so-called aneurysms of the vein of Galen belong to this category.

In the region of the diencephalon the segmental pial veins are dorsal and ventral diencephalic veins, crossed by the corresponding pial arteries.

For instance, if we look at the combination of posterior cerebral artery and dorsal diencephalic vein producing an arteriovenous fistula, at 20-mm stage the shunt is into the tentorial sinus and transverse sinus. Please note that the dorsal diencephalic vein (green) . At 60 mm there is a backward shift with the rest of the brain, and at 80 mm the shunt changes into basal vein as the tentorial sinus attenuates because of elongation. The arteriovenous fistula occurres between the posterior cerebral artery and the dorsal diencephalic vein. The drainage is into the great cerebral vein.

The mesencephalic segment the mesencephalic artery and vein cross each other. The initial drainage into the tentorial sinus is later shifted to the great cerebral vein. The mesencephalic vein is shown in green. Kindly note the independent origin of mesencephalic artery at 20-mm stage, which is gradually incorporated into the posterior cerebral artery. This is often not appreciated and is classified under posterior cerebral malformation.

The following is an example borrowed from the post-mortem report by Alpers and Forrester (Figures 7.2 and 7.13). The point or origin of the mesencephalic artery on either side is clearly seen. The mesencephalic vein is represented by means of venous channels draining into the vein of Galen.

It is perhaps relevant to quote the authors' original description here: 'The basilar artery divided normally into two posterior cerebral arteries, but a branch from each posterior cerebral vessel could be followed coursing around the mesencephalon sending branches into the aneurysm. On the tectum of the midbrain lay a large mass of vessels connected with the posterior cerebral artery sending many branches into the wall of the aneurysm.'

The mass of vessels on the tectum represents the persistent mesencephalic vein.

In the metencephalic (the cerebellum) and the myelencephalic (medulla oblongata) segments the segmental pial veins drain directly into the transverse sinus. They are therefore unaffected by the developmental changes in the embryonic tentorial sinus seen in other segments.

Therefore, persistent embryonic veins in the arteriovenous malformations of these segments drain into the transverse sinus in the adult (Schlesinger[289]). It is exceptional for these to drain into the cerebral vein.

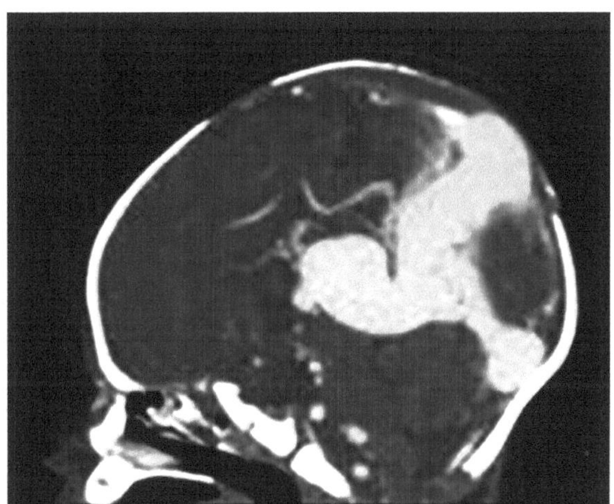

Figure 12.2 Vein of Galen Malformation (Radiopedia).

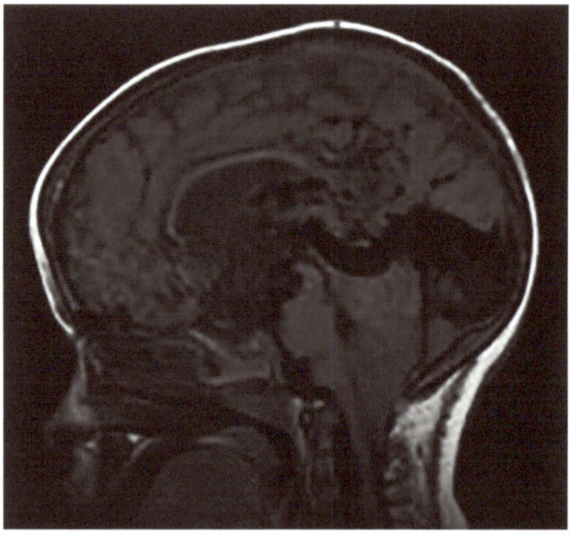

Figure 12.3 Vein of Galen Malformation (Radiopedia).

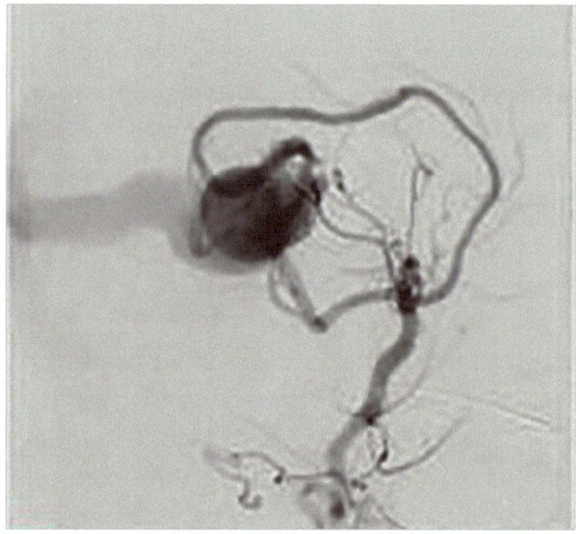

Figure 12.4 Vein of Galen Malformation (Radiopedia).

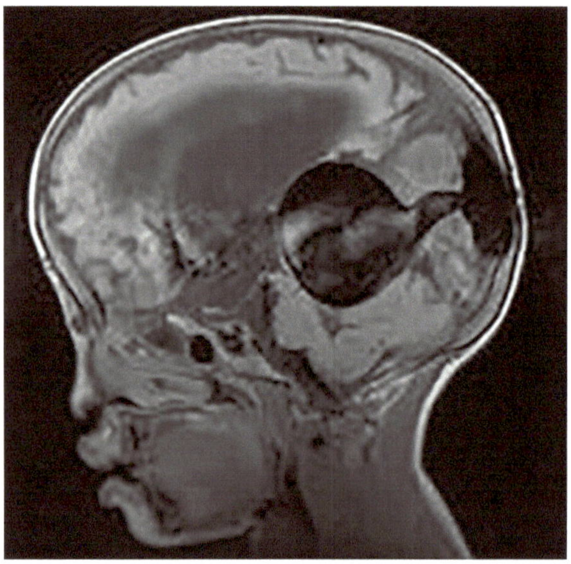

Figure 12.5 Vein of Galen Malformation (Radiopedia).

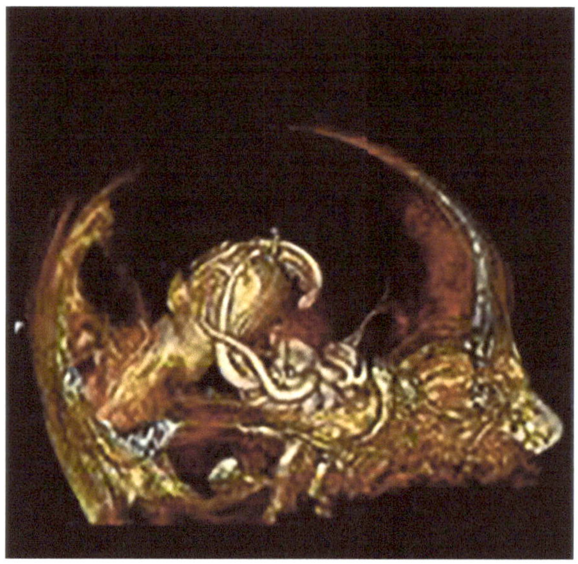

Figure 12.6 Vein of Galen Malformation (Radiopedia).

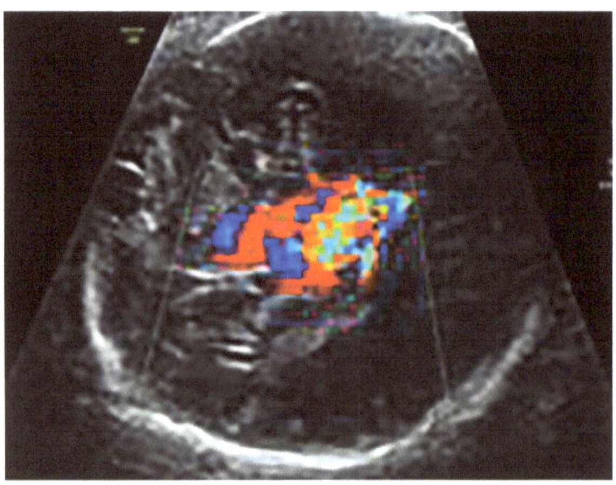

Figure 12.7 Vein of Galen Malformation (Radiopedia).

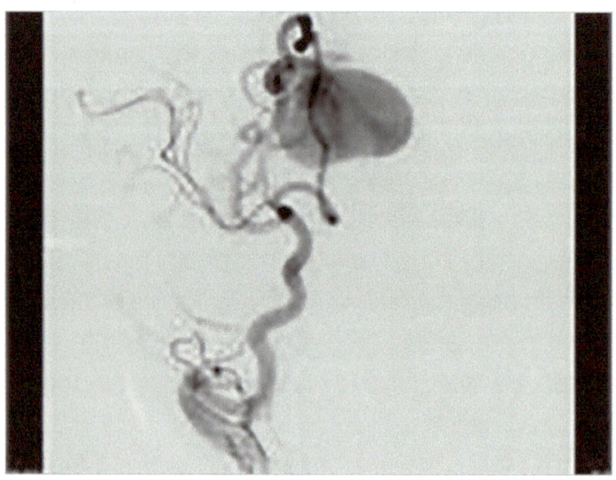

Figure 12.8 Vein of Galen Malformation (Radiopedia).

13

Histology of Persistent Embryonic Veins

Arterialised venous channels in arteriovenous malformations of the brain represent persistent embryonic veins. The anatomy of these veins resemble embryonic venous channels. Their microscopic features also resemble those of the foetal cerebral veins. The endothelial lining of these veins indicates the age of the foetus when the fistulae are likely to have occurred.

Histology of the Persistent Embryonic Veins in Arteriovenous Malformations of Brain

D. H. Deshpande and Vidyasagar Casikar[64]

Arterialised venous channels in the arteriovenous malformations of the brain represent persistent embryonic veins. The configuration of these veins resembles embryonic venous channels. Their microscopic features also resemble those of the foetal cerebral veins. The intimal lining of the persisting embryonic veins suggests the approximate age of the foetus at which the arteriovenous fistula is likely to have occurred (Bloom[23]).

Introduction

Arteriovenous malformation (AVM) of the central nervous system is a congenital vascular lesion. The abnormal veins in this malformation represent a segment of the foetal vasculature, which has persisted into post-natal life. It is clear from the available literature that the veins alone retain the embryonic character, whereas the arteries undergo normal developmental maturation. (Garner[72])

The configuration of the draining veins in AVM follows an embryonal pattern. Hence these abnormal veins have been labelled as persistent embryonic veins. Do these persistent embryonic veins have a structure similar to the foetal cerebral veins? We realised that, since we do not know the structure of foetal cerebral veins and since the standard textbooks on human histology and embryology. (Garner[86], Hamilton[115], Hedon[119]) do not mention the histological appearance of these veins, it was necessary for us to study the microscopic structure of the cerebral veins in different stages of development of the human foetus.

Material

The material for this study consisted of the following:

1. Ten human foetuses selected at random, varying from 17–110 mm and collected soon after natural abortion or hysterotomy
2. Ten biopsy specimens of adult human AVMs

Method

The human foetuses were fixed in 10 per cent formalin saline. Forty-eight hours later, the head of the foetus was severed from the neck with a sharp knife. The head was processed for paraffin embedding. Eight-micrometre-thick serial coronal sections of the entire head were cut. Two paraffin sections were collected at each one millimetre depth of the block. One set of sections was stained with hematoxylin and eosin and the other with Verhoeff's elastic tissue stain.

The ten biopsy specimens of AVMs sent to our laboratory were fixed in formal saline immediately after excision. Tissues were processed for paraffin embedding. Eight-micrometre-thick section selected at random were stained in the same way as were the sections of the human foetuses.

Observations

Structure of Cerebral Veins in the Human Foetuses (Table 13.1)

Marginal, segmental, and telencephalic veins in the brains of the human foetuses in all the serial sections were examined carefully under a light microscope. In human foetuses, which varied in size from 17–45 mm, the intracranial vessels were made up of a thin collagenous wall. Endothelial cells were not prominently seen. Their lumens contained nucleated erythrocytes. It was not possible at this stage to differentiate the vascular channels into arteries and vein, based on the microscopic features (Figure 13.1).

Between the 45-mm- and 80-mm stage, the vessels could be differentiated into arteries and veins. The arterial channels had thicker walls and cellular tunica media. The veins had thinner collagenous walls. Their intima was lined by prominent low cuboidal endothelial cells. The cell lining was continuous with shorter internuclear space (Figure 13.1b).

At the 95-mm stage and above, the intimal endothelial cell lining was still prominent, but the cells were flat and fewer. The tunica media and adventitia were blended into one layer and were made up of collagenous tissue (Figure 13.1c).

Histology of the Persistent Embryonic Veins

In Foetuses of 110 mm the walls of all the veins were relatively thick. The intima was lined by a few flat endothelial cells. There were no elastic tissue fibrils as in the arteries. The veins at this stage resembled mature adult cerebral veins (Figure 13.1c).

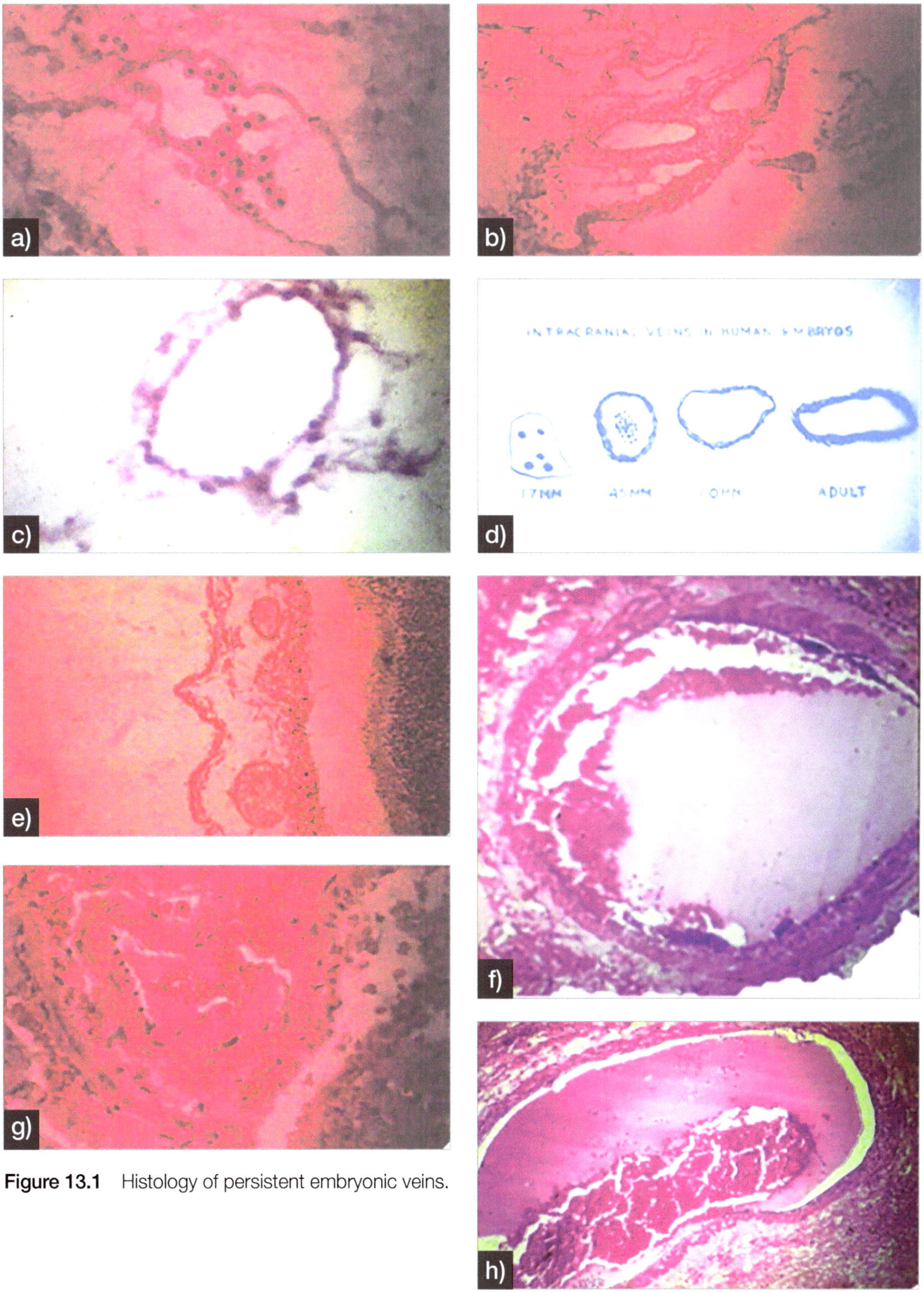

Figure 13.1 Histology of persistent embryonic veins.

Table 13.1 Structure of the cerebral veins in human foetuses.

S. no.	Size of the foetus (mm)	Intima lined by	Media and adventitia	Remarks
1	17	flat endothelial cells	Thin rim of collagen	Undifferentiated vascular channels
2	20	flat endothelial cells	Thin rim of collagen	Undifferentiated vascular channels
3	45	cuboidal endothelial cells Short internuclear space	Thicker collagenous	Differentiated venous structure
4	55	low cuboidal plump cellular endothelial cells, continuous cell lining	Collagenous, thin but	Differentiated venous structure
5	60	cuboidal cells, continuous lining	Collagen, fibroblasts, and smooth muscle cells	Differentiated venous structure
6	80	cell lining projecting into the lumen, plump cuboidal, fewer cells	Collagen, fibroblasts, and smooth muscle cells	Differentiated venous structure
7	95	flat but prominent endothelial cells	Collagen, fibroblasts, and smooth muscle cells	Differentiated venous structure
8	100	flat and scanty endothelial cells	Collagen, fibroblasts, and smooth muscle cells	Differentiated venous structure
9	110	flat and very few endothelial cells	Collagen, fibroblasts, and smooth muscle cells	Differentiated venous structure
10	110	flat and very few endothelial cells	Collagen, fibroblasts, and smooth muscle cells	Differentiated venous structure

Structure of Persistent Embryonic Veins in AVMs (Table 13.2)

The abnormal veins in all the biopsies consistently showed evidence of arterialisation (Figures 13.1d–13.1f). The walls of these vessels were irregularly thick because of an increase in the connective tissue and smooth muscle cells. However, no elastic tissue fibrils were noted in the media. Vascular lumen was dilated, and the dilatation was proportionate to the thickening of the wall.

In seven of the ten biopsy specimens studied the intimal lining of the arterialised veins showed prominent endothelial cells (Figures 13.1d and 13.1e). The nuclei of the endothelial cells were plump and placed close to one another.

In three specimens, however, veins were arterialised, but the intima did not show prominent endothelial cells (Figure 13.1f).

Discussion

Intracranial vascular channels in a human foetus differentiate into arteries and veins when it is about 20 mm. Later the cerebral veins undergo considerable alterations in their organisational pattern before attaining maturity. Thus in foetuses of more than 80 mm, several veins undergo atresia.[334] As a result, the foetal and postnatal cerebral venous patterns are dissimilar.

So far, little attention has been paid to the structure of the foetal veins. Our own observations indicate that the cerebral veins in the human foetus undergo a series of structural changes before they attain maturity. The changes take place mainly in the pattern of endothelial cell lining of the intima. As seen in Figure 13.1g, the endothelial cells are fewer and flat up to the 45-mm stage. Later the venous channels, including the marginal veins, show

Table 13.2 Structure of the persistent embryonic veins.

Reference no.	Intimal endothelial cell pattern	Media and adventi	Remarks
137/73	few flat endothelial cells, collagenous	Thick fibromuscular vein	Mature arterialised
252/75	cuboidal, nuclei closely spaced	Irregular collagenous thickening	Embryonic vein
270/75	cuboidal, projection into the lumen	Irregular collagenous thickening	Embryonic vein
115/76	flat but prominent nuclei number than normal, normal after the 80-mm stage	Thick, fibrocollagenous and heyline	Embryonic, but the more in shunt has occurred
118/76	low cuboidal but few cells	Irregular collagenous thickening	Embryonic vein
138/76	continuous cuboid cell lining	Fibrocollagenous thickening	Embryonic vein
178/76	flat, interrupted	Fibromuscular thickening	Mature arterialised vein
204/76	cuboidal cells butdiscontinuous cell lining	Irregular fibromuscular thickening	Embryonic vein
234/78	plump endothelial cells, nuclei placed closer to one another	Fibromuscular thickening	Embryonic, but the shunt has occurred after the 80-mm stage
267/79	very few flat endothelial cells, nuclei are inconspicuous	Fibrocollagenous thickening	Mature arterialised veins

prominent low cuboidal endothelial cells. Their nuclei make a continuous lining of the intimal surface. At the 110-mm stage and after, the veins structurally resemble adult veins. Cerebral veins in a foetus do not have elastic fibrils at any stage.

The persistent embryonic veins of adult AVMs in our material show two significant alterations:

A. The abnormal veins are remarkably dilated and thickened. The smooth muscle cells show hypertrophy. The total change in the veins has been described as an arterialisation of the veins. However, unlike true arteries, the persistent embryonal veins lack elastic fibrils in their media. The structural changes in the vessels result from the hydrodynamic alterations following arteriovenous shunts. The reactive hypertrophy of the media and the addition of layers of fibrocollagenous adventitia are part of nature's attempt to withstand the high arterial pressure in the embryonic veins.

B. The other change that has been noted by us is the prominent endothelial cell lining. Normal adult cerebral veins show an occasional flat endothelial cell in their intima. A majority of the persistent embryonic veins have shown prominent endothelial cell lining similar to that of the (telencephalic) veins of our human foetuses, which were between 45 and 110 mm. On the basis of our experience of the histological structure of the foetal veins and of the persistent embryonic veins, we believe that there is a strong structural resemblance between the two.

It has been argued earlier that AVMs occur in an embryo following a developmental defect in the wall of the vessels at the point of intersection between an artery and a vein. This in turn leads to the shunting of the arterial blood directly into the veins that drain into the venous sinuses.

Once the shunt is established between an artery and a vein, these venous channels perhaps remain unchanged at that stage of development. The structure of a persistent embryonic vein in terms of endothelial cell lining probably depends on the stage of the foetus at which arteriovenous shunting beings. In other words, if the shunt is formed between the 20–80-mm stages, as it does in the majority of instances, the embryonic character of the veins is well seen. However, in those cases where the shunt is formed at a later stage, the persistent vein would show a greater maturity of structure. The structural resemblance of the endothelial cell lining of the veins in AVMs to that of normal cerebral veins in human embryo is yet another proof of its persistent embryonic character.

In three cases, the persistent embryonic veins of the AVMs showed an intimal lining similar to that of mature adult cerebral veins. We can offer two possible explanations for this: a) The shunt might have developed in the foetus around the 80-mm stage, or b) the shunt might have occurred in a segment of a developing brain where the veins are more mature than in the other segments. It is known that in a foetus the veins show different stages of developmental maturity.[11]

In either event the embryonic veins will resemble an adult mature vein, as observed in three of our cases.

Acknowledgements

This research on the anatomy of the persistent embryonic veins was started at the suggestion of Prof. B. H. Dawson, consultant neurological surgeon at the Salford Royal Hospital, UK.

Our sincere thanks are due to Dr (Mrs) Sulochana Gunasheela and Dr (Mrs) Pushpa Srivnivas for supplying us the foetuses for our study.

Sincere thanks are also due to Mr K. M. James for his secretarial assistance, Mr Douglas A. Pleger for technical assistance, and Mr B. G. Rajaram for producing the illustrations for this work.

14

The Haemodynamic Properties of Arteriovenous Malformations: Experimental Findings

Vidyasagar Casikar, G S Ramaswamy and Vyshnavi Casikar[336]

The following chapter describes the observations made in the experimental ateriovenous fistulae, where the characteristics of the blood flo were measured in relation to the size of the fistula. Sharp predictable fluctuations were seen in the flow of blood, with very small changes in the relative diameters of the feeding artery and the fistula.The clinical implications of these findings are discussed.

Experiments on The Arterio-Venous Fistula

In the following chapter we describe the various experiments conducted on the arterio-venous Fistula. Herein is a brief background and the logical description that lead us to the conduct these experiments. We have presented results in various aspects of explaining the flow in AVF.

Background

The normal flow of blood in the living systems is that the artery and vein carry the blood from and to the heart as represented in Figure 14.1 (Lewis[165], Logue[169]).

The oxygenated blood is carried from the heart to the capillaries by the artery and its branches and the deoxygenated blood is carried back to the heart by the vein and its branches.

As one can see in Figure 14.1, normally there are no connections between the artery and vein excepting through capillaries.

In an arteriovenous fistula a direct connection called shunt, occurs between the artery and the vein Figure 14.2.

Though the artery and vein have their normal connection, the new opening between them, through the SHUNT caused some arterial blood to move into the vein and proceed on to the heart. This is because the difference in pressure between the artery and vein and the shunt being available passage. Zur[358]

The experimental process was initiated to provide the solution for the fundamental question which has been unanswered even after the extensive clinical and experimental investigations in the management of Cerebral Arterio-Venous Malformation(AVM). The results obtained from the experiments were not capable of arriving at the required relation between the physiological factors which influence the blood flow in the AVM. Thus the fundamental question still remains, when does a clinically silent lesion declares its presence either by haemorrhage (can be due to a sudden increase in flow or pressure) or by neurological manifestation suggestive of deprivation of blood to normal areas of brain (steal phenomenon).

The experiments reveal that the generalization in the results of the previous experiments by different doctors can be false due to the highly complex nature of the flow in the fistula under varying conditions. To name a few, Krumhar[157] reported that a 2mm large fistula in the iliac artery and vein of a dog caused retrograde flow.

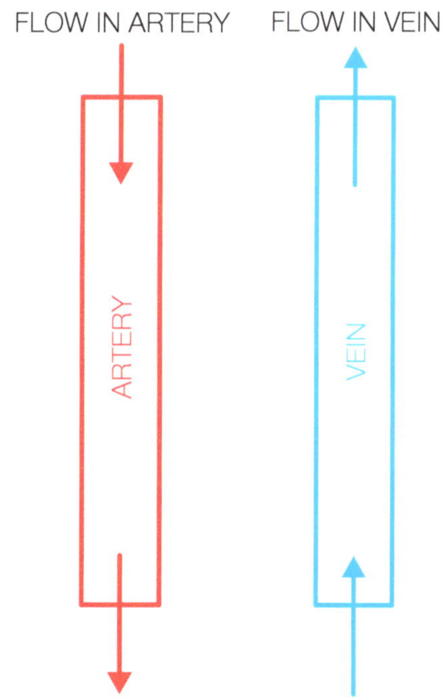

Figure 14.1 Normal flow pattern.

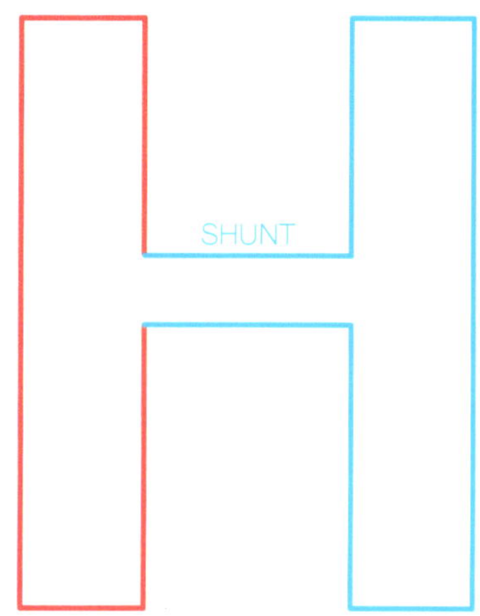

Figure 14.2 The shunt.

Louge[169&172] reported on the flow pattern in fistulae of different sizes, which he described as small, medium and large based on the length of the incision between the arteries and veins. Shi[246] graded AVMs based on the location, arterial supply and venous drainage. Pietelia[247] et.al., described an animal model by connecting a segment of temporal artery between the branches of middle cerebral artery and dorsal sagittal sinus. All such models do not reflect the complex flow pattern accurately. Vita[344]

The experiments performed have attempted to create an animal model incorporating as many biological conditions as possible, to assess the relative contribution of parameters such as size of the arterial feeder, the size of the fistula, systemic blood pressure, and volume and velocity of blood flow, to the flow in the fistula. The following sections elucidate the experimental procedure and the results have been analyzed.

Importance Of Finding The Flow Characteristics Of Blood In Avm

The percentage of flow of pure or the oxygenated blood being shunted back to the heart, without being utilized by the organs is to be known. By knowing the percentage of the blood being reverted back the amount of blood being deprived by the *shunt* can be known. The increase in the blood flow through the veins can also be calculated which would give a detailed report of when and under what conditions the veins would be punctured or lead to a haemorrhage. The study of the flow also gives a detailed picture of the present situation of the fistula and the importance of a treatment can be estimated.

Once the conditions which cause a greater blood flow into the shunt are known, care can be taken so as to avoid the occurrence of the conditions like an increase in pressure or even the size of the artery and vein can be altered to decrease the flow. To be able to perform alterations in size of the artery and the vein it is important that the effect of these factors on the flow be predicted with accuracy. The relation between the physiological factors on the flow of blood in the shunt should be known and the flow be predicted under various conditions accurately. The conditions can be changed to reduce the flow and regain the flow of oxygenated blood to the organ. The occurrence of steal can also be avoided.

In nature it is difficult to find AVMs whose limbs are as shown in Figure 14.2. The difficulties in accurately establishing the flow pattern in an AVF lead us to first try with **glass AFS**. Though the sizes could be correctly gauged, the difficulty in achieving the small differences in the size of the Shunt made us look for different materials.

AVFs made of acrylic proved to be the best. First the acrylic piece 6mm thick is taken (Figure 14.3) and TWO holes of the same diameter (viz.2.0mm, 2.1mm, 2.2mm or 2.3mm) were drilled. These two form the artery and vein both the H type AVF (Figure 14.3). The choice of the sizes is due to the fact that the intra-cranial vessels are in the range of 2.0mm to 2.3mm. Now the outer edges are rounded to 1.5mm more than the diameter of the holes drilled for the artery and vein. (Figure 14.3).

The next step is to drill the horizontal hole to create the SHUNT (Figure 14.4). The size of hole was in the range of 1.5mm and 3.0mm. We made FOUR sets of AVFs with artery/vein diameter of 2mm, 2.1mm, 2.2mm and 2.3mm. The shunt diameter was in the range of 1.5mm to 3.0mm in each set.

The extra material between the artery and vein was removed carefully to get the AVF (Figure 14.5).

In the next step the opening on the side of the vertical limb was closed (Figure 14.5) to get the AVF. Every 5th fistula was sliced open to confirm the sizes. Totally 72 units of the fistulae were made for the experiments.

The Experimental Setup and Process

The dogs were starved and sedated the previous night (Pietila[248],Qian[258]). The anaesthesia was maintained on spontaneous respiration intravenous with Nembutal as and when required. The animals were positioned in prone position. Femoral artery and vein were exposed in the groin. The magnetic blood flow meter was calibrated with an excised artery (preserved from the animal sacrificed after the previous experiment) for flow of saline as recommended by the manufacturer (Micron Instruments, USA).

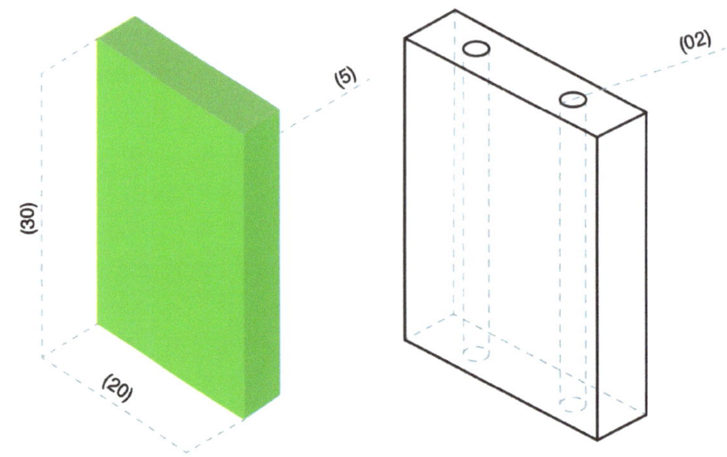

Figure 14.3 The acrylic shunt.

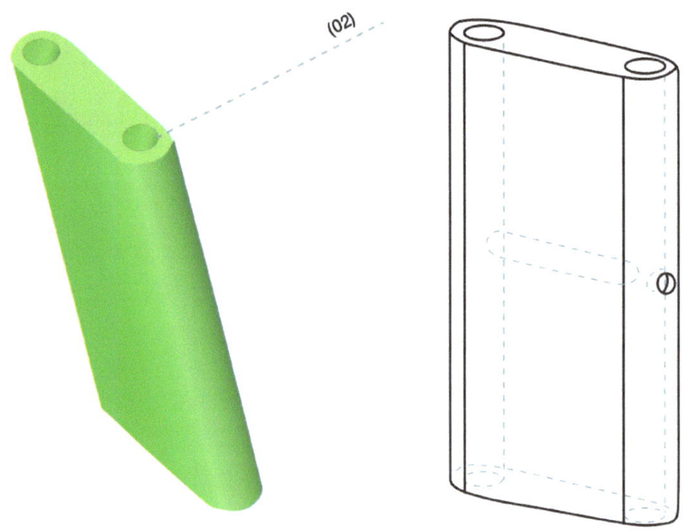

Figure 14.5 The acrylic shunt.

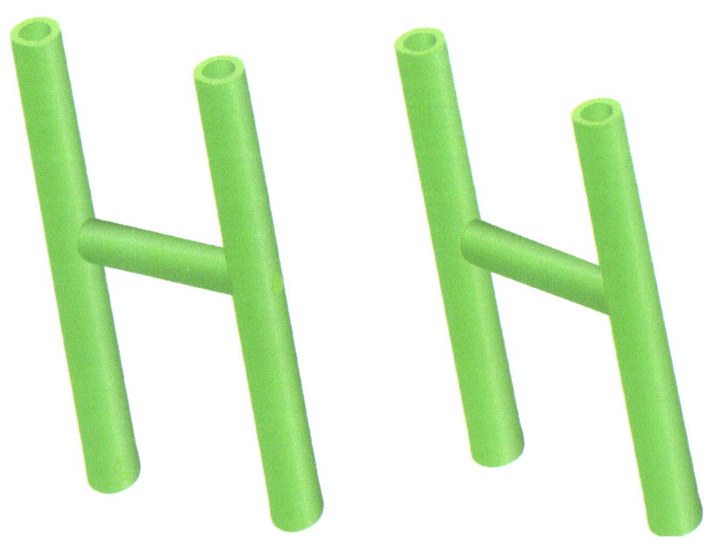

Figure 14.4 The acrylic shunt.

Calibration was also checked for flow of blood after the experiment before sacrificing the animal. If there was an error in excess of 10% between the calibrations, the data of the experiment was rejected.

The shunt was opened to the circulation by releasing the vascular clamps. A period fifteen minutes was allowed to stabilize the circulation. Systemic arterial blood pressure (SAP) and heart rate were not corrected to any specific level, except when SAP and blood flow were manipulated as deliberate procedures. Regional decrease in blood flow was achieved by partially occluding the femoral artery in the groin. Thus the flow through the fistula was controlled. Otherwise the circulatory disturbances occurring when the A.V. fistula was opened were allowed to stabilize on their own. This was intended to simulate biological conditions.

The following values were recorded after deliberate manipulations of blood flow, diameter of feeding artery and diameter of the Shunt.

1. Diameter of feeding artery(DFA)
2. Diameter of the shunt(DFS)
3. Flow in PA before introduction of the shunt (FPAB)
4. Flow in PA after introduction of the shunt and stabilised for 15 minutes (FPAA)
5. Flow in distal artery (FDA)
6. Fraction of PA flow in shunt (FRPA)
7. Systemic venous pressure after opening the shunt at artery fistula junction (SAPA)
8. Systemic venous pressure after opening the shunt at vein fistula junction (SVPA)

In addition to the length and diameter of the limb of the fistula the blood flow in the artery and in the vein at proximal artery (FPA), distal artery (FDA), proximal vein (FPV), distal vein (FDV), intra luminal pressure at AFJ and VFJ, were recorded. Each parameter was recorded three times at intervals of fifteen minutes and the average values were taken into consideration. The flow values at the arterial and venous limbs were calculated using the following equations.

Flow in the shunt = (Flow in the proximal artery) – (Flow in the distal artery).

Or

$$FS = FPA - FDA \qquad (1)$$

Flow in the shunt = (Flow in the distal vein) – (Flow in the proximal vein).

Or

$$FS = FDV - FPV \qquad (2)$$

This is represented in the Figure 14.6

Only those experiments where the difference in the values of FS computed using equations 1 & 2 was less than 5% have been included. Others were rejected.

After the experiment was over the shunt was removed and examined for evidence of any clot /occlusion in the lumen. If this was present, the *observations'* of the experiment were rejected.

Hemodynamics Theory

Before we proceed to the presentation of the data, we propose to refresh some aspects of hemodynamics for the sake of clarity of the terms being used there of below (Schenk[287&288]):

Newton's First Law Of Motion

Everybody persists in its state of being at rest or of moving uniformly straight forward, except in so far as it is compelled to change its state by force impressed.

Liquids too show similar properties.

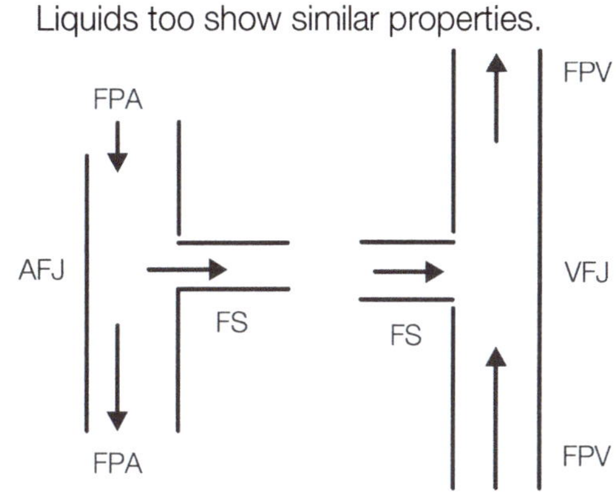

Figure 14.6 The flow pattern.

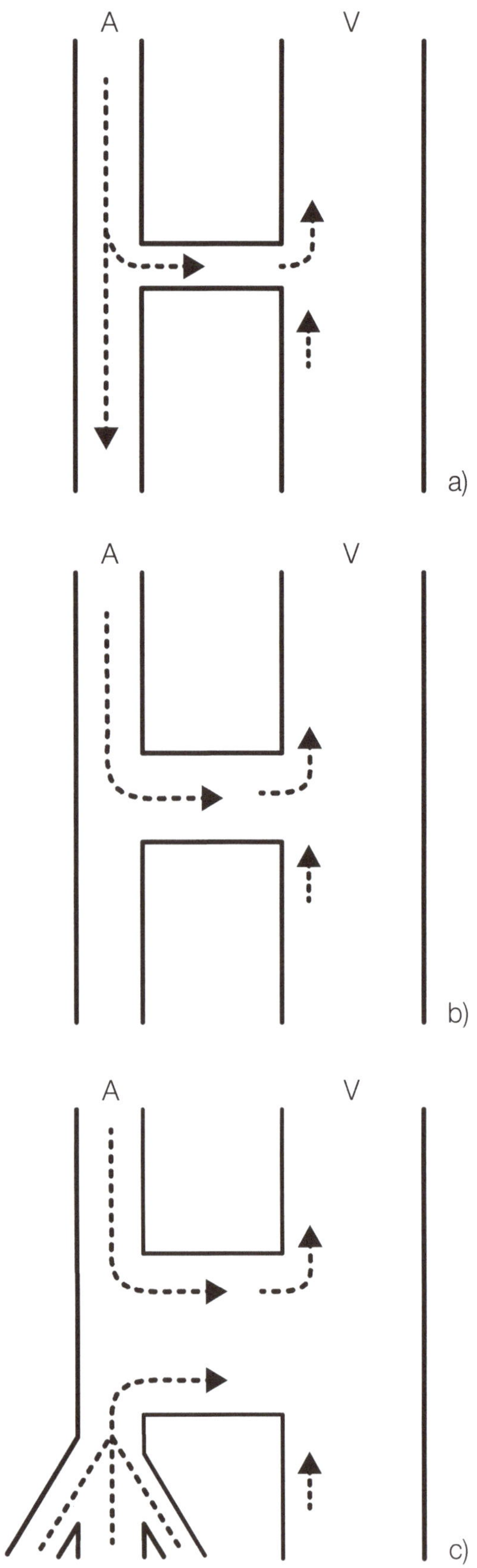

Figure 14.7 Please provide a caption.

Fluid: Fluid is a matter which, if subject to an unbalanced external force, suffers a continuous deformation. Fluids can withstand large compressive forces (pressure), but only negligibly small tensile forces. Fluids at rest cannot sustain shear forces; however fluids in relative motion do give rise to shear forces, resulting from a momentum exchange between the more slowly moving particles and those which are moving faster. The momentum exchange is made possible because the molecules move relatively freely.

Density: Density (ρ) is the mass per unit volume.

Newton determined the shear forces on the fluid under movement. Considering the movement of Newtonian fluid in a pipe, the velocity of the fluid varies from the wall to the centre of the pipe. It can be diagrammatically shown as below.

Fluid Flow

All fluids flow under the influence of the pressure. Flow is directed from the point of higher pressure to a point of lower pressure. The pressure lost due to flow has been illustrated in the Bernoulli's equation

$$\frac{p_1}{w} + \frac{v_1^2}{2g} + Z_1 = \frac{p_2}{w} + \frac{v_1^2}{2g} + Z_2 + h_L$$

Where p_x is the pressure, v_x is the velocity, g the universal gravity, Z_x the elevation of the point of fluid under consideration, h_L the head loss due to friction and w the density of the fluid and x is the physical location of the fluid, say at point 1 and point 2 marked in the figure.

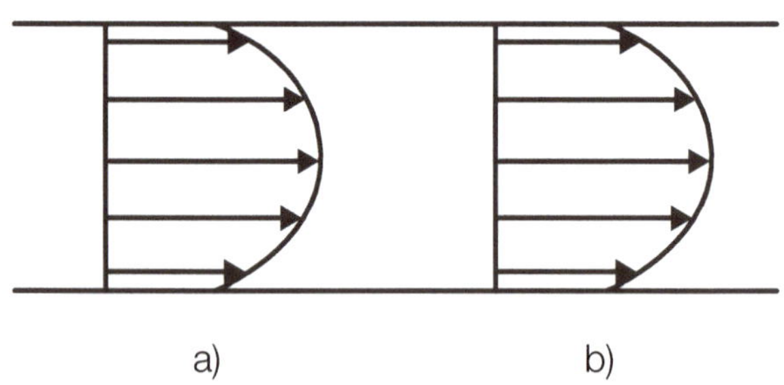

Figure 14.8 Newtonian fluid flow.

Though Blood has many components, each affecting the blood flow, for the present study it can be treated as a Newtonian fluid as the vessels involved are in the range of 0.16 to 0.20cm.

When we look at blood in the living systems, other than capillaries, the blood behaves no different than most fluids. The flow in the blood vessels in the human body may be treated as the flow through pipes.

The area available for the blood flow will be cross-sectional area of the vessel is a factor that affects the volume of blood flowing. Due to the blood pressure inside, the vessel assumes a circular shape. The inside diameter of the vessel through which blood flows is, say d. For a diameter, d cm, the cross sectional area will be

$$A = \frac{\pi}{4} d^2 cm^2$$

Supposing the volume of blood flow is q cubic centimetres/second.

The velocity of blood (**v**) (in cm/second) will be

$$av = {}^{q}\!/_{A}$$

The pressure difference being the cause for the blood flow, the quantum of blood flow can be expressed as

$$q = \frac{\pi}{128\mu} \frac{d^4}{L} h_L$$

Where

μ, is the viscosity of blood,

L, is the length of the vessel under study,

d, is the diameter of the vessel and

h_l, is the head loss.

The length of the arrow (in Figure 14.8 at position 1 & 2) indicates the speed of movement (velocity) of the fluid. As can be seen the velocity of the fluid near the wall is very low and the velocity is maximum at the centre of the tube.

In a generalised view of fluids the medium appears to have been made up of layers. Each layer gliding over the adjacent layer, to give the effect of total medium movement. The rate of change of velocity between adjacent layers is termed as **Shear rate**.

The Shear rate in terms of units is:

Shear stress is proportional to [the rate of change of velocity/distance from the periphery]

That is

$$\text{Shear stress} \propto \left(\frac{du}{dy}\right)$$

Where u is the velocity of fluid at the position atdistance from the wall.

This will be

$$\tau = \mu . \frac{du}{dy}$$

where, μ is the viscosity of the fluid.

Viscosity

If a moving mass of particles enables one fluid particle to move into a region of different velocity, there will be some momentum transferred and an apparent force or stress appears. This gives rise to viscosity.

Poise is the unit for viscosity, equivalent to dyne-sec/cm^2. Because one poise represents a high viscosity, 1/100poise, or one centipoise (cp), is used for measurements. One centipoises equals one millipascal-second. Viscosity must have a stated or an understood shear rate in order to be meaningful. The temperature, at which Viscosity Measurement is made, must be stated or understood clearly.

Kinematic Viscosity (V)

In resisting the applied forces the response of the fluid is proportional to the density ρ:

Total net force = mass × acceleration, so that

{ μ × (terms involving velocity gradient) + pressure terms} $\propto$ { ρ × (terms involving fluid accelerations)}.

It can be seen that dividing by density (ρ) shows that in the fundamental equation of motion the viscosity appears in the ratio μ/ρ. This is the *Kinematic viscosity V*:

$$\nu = \frac{\mu}{\rho}$$

An experimental AVF can be represented as an H-shaped pipe fixture.

In this the length of each limb is maintained to be more than SIX times the diameter, to remove the effects of entry and exit conditions for the flow of blood.

Here the terms
PA – the Proximal Artery,
DA – Distal Artery,
PV – Proximal vein,
DV – Distal vein,
AFJ – artery fistula Junction and
VFJ – the vein fistula Junction.

As we look at the arterial blood being shunted by the AVF, the same model can be applied to the H-type AVFs. The flow through the central limb is important.

Keeping the factors μ, L and h_l to be same, but increase the diameter of the shunt by say 20%, that is d_1=1.2*d*.

The flow q_1 will be

$$q_1 = \frac{\pi}{128\mu}\frac{d_1^4}{L}h_L = \frac{\pi}{128\mu}\frac{(1.2d)^4}{L}h_L$$

$$= \frac{\pi}{128\mu}\frac{2.0736d^4}{L}h_L = 2.0736q$$

This means that the flow in the shunt will increase TWO fold for a mere 20% increase of the vessel diameter.

Reynolds' number is the basis for determining the state of flow. It is important as it indicates the state of affairs in the vessel. The classification of blood flow being laminar or turbulent isdetermined by evaluating Reynolds' number (Re) by the equation

$$\text{Re} = \frac{Vd}{\mu} = \frac{qd}{\vartheta A}$$

Wherein the term
ρ is the density of blood,
V is velocity of blood,
d is the diameter of the vessel,
μ is the viscosity of blood,
q is the flow,
ϑ is the kinematic viscosity of blood,
A is the area of cross-section of the vessel.

The flow simulation of fluids through pipes is well documented. Any attempt to apply the simulation to the AVF will not work correctly for the following reasons.

1. The flow in the artery is pulsatile.
2. Emulating the flexibility of the biological condition of the vessels is tough.

Possible conditions of flow in an AVF is shown in Figure 14.10.

Condition A. The flow in the AVF in a normal situation is that there is feeding artery flow in PA to AFJ, some flow from AFJ to DA, some flow from AFJ–VFJ, some flow from PV–VFJ and flow from VFJ–DV returning to the heart.

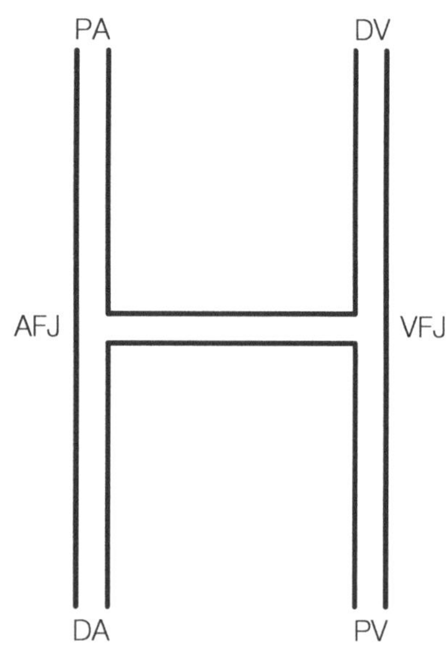

Figure 14.9 Locations where the flow were measured.

Condition B. As the diameter of the fistula AFJ–VFJ increases, the flow in the AJF–VFJ can sometimes be very large and there may not be ANY flow in the AFJ–DA section. In such case the AVF is said to be critical.

Condition C. Any further increase in the size of the fistula, flow capacity of the shunt is so high that all the blood from the feeding artery is drained to the AFJ–VFJ section and can also draw blood from the distal Artery (DA) causing retrograde flow (from DA to AFJ instead of the normal AFJ to DA) to satisfy the shunting capacity of the AVF. In such case the AVF is said to be in the Reverse flow.

The three conditions are represented below.

The monitoring system in the living system, being very sensitive and such conditions can occur. It also creates condition as seen above and controls the blood flow in the particular section, without affecting the flow in any other part of the body.

The Results Obtained from the Experiments On The Avfs

The following is the Table 14.1, showing the various data collected in our experiments:

To attain a relation between various variables present, each of them was varied and the observations made. The different factors which were changed are the diameter of the fistula, diameter of the artery, systemic arterial pressure(SAP), Flow in proximal artery(PA) and animals.

Figures14.13 to 14.18, show the plot of FRPA as percentage of blood shunted by the AVF for different artery diameters. The third order polynomial fits and the polynomial functions are also given. Though the curve fit is very good, the method to predict the FRPA for different artery diameters is still not achievable.

SAP Reduced, DFA and DFS Constant

Reduction of arterial pressure (SAP) did not always produce similar flow changes in the shunt, when the diameter of feeding artery and fistula were constant.

In the experiments 1&2 when the SAP was reduced, the flow in the PA reduced significantly. However the fraction off low in PA shunted did not reduce in all. The experiments 3&4, the fall in SAPA reduced the flow in PA, but the fraction of PA flow shunted was more than the total flow of

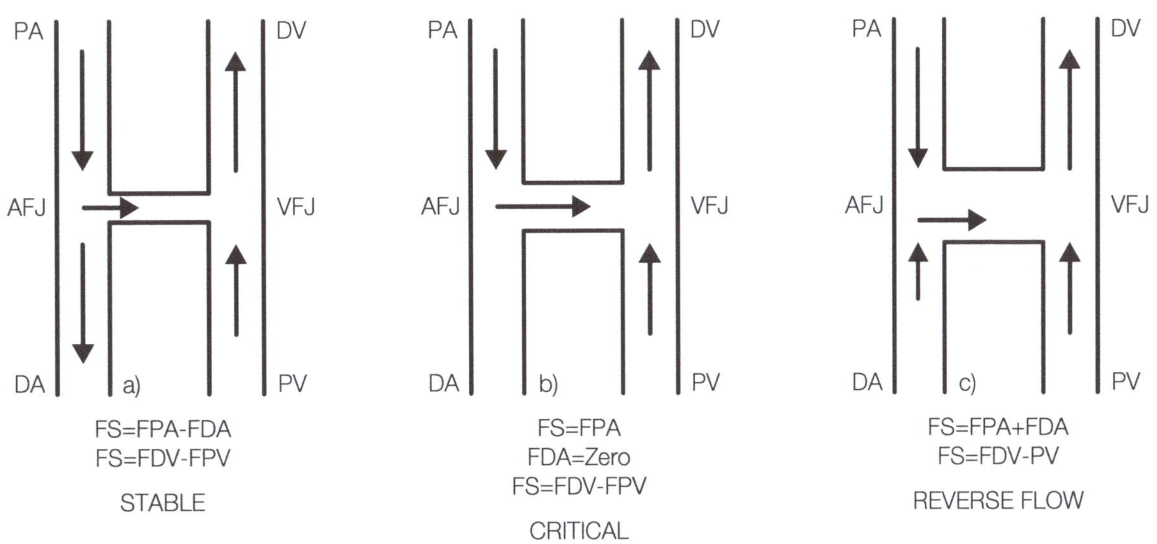

Figure 14.10 The possible variations in the diameters of the fistulae with reference to the diameters of the arteries and veins.

Table 14.1 Experiments data

Sl.no.	DFA	DFS	FPAB	FPAA	FDA	FRPA	SAPA	SVPA	FFSP
Units	mm	mm	cc/min	cc/min	cc/min	%	mmofHg	mmofHg	cc/min
1	2	1.1	67.5	56.25	4.5	51.75	92	99	47
2	2	1.1	20	31.5	-13.5	45	142.8	98	128
3	2	1.2	51	56.25	40.5	15.75	28	110	14
4	2	1.3	67.5	78.75	18.0	60.75	77.143	105	58
5	2	1.3	38	28.12	11.25	16.87	60	111	15
6	2	1.4	58.5	79.2	18.5	60.7	76.6	98	54
7	2	1.5	37.5	31.25	5.0	26.25	84	128	22
8	2	1.7	51.5	202.5	-22.5	225	111.1	128	177
9	2	1.7	21	213.75	19.0	194.75	91.1	117	172
10	2	1.7	106.5	101.25	4.5	96.75	95.6	73	201
11	2	1.8	63	317.5	-79.2	396.7	124.9	105	593
12	2	2	51	270.0	0.0	270	100	107	303
13	2	2	51	292.5	0.0	292.5	100	107	329
14	2	2.2	64	357.3	23.9	333.4	93.31	120	1222
15	2	2.3	67.5	168.5	11.25	157.25	93.3	93	351
16	2	2.3	21	87.4	-6.75	94.15	107.7	111	557
17	2.1	1.4	20.5	283.6	49.09	234.51	82.7	150	180
18	2.1	1.4	51.5	132.0	60.0	72	54.5	215	48
19	2.1	1.5	66.5	336.0	12.0	324	96.4	155	208
20	2.1	1.7	20.5	234.55	32.72	201.83	86	160	148
21	2.1	1.8	71	570.0	45.0	525	92.1	142	439
22	2.1	1.9	53.5	258.0	-18.0	276	107	160.	157
23	2.1	2	51	273.9	19.56	254.34	92.9	140	206
24	2.1	2.1	51.5	286.0	26.08	259.92	90.9	155	222
25	2.1	2.3	20.5	396.0	30.0	366	92.4	230	268
26	2.1	2.4	39	202.0	-27.75	229.75	113.76	115	295
27	2.1	3	30	258.75	22.5	236.25	91.3	100	227
28	2.1	3	30.5	236.25	28.12	208.13	88	64	1001
29	2.2	1.5	29	180	15.0	165	91.6	170	102
30	2.2	1.5	106	345	30.0	315	91.3	145	323
31	2.2	1.5	51.5	286.9	50.69	236.21	82.3	150	165
32	2.2	1.6	106	443.5	19.56	423.94	95.6	170	384
33	2.2	1.7	64	368.12	27.27	340.85	92.6	106	324
34	2.2	1.8	64	555	52.5	502.5	90.5	140	407
35	2.2	1.9	106	482.6	78.29	404.31	83.7	150	296
36	2.2	2	82	508	58.69	449.31	88.4	170	329
37	2.2	2.1	51	245.45	-27.27	272.72	111.1	180	168
38	2.2	2.3	66	337.5	-9.0	346.5	102.6	91	544
39	2.2	2.3	37.5	270	-13.5	283.5	105	80	661
40	2.2	2.4	24	167	6.4	160.6	96.1	100	263
41	2.3	1.3	21	61.9	9.0	52.9	85.5	123	78
42	2.3	1.5	24	168.75	11.25	157.5	93.3	111	220
43	2.3	1.5	39	202.5	-9.0	211.5	104.4	111	181
44	2.3	1.5	21	92.7	10.6	82.1	88.5	99	75
45	2.3	1.5	21	38.57	0.0	38.57	100	88	41
46	2.3	1.7	29	78.75	45.0	33.75	42.9	118	26
47	2.3	1.7	64	326.25	45.0	281.25	86.2	64	601
48	2.3	2	108	427	11.25	415.75	97.4	140	337
49	2.3	2	47	191.25	-18.0	209.25	109.4	110	283
50	2.3	2	57.5	258.75	-45.0	303.75	117.4	115	227
51	2.3	2.3	57.5	185.4	0.0	185.4	100	116	1784
52	2.3	2.4	55	258.75	11.25	247.5	95.7	99	251

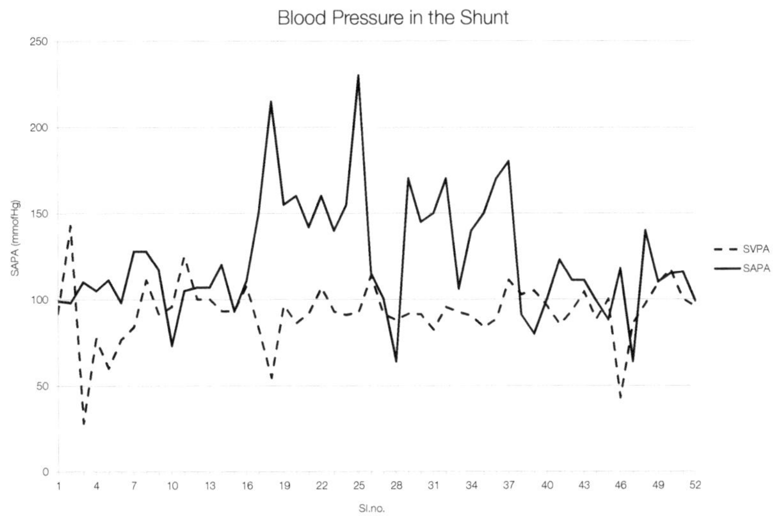

Figure 14.11 Blood flow in the Shunt Vs Shunt diameter.

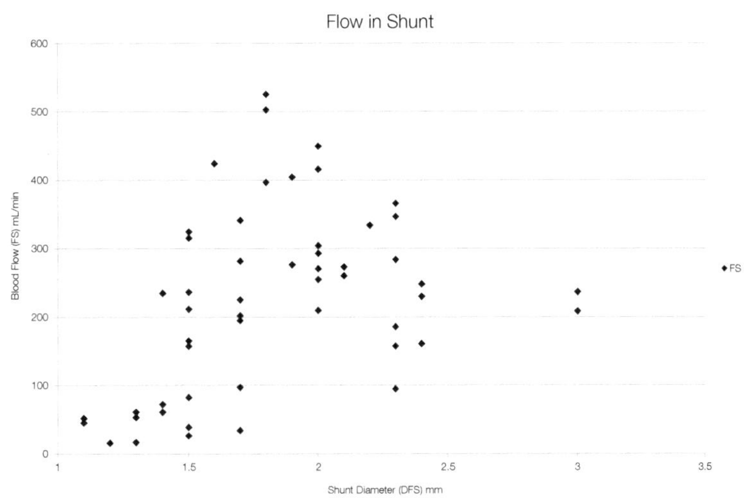

Figure 14.12 Correlation between SAPA and SVPA for all experiments.

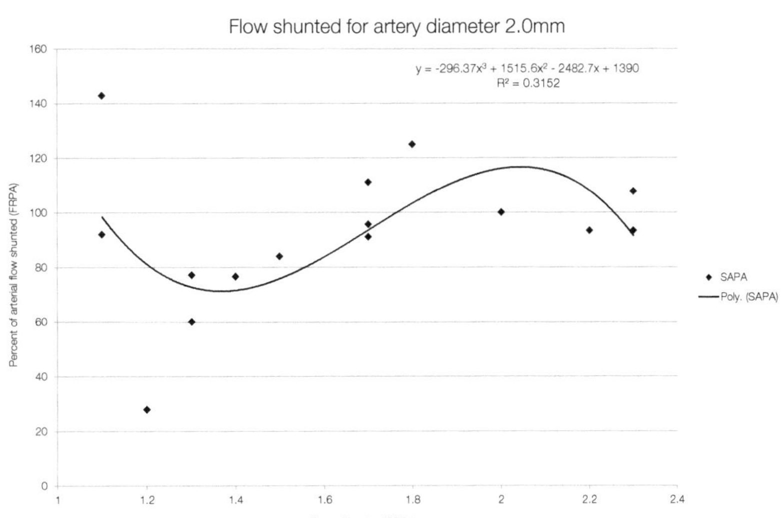

Figure 14.13 Percent of Proximal artery flow drained by shunt for artery diameter 2.0mm.

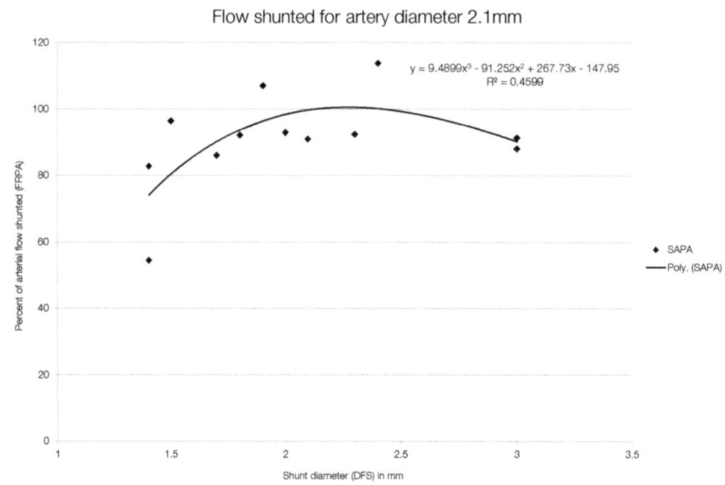

Figure 14.14 Percent of Proximal artery flow drained by shunt for artery diameter 2.1mm.

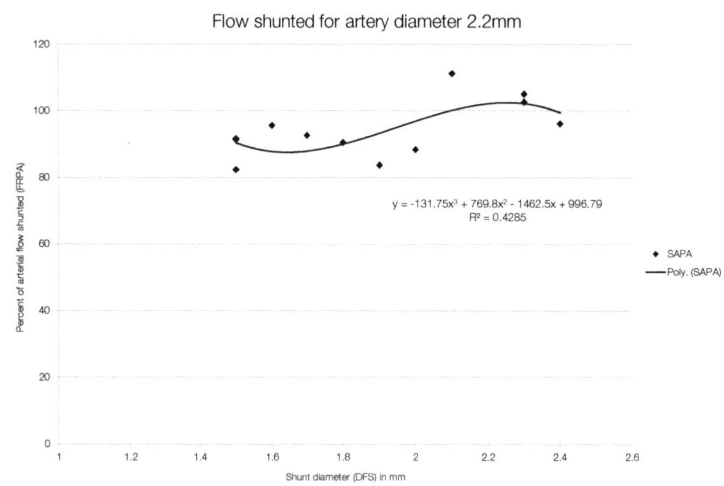

Figure 14.15 Percent of Proximal artery flow drained by shunt for artery diameter 2.2mm.

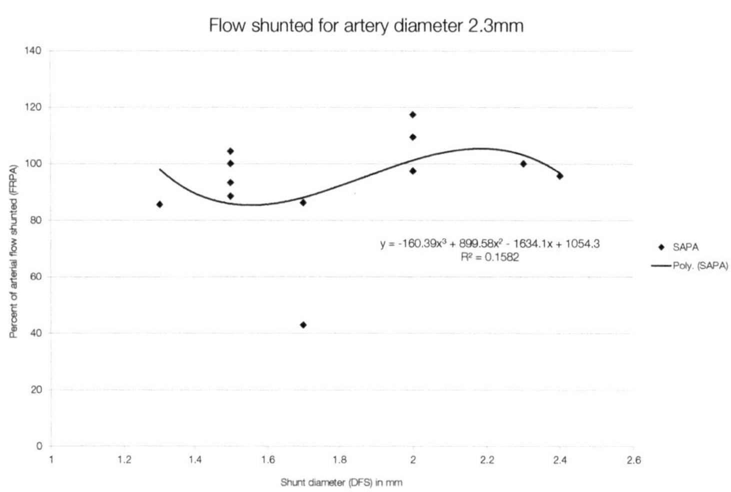

Figure 14.16 Percent of Proximal artery flow drained by shunt for artery diameter 2.3mm.

PA as evidenced by a significant reverse flow in the distal segment. Similarly in experiments 6&7 the fall in SAP from 91-80 mg of Hg increased the volume of reverse flow (steal flow).

Flow in PA Reduced DFA & DFS Constant

Diameters of the feeding artery and those of the fistulae were kept constant and the flow in the feeding artery (FPAB) was reduced in the following two sets of experiments. In experiments 10&11 there was no significant changes in the flow characteristics of the shunt. However a similar manipulation increased the fractionated flow in the shunt in the experiments 8&9 SAPA reduced with reduction of flow in FPAB.

Flow in PA Reduced. DFA Reduced. DFS Constant

However when the experiment was repeated when the diameter of the feeding artery was reduced to 2.0mm very different pattern of flow occurred.

A. Introduction of shunts of diameter of 1.1mm and 1.3mm did not alter the flow. However when the diameter of the shunt was increased to 1.7mm and 2.3mm there was very dramatic increase in the flow in the feeding artery (FPAA). SAPA did not show significant change.

B. In two out of four sets of experiment (12&13and16&17) a drop in the flow in the proximal artery produced reversed flow (steal) in the distal arterial segment.

Flow in PA Reduced. DFA Increased. DFS Constant

Instead when the diameter of the feeding artery was increased to 2.2mm and the flow in the feeding artery was reduced, there were no dramatic changes in the flow pattern of the fistula. SAPA remained unchanged.

Table 14.2 Experiments where SAP reduced keeing the DFA and DFS constant.

Expt No.	DFA mm	DFS mm	FPAB ml/min	FPAA ml/min	FDA ml/min	FRPA %	SAPA mm/Hg	SVPA mm/Hg
1	2	1.7	51.5	202.5	-22.5*	110	128	30
2	2	1.7	21.0	2.3	19	90	117	30
3	2.3	2	108	427	11.3	100	140	45
4	2.3	2	57	258.8	-45*	120	115	12
5	2.3	2	47	191.3	-18*	110	110	53
6	2.2	2.3	55	337	-09*	100	91	42
7	2.2	2.3	37.5	270	-13.5*	110	80	47

Table 14.3 Experiments where flow in the PA reduced keeping DFA & DFS constant.

Expt No.	DFA mm	DFS mm	FPAB ml/min	FPAA ml/min	FDA ml/min	FRPA %	SAPA mm/Hg	SVPA mm/Hg
8	2.1	1.4	51.5	132	60	50	215	100
9	2.1	1.4	20.5	283	49.1	80	150	50
10	2.1	3	39	258.8	22.5	90	100	20
11	2.1	3	20.5	236.3	28.1	90	64	48

Flowin PA Reduced. DFA Constant. DFS Increased

When the experiment was repeated by increasing the diameter of the feeding artery to 2.3mm by keeping the diameter of the fistula constant, with the drop in the proximal artery flow, reversal of flow occurred in the distal arterial segment. SAPA showed very little changes.

When the above experiment was repeated by increasing the diameter of the fistula to 2.7mm, drop in the proximal artery flow eliminated the reverse flow in the distal arterial segment.

Flow in PA Constant. DFA & DFS Changed

In the following set of experiments the flow and the diameters of the fistula were kept constant while the diameter of the feeding artery was reduced from 2.3mm to 2.2mm. They produced a significant reversal of flow in the distal arterial segment.

DFA and Flow in PA Constant. DFS was Increased

However when the experiments were repeated on different groups of animals by keeping the flow and diameter of the feeding artery constant and increasing the diameter of the fistula, the flow characteristics were stable in all except in two where there was a reversed flow in the distal arterial segment (Table14.9).

DFA, DFS and SAP Constant. Animals Changed

In the following set of experiments diameters of feeding artery, and the fistula were kept constant and the flow in the proximal artery was kept constant, while the animals were changed. Response of the animals varied very considerably.

Table 14.4 Experiments where Flow in PA and DFA reduced keeping DFS constant.

Expt No.	DFA mm	DFS mm	FPAB ml/min	FPAA ml/min	FDA ml/min	FRPA %	SAPA mm/Hg	SVPA mm/Hg
12	2	1.1	67.5	56.3	4.5	90	99	15
13	2	1.1	20	31.5	-13.5*	140	99	71
14	2	1.3	67.5	78.8	18	80	105	24
15	2	1.3	38	28.1	11.3	60	111	25
16	2	1.3	106.5	101.3	4.5	100	73	36
17	2	1.7	51.5	202.5	-22.5*	110	117	30
18	2	2.3	67.5	168.5	11.3	90	93	58.5
19	2	2.3	21	87.4	6.8	110	111	98

Table 14.5 Experiments where Flow in PA reduced with increase in DFA keeping DFS constant.

Expt No.	DFA mm	DFS mm	FPAB ml/min	FPAA ml/min	FDA ml/min	FRPA %	SAPA mm/Hg	SVPA mm/Hg
20	2.2	1.5	1.6	345	30	90	145	70
21	2.2	1.5	51.5	286.9	57	80	150	40
22	2.2	2.3	55	337	-27.3*	100	91	42
23	2.2	2.3	37.5	270	-13.4*	110	80	47

Table 14.6 Experiments wherein the Flow in PA reduced increased DFS keeping the DFA constant.

Expt No.	DFA mm	DFS mm	FPAB ml/min	FPAA ml/min	FDA ml/min	FRPA %	SAPA mm/Hg	SVPA mm/Hg
24	2.3	2	108	427	11.3	100	140	45
25	2.3	2	57	258	-45*	120	115	12
26	2.3	2	47	191.3	-18*	110	110	53

Table 14.7 Experiments wherein the Flow in PA reduced increased DFS and DFA.

Expt No.	DFA mm	DFS mm	FPAB ml/min	FPAA ml/min	FDA ml/min	FRPA %	SAPA mm/Hg	SVPA mm/Hg
29	2.3	2.3	57.5	185.5	0	100	116	108
30	2.2	2.3	55	337.5	-9*	100	91	42

Table 14.8 Experiments DFA and flow in PA was constant, the DFS was increased.

Expt No.	DFA mm	DFS mm	FPAB ml/min	FPAA ml/min	FDA ml/min	FRPA %	SAPA mm/Hg	SVPA mm/Hg
31	2.0	1.1	67.5	56.3	4.5	90	99	15
32	2.0	1.2	67.5	78.9	18.0	60	105	24
33	2.1	1.4	51.5	132	60.0	70	215	100
34	2.1	1.9	53.5	258	-18*	90	160	25
35	2.1	2.1	51.5	286	26.1	90	155	65
36	2.1	1.4	20.2	283.6	49.1	90	150	50
37	2.1	2.3	20.5	396	30.0	90	230	125
38	2.1	3.0	20.5	236	28.1	90	64	48
39	2.2	1.5	51.5	286.9	50.7	90	150	40
40	2.2	2.1	51.0	244.5	-27.3*	100	180	55
41	2.2	2.3	55.0	337.5	-13.5*	110	91	42
42	2.2	1.7	64	368.1	27.2	90	106	25
43	2.2	1.8	64	555	52.5	90	140	45
44	2.2	2.4	24	167	6.4	100	100	53
45	2.2	2.5	29	180	15	90	170	45
46	2.3	1.3	21	61.9	9	90	123	71
47	2.3	1.5	21	38.6	0	100	88	15
48	2.3	1.5	21	92.7	10.6	90	99	15
49	2.3	2	57	258.8	-45*	120	115	12
50	2.3	2.3	57.5	185.4	0	100	116	108

Table 14.9 Experiments with DFA, DFS and SAP constant but on different animals.

Expt No.	DFA mm	DFS mm	FPAB ml/min	FPAA ml/min	FDA ml/min	FRPA %	SAPA mm/Hg	SVPA mm/Hg
51	2.3	1.5	39	202	0.9	100	111	21
52	2.3	1.5	21	38.6	0	100	88	185
53	2.3	1.5	24	168	11.3	90	111	56
54	2.3	1.5	21	92.7	10.6	90	99	15

Discussion

Model

The present experiment was designed to identify the physiological factors, which influence the flow of blood in an AVF. Ananimal model was preferred to a bench top model with a pulsatile pump. Though the latter would have allowed more strictcontrol over parameters like pressure and flow, it would not have represented the in-vivo condition where two fluid systems of very different pressures and flow are inter connected as seen in an AVF. When a fistula is introduced in the circulation a number of physiological adjustments occur before the flow is stabilised. AVF is equivalent to an arterial bleed except that there is no loss of fluid to the outside. To maintain this internal loss the circulatory compensations such as cardiac output and heart rate occur. The efficacy of this mechanism varies in the biological models. We feel that these changes are important and are not possible to include in in-vivo models. There was a significant animal variability when the parameters were constant and animals were varied (Table 14.9).

This highlights the biological variability. The observations of Djurbeg[67] the hemodynamics of a cerebral AVM is complex and varies from patient to patient as well as same patient when cardio-vascular parameters change" summarise the superiority of an animal model which includes this very important variable.

The theoretical models described by Gao[87&88] and Hademenos[107 110] do not contain the diameters of the fistulae and are therefore inadequate.

We feel all these models attempt to extend the concept of flow through a linear tube by certain assumptions. We accept that certain assumptions are necessary in any evaluation of flow. However our model has shown that assumption of the diameters is likely to obscure the very essence of AVF dynamics.

Experimental Errors

As in any experiment of this nature where the flow of fluid is measured in pipes, there are some potential errors in the methodology. An error of about 10% is likely to have crept into our values, which is inherent in any measurement of fluid flow. The actual fistula was rigid (unlike in the biological state) and it was impossible to estimate the influence of this non-pulsatile structure on our values. The dogs though were of nearly same the weight, could not be expected to behave uniformly to the physiological manipulations.

The clip-on magnetic probes has a tendency towards baseline drifts and in spite of intense efforts some errors in calibration are likely to have occurred.

The influences of turbulence on the flow characteristics (flow measurement) under such conditions were unavailable to us. We concede that these various errors have crept into our experimental data. However, we are of the opinion that while the errors may be considerable for actual individual values, since we are looking at the overall pattern of flow over a large number of experiments, the observations are still valid.

Pressure Changes

Pressure changes at the arterial and venous segments of the fistulae showed good correlation. These findings add credibility to our model and the experimental procedure. Estimation of pressures does not reflect the unpredictable behaviour of these lesions. We feel that the pressure gradient is maintained by the flow. Flow is sensitive to the diameter of the vessels. Over a period of time the vessel diameters change due to dilatation or thrombus formation and upset the pattern. Our model has demonstrated that the flow in the fistulae is very sensitive to small changes in the diameters.

Feeding Artery Pressure

In all our experiments the flow in the feeding artery increased after the fistula was opened. This was as expected. Batger[16] reported changes in AVF with relation to cerebral perfusion and opined that reduction of blood pressure as an effective measure of reducing the flow in the fistula. Quick et al[259&260] concluded from their mathematical model that the increase in the feeding artery pressure secondary to adaptation in the external system increases the risk of hemorrhagic stroke. Nornes[217&219] recorded a lower pressure in the feeding arteries at their entrance to the fistula than the SAP. Nornes does not mention vessel diameters. His observations on pressure ranges between 40-77mmof Hg are in our opinion over-simplification of the problem.

In our model reduction of SAPA produced corresponding reduction of the FPAA. However the flow in the fistula did not reduce on all occasions. (Table 14.2) In experiments 1&2 when the SAP was reduced, the flow in the shunt FRPA decreased. When the SAP was reduced in experiments 3&4 and 6&7 the FRPA was more than the PA flow. This was because of contribution from the distal arterial segment (steal).

Proximal Artery Flow

Table 14.10 shows the fraction of PA flow that flows across the shunt for diameters of the fistulae. When the flow in the PA was reduced in six of the experiments there was actually an increase in the fraction (more than the total flow in the PA), due to reverse flow in the distal arterial segment. If the flow in the PA is reduced in certain situations the fistula draws blood from other sources to maintain the pressure gradient.

Duonget.al[71&72] concluded that high arterial input pressure (measured) and venous drainage pressure were principal risk factors for haemorrhage. In our experiments there was a good correlation between the systemic arterial pressure and the pressure at the arterial end of the fistula. The assumption by these authors that a deep venous drainage has higher pressure is unacceptable without actual measured values at the venous end of the fistula (see below–venous pressures).

While describing AVM in the brain it was observed by Deutch[65], Holman[126-135] Luessenhop[173-175] and Spetzler[307-310] that occlusion of the feeding arteries in a fistula reduces the flow in the fistula proportionately. In our experimental model the proximal arterial segment represented the sum total of all the feeding arteries. Reduction of blood flow in the feeding artery produced inconsistent flow pattern. In the experiments where the diameter of the feeding artery was 2.1mm & 2.2mm drop in the arterial flow did not produce any significant flow changes. However when the diameter of the feeding artery was changed to 2mm and 2.3mm, there was reversed flow in three instances in the distal arterial segment. It is possible that in addition to the volume of blood flow, the diameter of the feeding artery has very unpredictable contributions to the flow in the shunt (Table 14.2).

Manchola et al[177] have demonstrated a significant high flow in the AVM feeders compared to the non feeding arteries. There is no mention of either the sizes of the fistula nor were the

Table 14.10 Fraction of the PA flow shunted across various sizes of DFA and DFS.

Expt No.	DFA mm	DFS mm	FPAB ml/min	FPAA ml/min	FDA ml/min	FRPA %	SAPA mm/Hg	SVPA mm/Hg
8	2.1	1.4	51.5	132	60	0.5	215	110
9	2.1	1.4	20.5	283	49.1	0.8	150	50
10	2.1	3	39	258.8	22.5	0.9	110	20
11	2	3	20.5	236.3	28.1	0.9	64	48
12	2	1.1	67.5	56.3	4.5	0.9	99	15
13	2	1.1	20	31.5	-13.5*	1.4	99	71
14	2	1.3	67.5	78.8	18	0.8	105	24
15	2	1.3	38	28.1	11.3	0.6	111	25
16	2	1.7	106.5	101.3	4.5	1	73	36
17	2	1.7	51.5	202.5	-22.5*	1.1	117	30
18	2	2.3	67.5	168.5	11.3	0.9	93	58.5
19	2	2.3	21	87.4	6.8	1.1	111	98
20	2.2	1.5	106	345	30	0.9	145	70
21	2.2	1.5	51.5	286.9	57	0.8	150	40
22	2.2	2.3	55	337	-27.3*	1	91	42
23	2.2	2.3	37.5	270	-13.4*	1.1	80	47
24	2.3	2	108	427	11.3	1	140	45
25	2.3	2	57	258	-45*	1.2	115	12
26	2.3	2	47	191.3	-18*	1.1	110	53

fractions of feeding artery flows that shunted. We feel from our experimental findings that these are important issues. The problem is more complex when the flow values in a fistula are evaluated. While our experiments showed (Figures 14.11,14.12) that the flow in the FA followed the trend of flow in the fistula, it was not possible to assume that the volume of flow was an indicator of the size of the fistula. In our experiments in certain areas increase in the size of the fistulae were associated with a decrease in the PA flow. Therefore it would be an error to assume that PA flow reflects the events in the fistula fully.

Flow in Shunt And Pressure Drop

No relationship could be established between the shunt flow and pressure drop (Figure 14.11). One would have expected same relationship between the set of parameters, although not necessarily a linear relationship. We believe that this is due to the fact that when there is a drop in the pressure in the shunt, flow (in the shunt) actually increases by the contribution from the distal arterial segment, (steal flow), to maintain the flow in the fistula (Constantino[49]). This phenomenon we believe is peculiar to AVF not seen in other types of fluid flow systems. It is because of this lack of relationship between flow and pressure drop, manipulations of systemic arterial pressure and volume of blood flow in PA do not necessarily produce corresponding flow changes in the shunt. In our experiments, drop in the SAP reduced flow in PA as expected, but for reasons mentioned above a similar reduction was not seen in the shunt consistently. The scatter in the data could be either due to errors in the measurements or due to inherent character of the fistula. As explained earlier all standard precautions were taken to obtain as accurate data as possible, and to minimise the inherent inaccuracies of any fluid flow measurements. Therefore, it is necessary to speculate that the linear type of relationship that is normally seen between flow and pressure drop in a laminar flow in a tube is not seen in an AV-fistula, where two fluid systems under different pressures are inter-connected.)

Retrograde Flow

We feel that there are three possible conditions of AVF. Figure 14.10A shows a situation where the feeding artery is capable of delivering required amount of blood to areas beyond the AVF in spite of some loss across the shunt. As long as this condition exists, the situation is stable. This condition is represented on Figure 14.17 as the region below the horizontal line.

The region **A** represents the example of AVM where the fraction of proximal artery flow across the shunt is less than1.0 (algebraic).

The second possibility is when the feeding artery is able to feed the quantum of blood just adequate to meet the ability of the fistula to shunt (Figure 14.10B). Thus, the entire flow in the feeding artery is shunted into the venous system and the regions beyond the shunt do not receive any blood flow). Such an AVF is critically poised. Any further change in flow could alter the pattern. The condition is represented in Figure 14.17 as the horizontal line (position **B)**. In this condition all the flow in the feeding artery is being shunted into the venous system, across the fistula.

The third possibility is that of the fistula being capable of shunting quantities over and above the capabilities of the feeding artery (Figure 14.10C). The segment of blood vessel distal to the shunt will draw blood from other sources to satisfy the demands of the shunt and thus create an unstable condition. This condition is represented in Figure 14.17 as the region **C** above the horizontal line. In this region, the flow in the shunt is greater than that in the feeding artery implying that there is more than one feeder or that there is retrograde flow in the distal artery.

In our experimental setting reversal of flow in the distal arterial segment represented steal phenomenon. This occurred on 16 occasions. We could not find any definite combination of experimental conditions that induced this flow pattern. The fluctuating neurological deficits associated with steal phenomenon are due to disparity in the feeding artery flow and the fraction of this flow that shunts across Spetzler[251&252].

Diameter of the Fistula

The diameter of the shunt determines the volume of the arterial blood that is shunted. In most of our experiments there was increase in the flow across the shunt with incremental increases in the diameter of the latter. The anomalous decline in the flow for certain values of the shunt diameter did not suggest any pattern (Table 14.5).

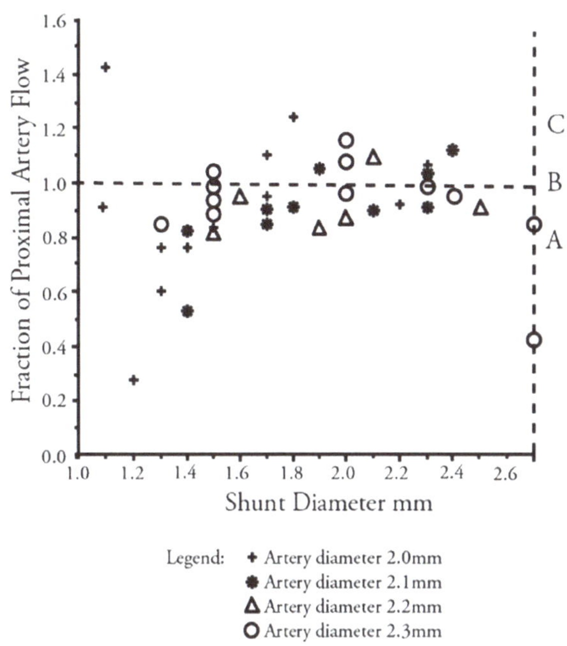

Figure 14.17 Fraction of Proximal artery flow and the diameter of the shunt.

There have been many reports of spontaneous regression of AVMs Buis[34]. Occlusion or thrombosis of the feeding arteries was not seen in all these reports. It is possible with passage of time due to constant high flow the diameter of the fistula increases and may induce an anomalous decline in the flow. The magnitude of change in the diameter of 0.1mm could induce major changes in the flow. 50% of the patients in this study had either a single arterial feeder. This supports the sensitivity of the flow to small changes in the size of the fistulae.

Fraction of Arterial Flow and Shunt Diameter

No clear trend could be recognised between the fraction of PA flow and shunt diameter, except for periodic fluctuations in the flow as the diameter of the shunt increased. The fractional flow seemed to increase with the increase in the diameter of the shunt over a short range, followed by a drop with further increase in the diameter (Table 14.6). This pattern was seen in all the four groups of experiments with different diameters of F.A. (2.0-2.3). There was not sufficient consistency in these fluctuations to produce any meaningful predictions.

The fistula is an abnormality in the circulatory system. Pressure drop between the AFJ and VFJ is compensated by adjusting the flow. Beyond a certain level the compensation fails.

A fistula is similar to an arterial bleed perhaps more complex. The compensation is in the form of increased flow in the FA, reverse flow in the distal segment and perhaps other systemic circulatory corrections. We do not know the limits of this compensation. We feel an animal model like ours is more likely to reflect these features. Our experiments demonstrate that the diameters of the fistula play a significant role in these.

Venous Drainage Pressures

The flow values in the venous segment of the fistula are valid only if it is done close to the fistula. Murayama et.al[205] obtained pulsatile flow in the veins only when the probe was close to the site of the fistula. Duong et.al[71&72], concluded that the combination of raised systemic arterial pressure and deep veins have increased risk of bleed. We feel that assumptions of venous pressures are unacceptable. We were unable to measure the flows at the venous side of the fistula due to constraints of our acrylic fistulae.

The venous pressures had good correlation to the systemic arterial pressures even though they were measured at a distance of 1cm from the actual fistula. This is because the construct of the fistula was such that there were no branches before the pressures were recorded.

We feel that any evaluation based on the site and size of the nidus is likely to be inaccurate. Hademenos[107&110]. The flow characteristics in the venous segment change rapidly due to the elasticity of the veins and the presence of the plexus.

Our experiments have also indicated that pressures at the arterial and venous segments of the fistulae correlate. The various models and other observations reached on the assumption that pressures indicate the flow in the shunt are likely to miss the basic feature of AVM dynamics. (Smith[305] Quick[259&260])

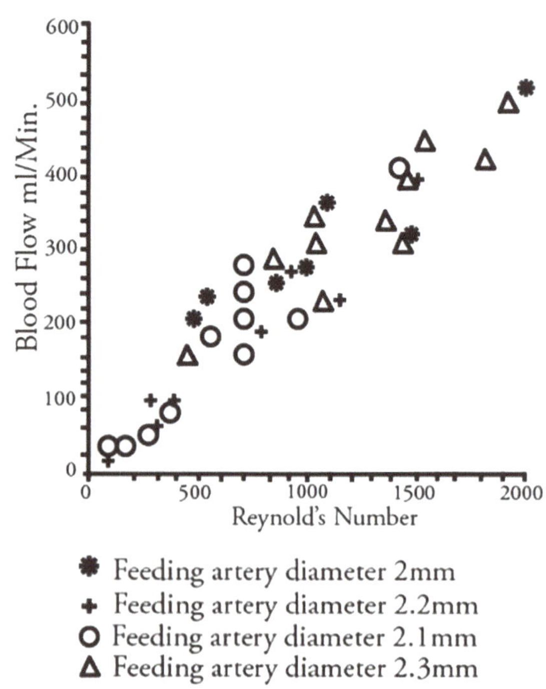

Figure 14.18 Reynold's numbers.

Statistical Validity

Statistical correlations are not difficult to achieve when derived values are used. The theoretical models are based on derived values for flow in a linear tube and are likely to show statistical validity. In our study we could demonstrate similar correlation between blood flow and Reynolds number Figure 14.17). The actual measured experimental values often show a greater variation. (Tables 14.11 and Table 14.12). Regression analysis of the experimental values (Tables 14.41 &14.12) do not show good correlation.

Mechanical Properties Of Vessels

We acknowledge that the mechanical properties of the vessels influence the flow. Monson[200] studied the biaxial response of passive cerebral arteries. They concluded that the behaviour of the arteries was nonlinear and anisotropic. They also observed that there was greater deformation in the axial direction than in the circumference. Their experiments do not take into consideration the influence of vessels with varied diameters. They have assumed that the circumference of the end of the vessels from where the measurements are made is the same as that in the middle of the vessel. This is not accurate. Our findings demonstrate the sensitivity of the flow to very small changes in the diameter of the vessels. Changes in the diameter of the arteries in a given individual over a period of time are well known. Bushby and Burton[36] demonstrated that with increased pressure both the length and diameter increases. However they observed that diameter was less sensitive to pressure changes than the length. Their experiments were with large carotid arteries. We do not believe that this is necessarily applicable to vessels with smaller diameters as well. Hayashi et.al[118] have observed that the stress on the vessel wall due to pressure is less significant for normalized parameters such as stress. Stephanis et.al[313] have observed that the coefficient of elasticity of the arterial wall is dependent on the thickness and that it is very difficult to estimate this accurately in-vivo.

Table 14.11 Multiple regression values for Proximal arteryflow vs Various parameters.

Parameter	All Cases					Cases with Retrograde Flow				
Artery Diameter	+	-0.0476	+	+	+	+	-0.1711	+	+	+
Shunt Diameter	+	-0.0156	+	+	+	+	-0.1916	+	+	+
Pressure at AFJ	+	-0.0015				+		+		+
Pressure at VFJ										
Flow thru Shunt	+	0.00016	+			+		+	+	
Reynolds' No.	+					+				
Shear Rate	+					+				
Intercept	1.11						1.811			
F Value	1.97	2.58	0.58	2.01	0.51	1.61	3.77	2.21	3.13	3.36
Probability	0.080	0.049	0.634	0.125	0.676	0.338	0.059	0.169	0.087	0.075
Significant at 5% level										

Table 14.12 Stepwise regression of various parameters controlling the flow through AVF.

Variable	R2	1-R2	N-K-1	(1-R2) / (N-K-1)
Artery Diameter	0.002	0.998	50	0.01196
Shunt Diameter	0.015	0.985	49	0.02010
Proximal Artery Flow	0.038	0.962	48	0.02004
Distal Artery Flow	0.618	0.382	47	0.00813
AFJ Pressure	0.621	0.379	46	0.00824
VFJ Pressure	0.662	0.338	45	0.00751
Reynolds Number	0.663	0.337	44	0.00766
Shear Rate	0.691	0.309	43	0.00719

K is the number of parameters entered into analysis
N is the number of data points

It is also important to understand that in-vivo vessel tries to maintain homeostasis. Vasoconstriction due to vasospasm is very active in cerebral vessels (Nagasawa et.al.[206]). This factor is difficult to reproduce in experimental models. Venous channels offer flow limiting resistance to arterial flow (Pang[237]). This is dependent on the histological characteristics of the vessel wall. In a cerebral AVF over a period of time veins tend to develop more deposition of fibrous tissue, and therefore may influence the flow dynamics. The various observations on the mechanical properties of the vessel (reported in the literature) are based on single segments of the arteries. (Vita & Dixon[342]). As we have mentioned earlier we are not sure if these observations are applicable to an AVF where the flow characteristics are very different.

Spontaneous regression of AVMs (Kushner[158], Steal phenomenon causing neurological manifestations distant to the site of the lesion and unpredictable results from procedures designed to reduce the flow by reducing the systemic hypertension or occluding the feeding vessels indicate the importance of the diameter of the fistula. We have demonstrated significant changes in the flow with very small alterations to the diameters of the fistulae. Anomalous flows and retrograde flow that occur with very small changes in the diameters of the FA and the fistulae are the principal reasons for the unpredictable behaviour of these lesions. We feel that this phenomenon is the primary nature of AVF. Unlike in a linear pipe where the volume of flow is dependent directly to the pressure, velocity and the diameter of the tube, the flow in an AVF is dictated by more complex combination of factors due to the fact that in an AVF we have a system where two fluid systems under very different pressures are interconnected. Simple manipulations of SAP or blood flow in the feeding artery may create more problems by destabilising the flow patterns. We were unable to demonstrate any definite predictable patterns. Our experiments in spite of their inherent defects strongly suggest that the flow characteristics of an AVF are too complex, to be influenced entirely simple physiological parameters such as blood pressure, velocity of flow and volume of blood flow in the feeding arteries. Our model has demonstrated that pressure studies alone do not reflect the flow characteristics of the fistula and that the diameters of the fistula and the feeding arteries play a very significant role in the hemodynamics of the malformation. Perhaps there is a very significant relationship between the shunt diameter and a non-dimensional factor such as the fraction of arterial flow shunted across. (Goldberger[98&99]) More experimental work with a model that incorporates the diameters of the fistula and FA is needed to elucidate this very complex problem.

15

Cerebral Arteriovenous Malformations: A Computational Study

Minal Bhagwat, Vidyasagar Casikar*, Karkenahalli Srinivas
School of Aerospace, Mechanical and Mechatronics Engineering University of Sydney. Australia.

Introduction

There are many published reports of studies of blood flow in an Arterio- venous fistula. One such is the experiments by Casikar and Ramaswamy[41] which has clearly demonstrated the unexpected relationship among vessel diameter, blood pressure and steal phenomenon. The model utilised in the experiments were made of acrylic. 'H' shaped prosthesis with a wide range of diameters were generated by drilling into a solid block of acrylic sheet. They inserted these into femoral vessels of dogs. This model was limited as the natural vasculature of the dogs were not controlled – the collateral artery and collateral vein were not control variables. The results from these models were not able to identify a clear relationship between the physiological factors influencing blood flow in the AVM. The models did indicate some connection between these factors, exemplifying the complexity of blood flow through the AVM and the disordered vessel structure itself.

On the other hand, the theoretical studies have applied the principles of flow in a linear tube and drawn conclusions. We believe this type of study does not illustrate the complex flow pattern of a fistula where two fluid systems with very different pressures are interconnected.

The present research was designed to create a computational model to critically analyse the experimental findings. In addition, due to the difficulty of measuring any values in vivo, a computational model is the most feasible response to enhance the current understanding of this vascular malformation in the medical and engineering communities. The present work is a continuation of the previous work conducted by Prattipati[256] and Brady[29]. Prattipati computed the governing equations of motion and observed artery diameter as affecting blood flow and velocity, alongside fistula diameter. He maintained a pre-determined pressure throughout the AVM and its components and thus pressure could not be analysed separately. The research also indicated the ability to simulate pressure calculations over a pre-determined flow velocity model.

Many published models have used two-dimensional analysis models, each with different aims and geometry. A review of these models, however, indicates that AVM blood flow through real patient geometry has not been replicated.

Methodology

Test 1: Buckingham Pi Analysis

To initiate this examination of the factors leading to arteriovenous malfunction development and progression, a Buckingham Pi analysis was conducted in order to identify some dimensionless value connected with the specific blood flow found in the AVM network. Various assumptions were incorporated into the calculations. Critical variables (based on the assumptions made in this analysis) were identified.

ANSYS Workbench, version 16.2 was employed along with its various functions. ANSYS Meshing, ICEM, and CFX Solver were utilised. A model was generated through SolidWorks, version 2013 and imported to the ANSYS modules.

Model Development

The initial workings of this thesis were through the application of a two-dimensional model. The first model drawn matched the dimensions used in both Brady[29] and Prattipati[256]. The figure 15.1 indicates the 'H' configuration that was used. Table 15.1 indicates the various values used for the diameter of the fistula.

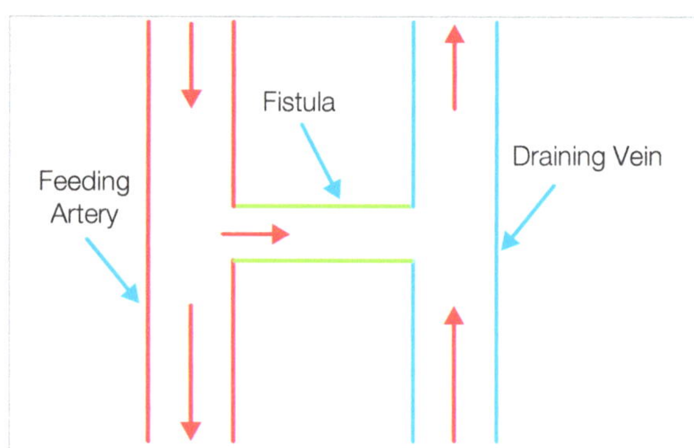

Figure 15.1 Simplification of flow through an AVM.

Model Geometry and Generation

The drawing tools were employed in *SolidWorks* in order to generate the models for analysis in a computational fluid dynamics software. A rectangle was drawn from the origin with length 0.035m and width of 0.002m. Another rectangle was positioned 0.012m from the top of the first rectangle placed perpendicular and coincident to it. Finally, a third rectangle was drawn parallel to the first one to generate the 'H' shape, skewed at two ends. Once all nine models were generated, with differing fistula diameters, these were exported as IGS files to enable working in *ANSYS Workbench*.

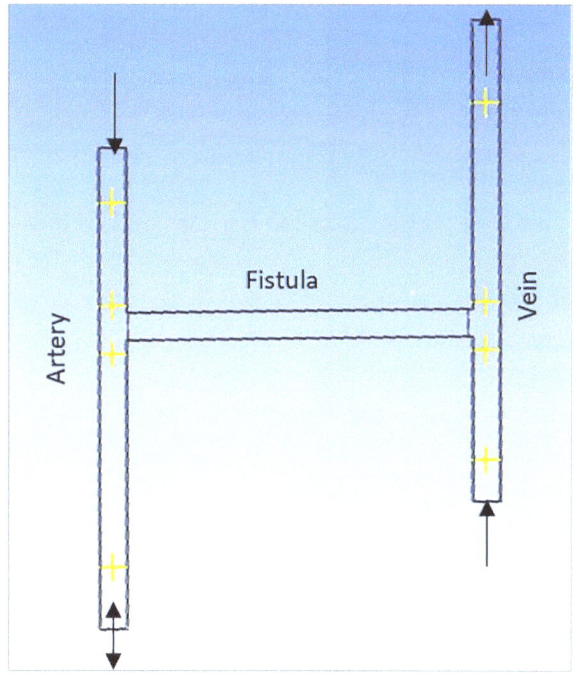

Figure 15.2 Geometry of model used.

Table 15.1 Buckingham Pi variables and units.

Variable	Algebraic Variable	Units	Measurement Variable
Inlet Velocity	$\overline{V_{in}}$	$m.s^{-1}$	$L.T^{-1}$
Artery Diameter	D_{artery}	m	L
Vein Diameter	D_{vein}	m	L
Fistula Diameter	$D_{fistula}$	m	L
Length of Fistula	$l_{fistula}$	m	L
Change in Pressure across Fistula	$\Delta P_{fistula}$	$Pa = kg.m^{-1}.s^{-2}$	$M.L^{-1}.T^{-2}$
Dynamic viscosity	μ	$kg.m^{-1}.s^{-1}$	$M.L^{-1}.T^{-1}$
Density	ρ	$kg.m^{-3}$	$M.L^{-3}$
Artery outlet Velocity	$\overline{V_{artery\ out}}$	$m.s^{-1}$	$L.T^{-1}$
Vein outlet Velocity	$\overline{V_{vein\ out}}$	$m.s^{-1}$	$L.T^{-1}$

Meshing

The geometry generated (Figure 15.2) in *SolidWorks* was imported into the *ANSYS Meshing* module within *ANSYS Workbench*. To identify the most suitable mesh for application to the models, a mesh convergence test was conducted. This entailed the procedure of testing various mesh sizes, evaluating the time taken, and the accuracy of the data obtained. To do so pressure was measured at a selected point, through a standard probe used in all models. This analysis was facilitated by multiplying the number of nodes by the three, or the individual degrees of freedom each node has, and identifying some convergence points.

For this analysis, a tetrahedral mesh was utilised allowing refined elements to be used for examination, with 4 nodes per element. Each element, furthermore, had 3 degrees of freedom along the three dimensional planes (x, y and z) Jo-YU[4]. A convergence test was conducted and the following mesh convergence graph was generated. (Figure 15.5)

The tests indicate convergence of the degrees of freedom and pressure at the predetermined probe occurs in the region of mesh size between 0.000140.00005. The denser

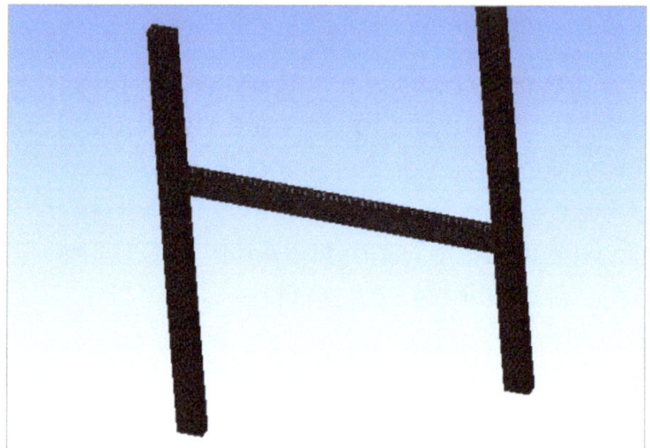

Figure 15.3 Mesh sizing 0.00013 convergence test.

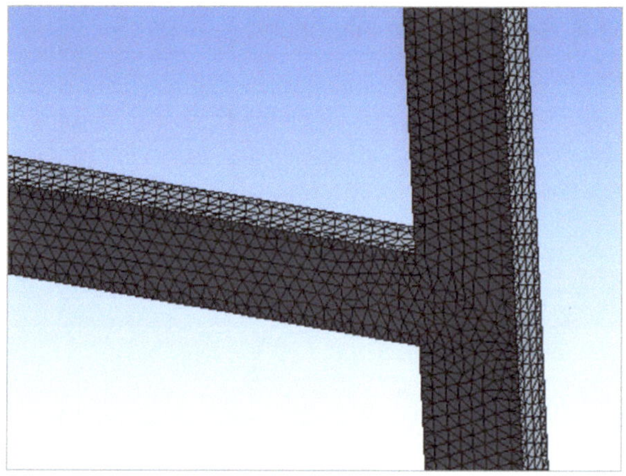

Figure 15.4 Close view of Mesh sizing 0.0013 convergence test.

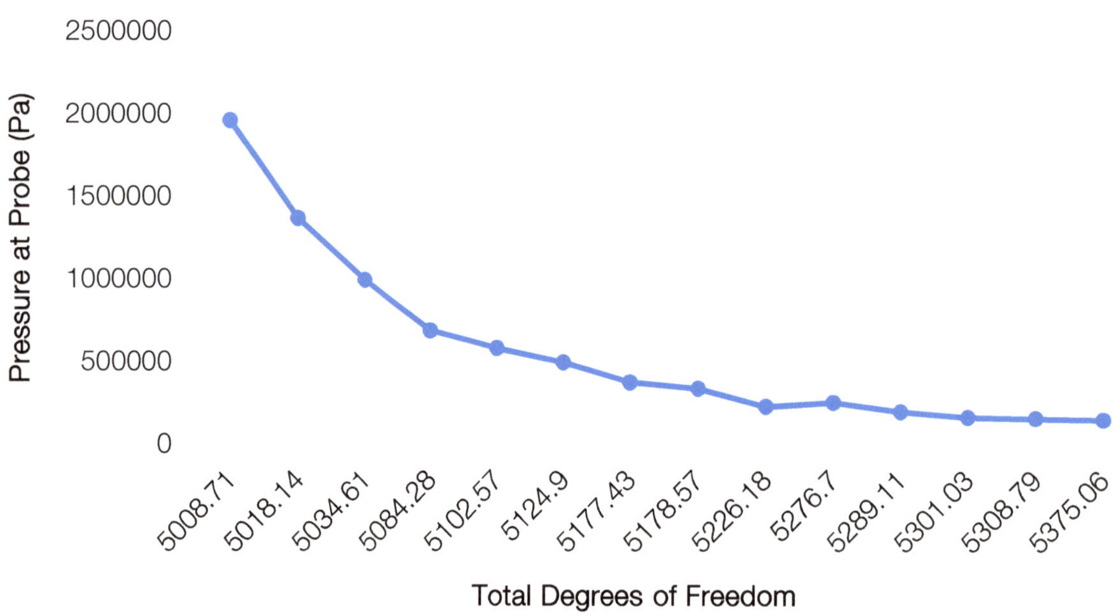

Figure 15.5 Mesh Convergence Test.

mesh followed a particularly lengthy solution, however generated solutions with greater accuracy.

A finer mesh produced a faster solution, however with a greater level of inaccuracy. With consideration of mesh quality and time taken, the mesh size 0.00013 was selected using the patch conforming method. This mesh was exported as an *ANSYS Mesh* file for application within the *CFX module*. The final mesh that was utilised is shown in Figure 15.3 and 15.4.

CFX Module

After the mesh was generated, the mesh data was imported into the *CFX module* setup using *ANSYS Meshing* software. To conduct a computational solution, this mesh data and geometry were required to have boundary and flow conditions.

Boundary Conditions

The boundary conditions detailed by Prattipati[255] are utilised in this examination to perform various calculations and measurements. Maintaining conditions that represent true blood flow in the brain enables a more accurate study. The initial values utilised were drawn from the measurements used by Prattipati[255] which match those identified by Casikar[41]. Extending upon the examination by Brady[29] of AVM blood flow as adequately represented as pipe flow, in addition to the models developed by researchers, various pipe flow assumptions were utilised in this study [Vignon[341] & Venkateshan[331]].

Examining regular blood flow, the blood travels from artery through to the veins via the capillary bed whereby nutrients are absorbed by the body [Blair[22] & Ornstein[231]]. Thus, the quantification of velocity or mass flow rate at the venous inlet or outlet is not based solely on the incoming flow from the feeding artery of the AVM, but is greatly affected by the capillary action. Additionally, with lack of sufficient data to quantify cerebral venous blood flow, it was essential to assume some value for this flow rate. To simplify the model, without excessive application of further theorems and to improve the applicability to the results, venous flow was considered as equal to arterial blood flow. Figure 15.6.

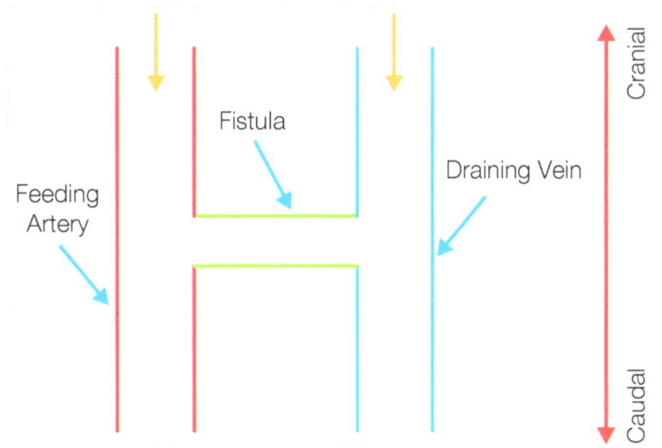

Figure 15.6 Anatomical orientation of AVM.

The inlet and outlet conditions were fixed for each trial to enable reliable and valid data to be measured from each test. These conditions however were varied in literature, with many articles in contention with one another [Cipolla[44] & Krauss[152]].

Finally, as a result of the setup requiring a flow rate applied to the inlets, the outlet pressures had to be measured. The equation was as follows:

$$P = P_{inlet} - \rho g \Delta h$$

$$P_{artery\ outlet} = 100 \text{ mm Hg} - 1280(9.81)(0.035)$$

$$P_{artery\ outlet} = 96.7 \text{ mm Hg}$$

$$P_{vein\ outlet} = 30 \text{ mm Hg} + 1280(9.81)(0.35)$$

$$P_{vein\ outlet} = 33.296 \text{ mm Hg}$$

These conditions were applied to the geometry. The solver controls were set for 200 iterations and a convergence point of 0.000001. Additionally, the material was set to water, after editing the fluid properties of water to match that of blood. These changes are summarised in Table 15.2.

Table 15.2 Changing Fistula Diameter.

Model Number	Artery Diameter (m)	Fistula Diameter (m)	Fistula Length (m)
1	0.002	0.0012	0.014
2	0.002	0.0014	0.014
3	0.002	0.0016	0.014
4	0.002	0.0018	0.014
5	0.002	0.002	0.014
6	0.002	0.0022	0.014
7	0.002	0.0024	0.014
8	0.002	0.0026	0.014
9	0.002	0.0028	0.014

Test 2.1: Okell,[228] assumption Q_{inlet} = 0.00576 kg/s

The arterial outlet assumption was based on research conducted by Okell and Chappell [[228]]. This study found the value to be equal to 4.5 mL/s, or 0.00576 kg/s, which quantified middle cerebral artery blood flow.

Test 2.2: Stock[316] Assumption Q_{inlet} = 0.0048 kg/s

A value of 0.0048 kg/s was selected as both arterial inlet and venous outlet flow based on the research conducted by Stock et.al[316], who also aimed to quantify middle cerebral arterial blood flow.

Test 2.3: Changing Diameter with Q_{inlet} = 0.003 kg/s

Following the above tests, an assumed value of 0.003 kg/s was tested as the mass flow rate at both arterial and venous inlet. The test was conducted to provide further insight into the effects of changing inlet flow rates on the blood flow. This offered more comparison points.

Test 2.4: Changing Diameter with Q_{inlet} = 0.0025 kg/s

Another assumed value of inlet blood flow rate of 0.0025 kg/s was tested. The test was another comparative test exploring the overall effects of mass flow rates.

Test 3: Controlled Flow Test

Test 3 was conducted to observe the flow characteristics using fixed flow conditions, which included a model for steal phenomenon. For this trial, measurement of the wall shear stress and pressure were essential to the determination of the effects of changing flow (ignoring autoregulation). A standard model of 0.002m fistula

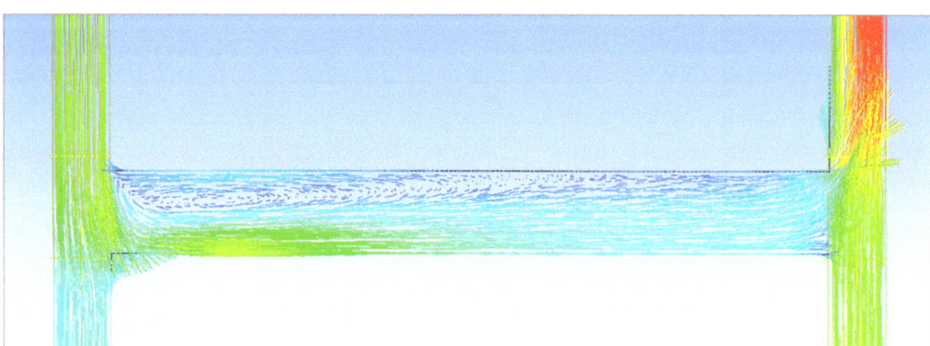

Figure 15.7 Blood Swirling through fistula D = 0.0028m Test 2.1.

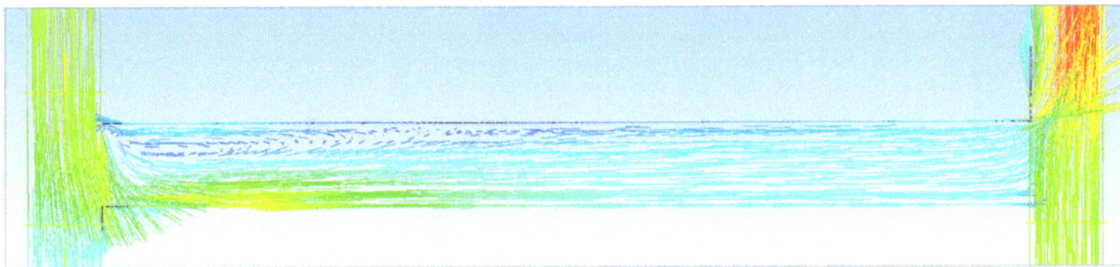

Figure 15.8 Blood Swirling through fistula D = 0.0022m Test 2.2.

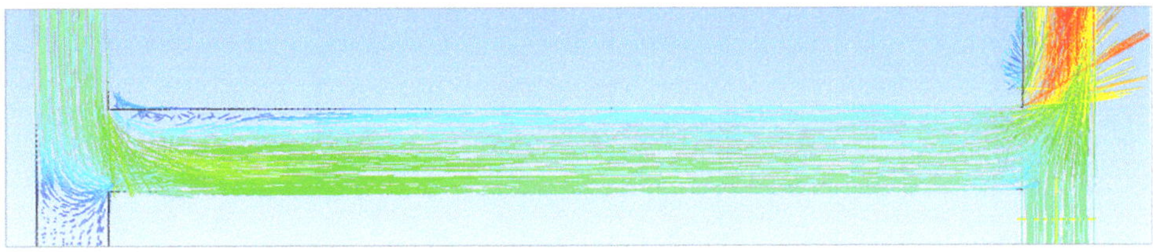

Figure 15.9 Blood Swirling through fistula D = 0.0022m Test 2.3.

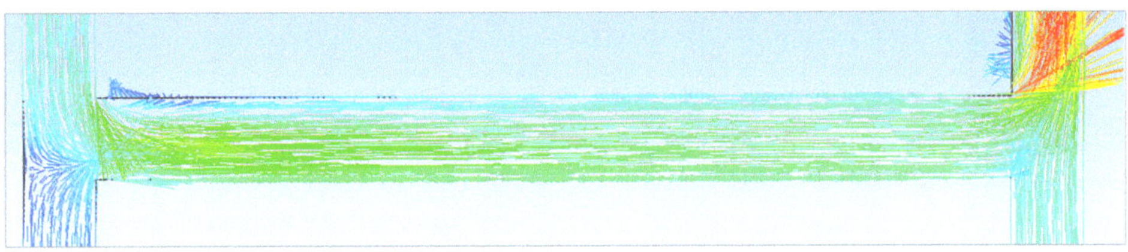

Figure 15.10 Blood swirling through fistula D = 0.0022m Test 2.4.

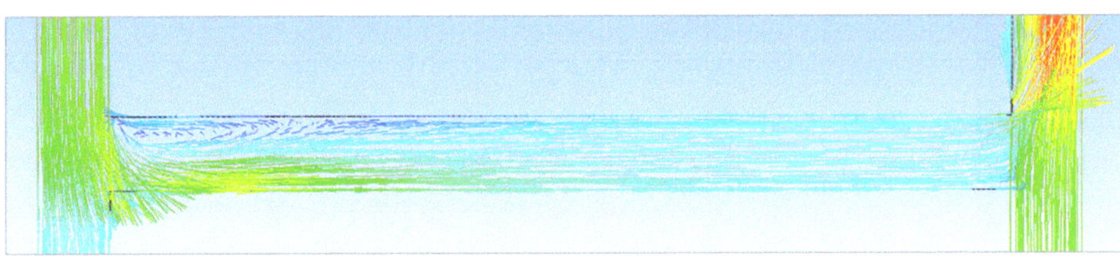

Figure 15.11 Blood swirling through fistula 50% flow shunted Test 3.

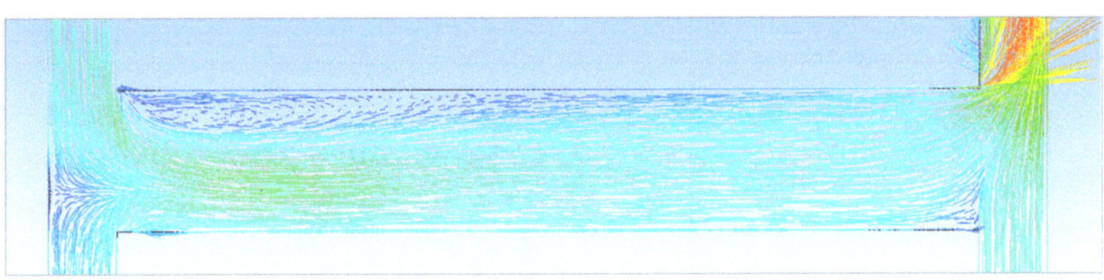

Figure 15.12 Blood Swirling through fistula ratio = 1:2 Test 4.

Figure 15.13 Blood swirling through fistula ratio = 2:1 Test 4.

diameter was utilised and venous outlet flow was controlled. Similar to Test Two, pressure conditions were maintained at calculated values. Each trial involved adjusting the venous outlet blood flow which comprised of 10% arterial blood through the fistula to greater than 100% of arterial blood flow, thereby simulating steal phenomenon.

Test 4: Examination of Ratio of Artery and Fistula

Following hypothesis generated by Casikar[41], a final test regarding the ratio between artery diameter and fistula diameter was conducted. These authors postulated that the ratio between the diameters of the feeding artery and the fistula artery could be a significant factor in the development of the AVM in the brain, and may also provide some explanation for the flow patterns observed in their animal models. To conduct this test, the ratio between feeding artery diameter and fistula were set and thus new models were generated to facilitate this examination. Table 15.3 identifies the geometries utilised.

Table 15.3 Summary of Blood properties applied to Water in Material Library.

Property	Value	Units
Density	1280	
Dynamic Viscosity	0.0027	

Testing Points

In order to provide reliability of results, several test points were maintained as constant throughout each AVM model. By applying probes and plane sections to the model, a comparison between each model could be made -approximately. Table 15.4 describes the x, y and z coordinates of these testing points, and Figure 15.11 indicates the XZ plane configuration and visual indication of measurement

Table 15.4 Feeding Artery Diameter to Fistula measurements.

Model	Ratio	Artery (m)	Fistula (m)
1	5:1	0.002	0.0004
2	4:1	0.002	0.0005
3	3:1	0.002	0.0006667
4	2:1	0.002	0.001
5	1:1	0.002	0.002
6	1:2	0.002	0.004
7	1:3	0.002	0.006
8	1:4	0.002	0.008
9	1:5	0.002	0.01

points. These points were selected based on the requirement to identify pressure at each inlet and outlet, and to further identify the flow characteristics closer to the fistula location. Planes, across XZ plane, were applied to the model in order to observe the flow patterns across the feeding artery opening to the fistula and exiting draining vein of the fistula.

Measurements and Calculations

Across each testing point, velocity and pressure were measured both at the probes and across the specific planes. These values were used to measure mass flow rate and wall shear stress at each of these points. These calculations were conducted using *Microsoft Excel (2013).* Line graphs were generated to provide a visual representation of the flow, pressure and stress patterns across the various models. Based on the values obtained, further models were generated to identify converging points of the changes occurring in the modelling AVM progression.

The physiological responses to stimuli have largely been ignored for this examination. These include the biological methods of cell renewal within the body, in addition to other body maintenance mechanisms. These responses are not easily modelled in a computational modelling system, and form the crux of the inaccuracies of this study. Standardised model, with a single independent variable was employed, to maintain testing validity.

Vessel thickness was assumed to be of 1mm based on prior models utilised to conduct computational studies, in particular by Brady[29] and Prattipati[255]. The assumption however is not reflective of true blood vessels in the brain, as vessels have geometry that changes and alters continually in response to the various stimuli (Cipolla[44]).As a result, this assumption reduces the accuracy with which these experiments were conducted. However, this was considered necessary in order to facilitate the examination. By setting the vessel thickness, the study maintained a level of improved validity, removing an additional changing factor in the analysis.

As identified in methodology, several values of cerebral blood flow were utilised in order to visualise blood flow. These tests were conducted to understand blood flow, and the factors affecting the flow rate through the system. Many researchers have previously identified the difficulty of measuring cerebral blood flow rates for such computational analysis [Brady[29], Cipolla[44] & Schaller[285]) . Blood flow in the body adjusts to stimuli and responses to vasculature (Shakur[297&298] & Schmid-Schonbein[290]). In this manner, the blood flow rate continually adjusts in order to maintain the same pressure levels across the vessels through the auto-regulation mechanism Spetzer[307&310]. The assumption is thus utilised to enable a visual representation of blood flow, not accurately depict flow in cerebral vessels.

The application of identifying the challenge in the quantification of venous flow, and understanding that this is highly dependent on the capillary action, the assumption is made that both arterial and venous flow could be compared with equivalence for purposes of simplification (Gao[87&88]).

The tests indicate convergence of the degrees of freedom and pressure at the predetermined probe occurs in the region of mesh size between 0.000140.00005. The denser mesh followed a particularly lengthy solution, however generated solutions with greater accuracy.

A finer mesh produced a faster solution, however with a greater level of inaccuracy.

With consideration of mesh quality and time taken, the mesh size selected was 0.00013 using the patch conforming method. This mesh was exported as an ANSYS Mesh file, ready for application within the CFX module. The final mesh utilised is shown in Figure 15.3 and 15.4.

Results

Test 1: Buckingham Pi analysis

The dimensionless groups are listed below.

$$\Pi_1 = \frac{D_{artery}}{D_{fistula}} \qquad \Pi_4 = [V_{in}]^{-2}[\rho]^{-1}\Delta P$$

$$\Pi_2 = \frac{D_{vein}}{D_{fistula}} \qquad \Pi_5 = \frac{V_{artery\ out}}{V_{in}}$$

$$\Pi_3 = \frac{l_{fistula}}{D_{fistula}} \qquad \Pi_6 = \frac{V_{vein\ out}}{V_{in}}$$

Test 2.1: Changing Diameter with Okell,[228] assumption Q_{inlet} = 0.00576 kg/s

The high flow of the Okell, provided results without modelling steal. The plots obtained however, indicate important flow characteristics pertaining to the various factors involved. It identified that as the fistula diameter increased, the blood flow through the venous outlet proportionally increased.

This was due to a decrease in blood leaving the modelled system via the arterial outlet, and is shown in Table 15.4.

Figure 15.14 consists of pressure plots across the measured locations of the AVM model. The plot indicates a consistent increase in the pressure measured at both the arterial

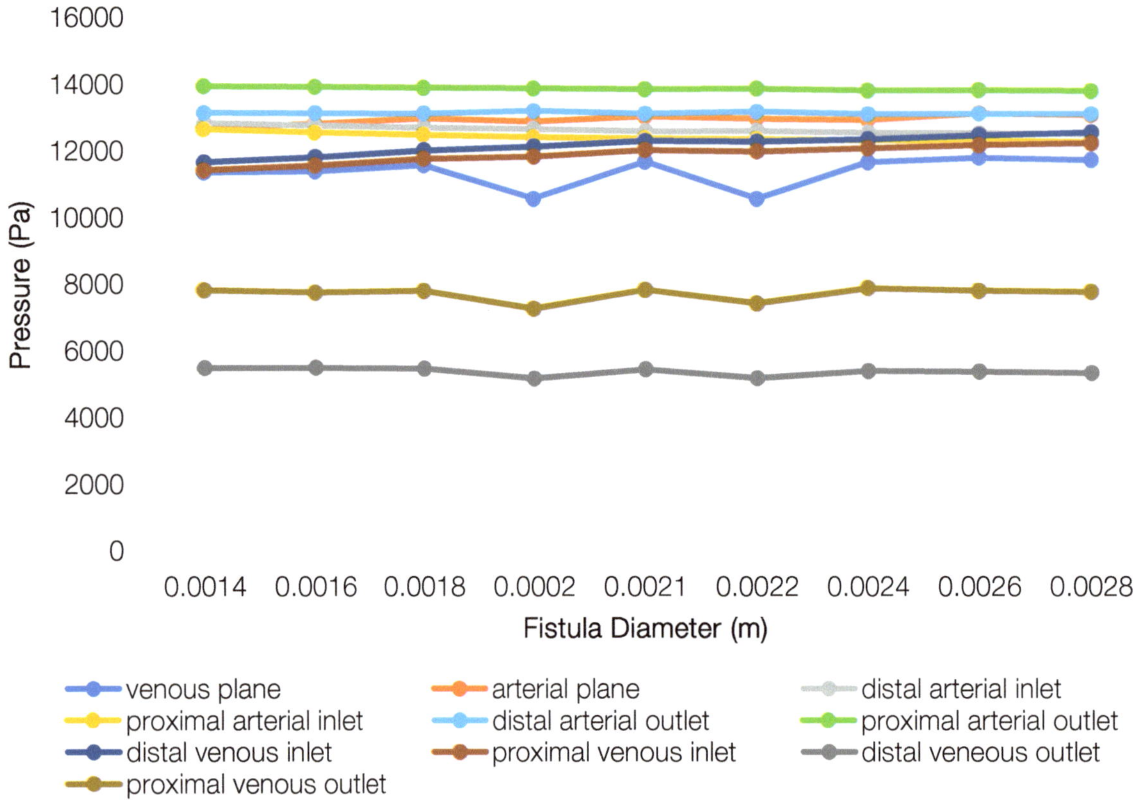

Figure 15.14 Test 2.1 Pressure Plot.

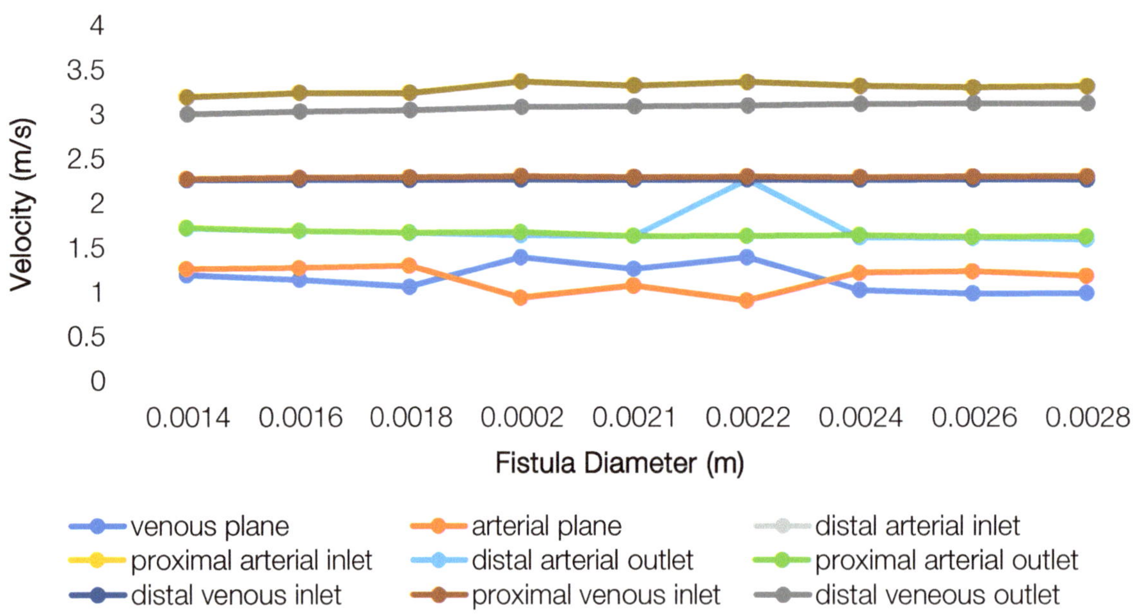

Figure 15.15 Test 2.1 Velocity Plot.

and venous inlet segments. Additionally, on average, the pressure at the venous and arterial planes increase with increased diameter also.

The velocity plots obtained, as shown in Figure 15.5, highlight very little change, on average, of velocity across all locations measured. There is some noise in the data obtained, also shown in the Graph below.

Wall shear stresses are shown in Figure 15.16.

Test 2.2: Changing Diameter with Stock,[316] assumption Q_{inlet} = 0.0048 kg/s

The Stock, Wetzel assumption provided results highlighting the importance of inlet mass flow rate on the flow through the AVM. In this set, cerebrovascular steal was not modelled. However the trial showed information pertaining to all other analysis factors. It was found that as diameter increases, the flow through the arterial outlet decreases.

The pressure curves obtained in Figure 15.17 are indicative of increasing pressure across the fistula, and at the venous inlet. The pressure across the other locations shows no indication of major change. As steal is not modelled in this trial, the effects of steal cannot be determined.

The velocity curves in Figure 15.18 show an overall decrease in velocity across the fistula, and arterial outlet. The velocity at the draining vein outlet steadily increases as diameter increased. Without cerebrovascular steal modelling, the way in which the velocity would change as a result at utilising inlet flows equal to 0.0048 kg/s, cannot be established.

Wall shear stress, the values of highlights the overall decreasing wall shear stress across all locations as fistula diameter increased. This is emphasised in Figure 15.19 from which indicates more significant increase in wall shear stress within the venous outlet locations.

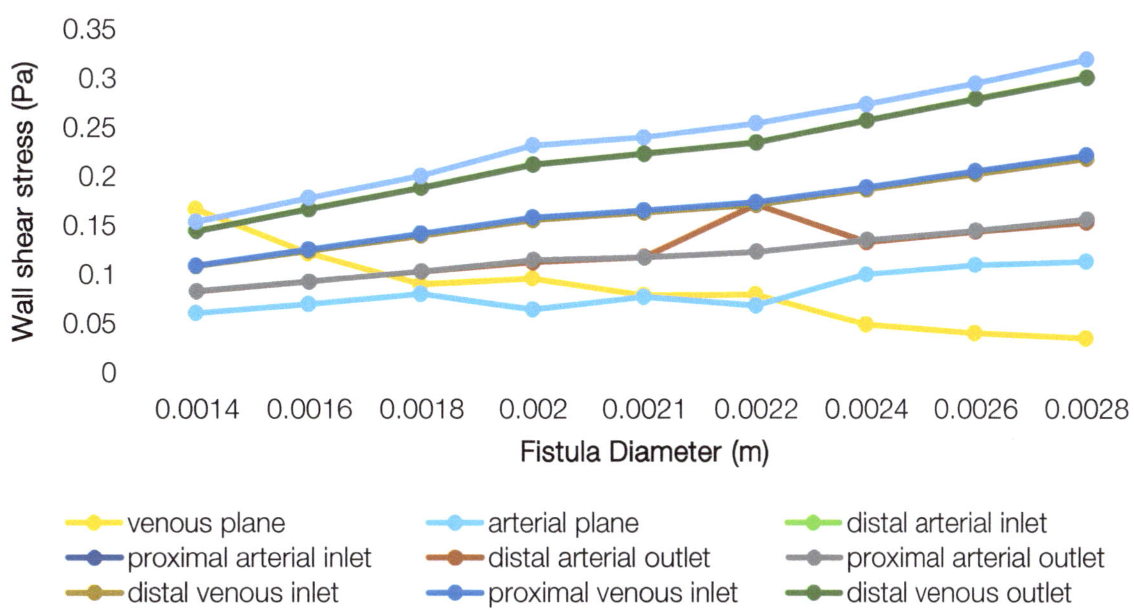

Figure 15.16 Test 2.1 Wall shear stress.

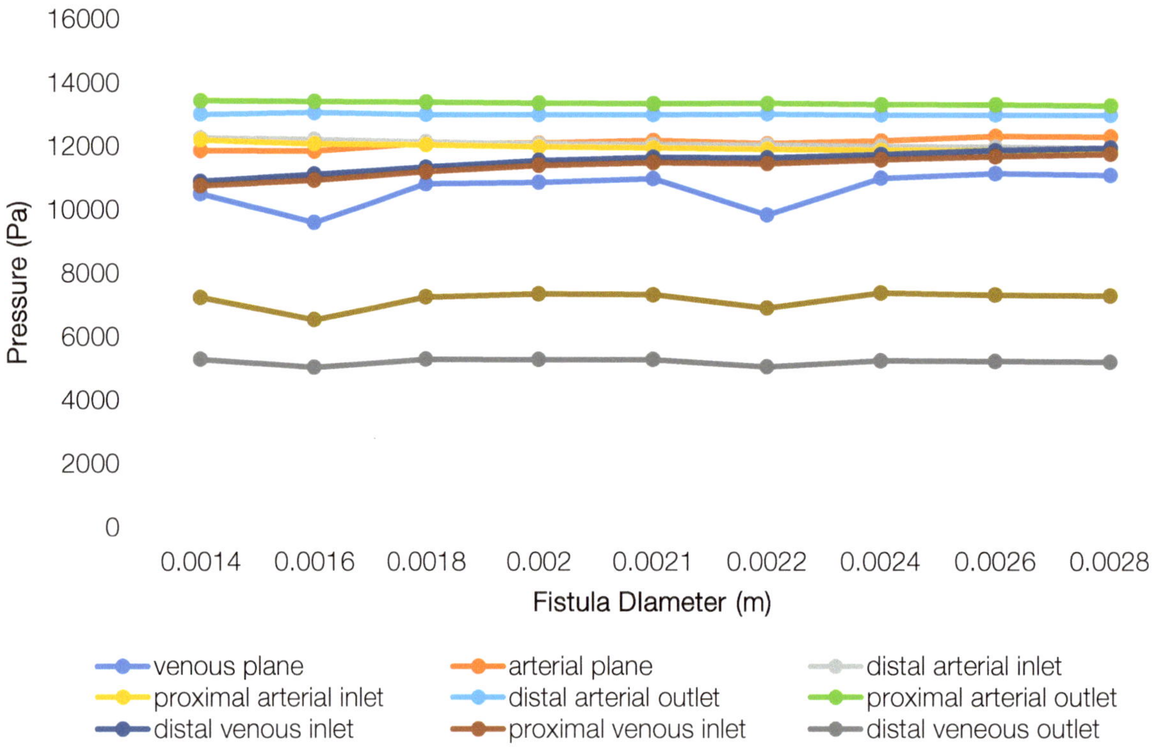

Figure 15.17 Test 2.2 Pressure Plot.

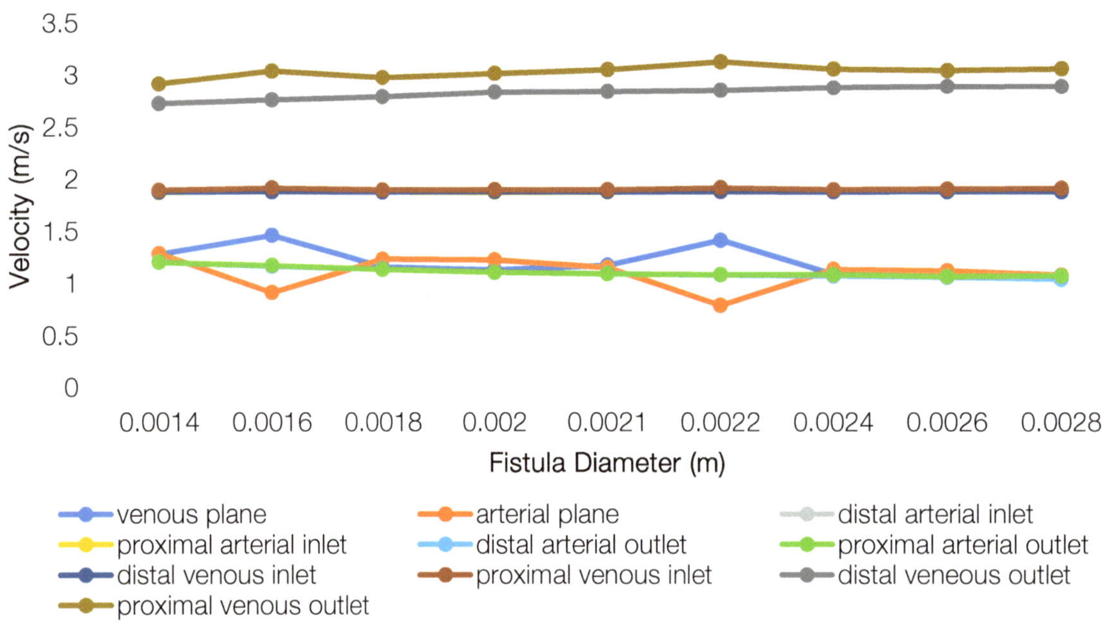

Figure 15.18 Test 2.2 Velocity Plot.

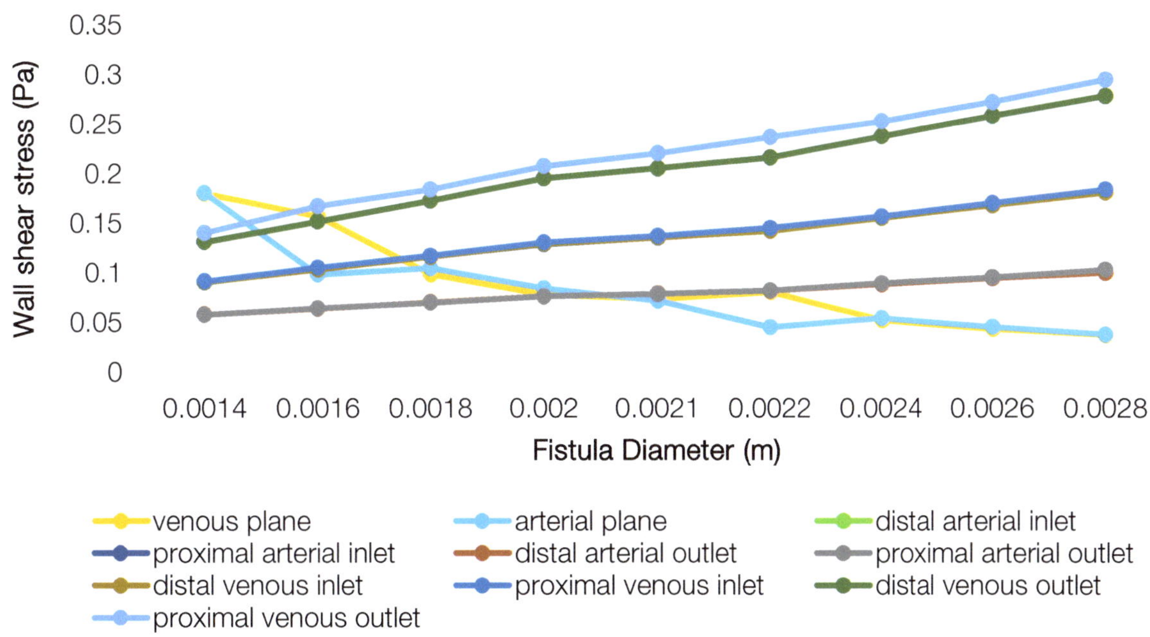

Figure 15.19 Test 2.2 Wall Shear Stress.

Test 2.3: Changing Diameter with Q_{inlet} = 0.003 kg/s

Utilising mass flow rate equivalent to 0.003 kg/s yielded different flow regime to that found in the previous tests conducted. Cerebrovascular steal was modelled between 0.002m and 0.0021m. Outlet flow rates are shown in Figure 15.20, the equations of which are illustrated in Table 15.5. Figure 15.21 indicates the pressure change occurring across each diameter model at the various testing points.

Table 15.5: Both proximal arterial outlet and the distal arterial outlet yielded similar pressure results, thus resulting in the overlapping lines in Figure 15.21. Additionally, there is a change in

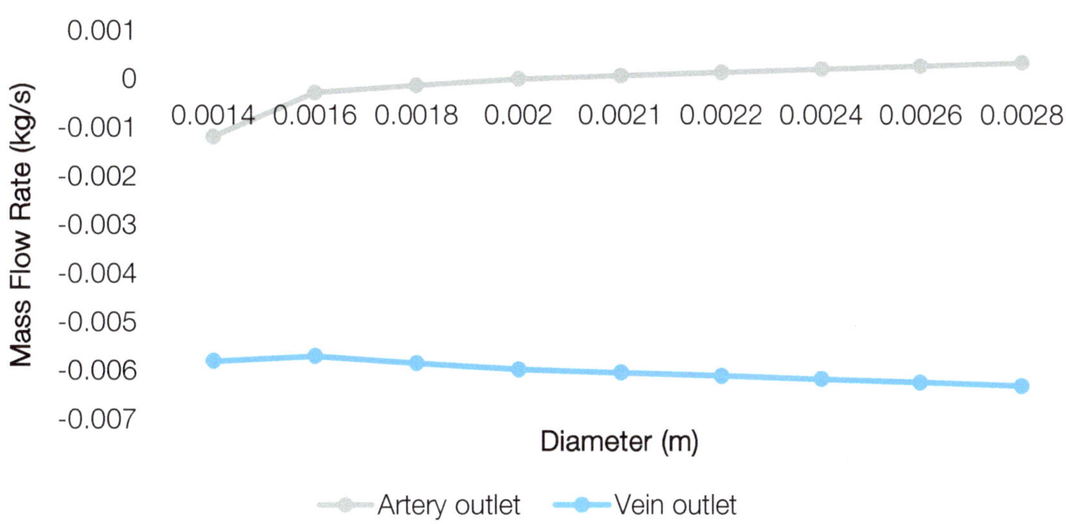

Figure 15.20 Outlet flow rates.

Table 15.5 Locations of measurement points.

Locations	Axis		
	X	Y	Z
Distal arterial inlet	0.0005	0.001	0.031
Distal arterial outlet	0.0005	0.001	0.0045
Distal venous inlet	0.0005	0.0283	0.012
Distal venous outlet	0.0005	0.0283	0.038
Proximal arterial inlet	0.0005	0.001	0.0235
Proximal arterial outlet	0.0005	0.001	0.02
Proximal venous inlet	0.0005	0.0383	0.02
Proximal venous outlet	0.0005	0.0283	0.0235
Arterial Plane		0.0021	
Venous Plane		0.027	

curvature of the pressure plot obtained for the arterial plane and venous plane as the fistula dilates. Since the venous outlet pressure condition is set within the CFX module, the venous inlet presents better information regarding the flow through the system. Figure 15.21 indicates an overall increase in venous inlet pressure.

Figure 15.22 shows the velocity of blood flow measure across the testing points for each model. The velocity of the arterial outlet changes direction between diameters 0.02m and 0.021m. The plot indicates that at diameters less than 0.02m the velocity is continually decreasing, while after the onset of steal, velocity steadily increases. This is illustrated in tables 15.6 and 15.7.

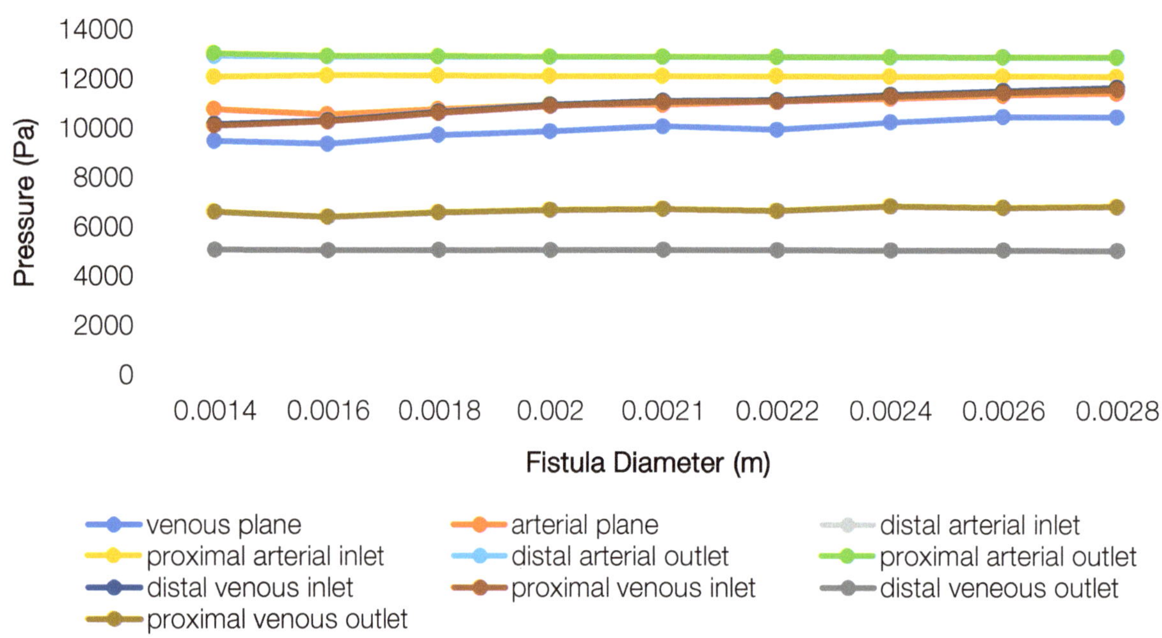

Figure 15.21 Test 2.3 Pressure Plot.

Table 15.6 Mass Flow Rate (kg/s) at model Outlets.

Location	Diameter (m)								
	0.0014	0.0016	0.0018	0.002	0.0021	0.0022	0.0024	0.0026	0.0028
Artery outlet	-0.00423	-0.00416	-0.00411	-0.00405	-0.00402	-0.004	-0.00398	-0.00396	-0.00393
Vein outlet	-0.00729	-0.00736	-0.00741	-0.00747	-0.0075	-0.00752	-0.00754	-0.00756	-0.00759

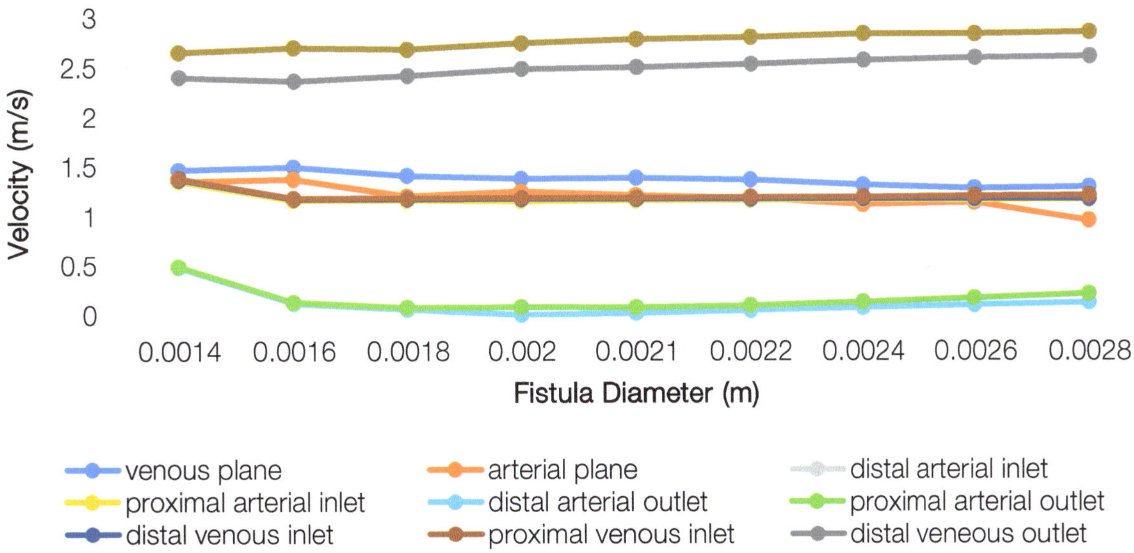

Figure 15.22 Test 2.3 Velocity Plot.

Table 15.7 Equations of Velocity (m/s) across all locations of AVM Test 2.1.

Location	Equation ($y =$)	$\frac{dy}{dx}$
Arterial Plane	-0.0105x + 1.1986	-0.0105
Venous Plane	-0.0225x + 1.2657	-0.0225
Distal Arterial Inlet	-6E-05x + 2.2617	-0.00006
Proximal Arterial Inlet	0.0011x + 2.2677	0.0011
Distal Arterial Outlet	-0.0036x + 1.7279	-0.0036
Proximal Arterial Outlet	-0.0113x + 1.7087	-0.0113
Distal Venous Inlet	0.0005x + 2.2574	0.0005
Proximal Venous Inlet	0.0027x + 2.274	0.0027
Distal Venous Outlet	0.0154x + 2.9995	0.0154
Proximal Venous Outlet	0.0137x + 3.2229	0.0137

Observing wall shear stress across the system, the following results are yielded. With increasing diameter, it is clear that wall shear stress within the vessels is continually decreasing. Additionally, highest wall shear stresses are consistently measured in the draining vein, as shown in Figure 15.23.

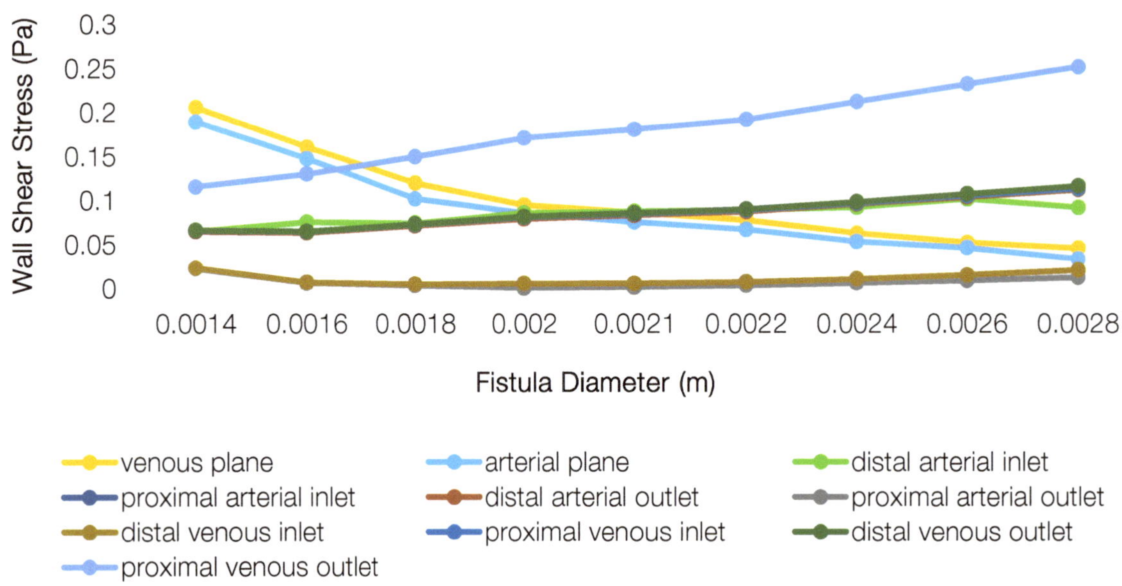

Figure 15.23 Test 2.3 Wall Shear Stress.

Test 2.4: Changing Diameter with Q_{inlet} = 0.0025 kg/s

This test successfully modelled cerebrovascular steal, as shown in Table 15.8, for the entire trial set. The inlet locations, along with the venous and arterial plane show continual increase in pressure as the fistula diameter increases in the models.

Figure 15.24 illustrates the pressure changes across the AVM modelling, utilising the assumption of mass flow rate at the inlets equal to 0.0025 kg/s.

Figure 15.25 shows the velocity curves obtained for all locations within the AVM model, and the equations governing these curves are included in Table 15.9.

Table 15.8 Test 2.2 Velocity (m/s) plot equations, and derivatives.

Location	Equation $(y =)$	$\frac{dy}{dx} =$	$\frac{d^2y}{dx^2} =$
Arterial Plane	-0.0138x + 1.173	-0.0138	
Venous Plane	-0.0319x + 1.3636	-0.0319	
Distal Arterial Inlet	0.00006x + 1.8832	0.00006	
Proximal Arterial Inlet	0.0009x + 1.8801	0.0009	
Distal Arterial Outlet	$0.0018x^2$ - 0.0368x + 1.2338	0.0036x – 0.0368	0.0036
Proximal Arterial Outlet	$0.0029x^2$ - 0.0448x + 1.2451	0.0058x – 0.04448	0.0058
Distal Venous Inlet	0.0003x + 1.8814	0.0003	
Proximal Venous Inlet	0.0011x + 1.9014	0.0011	
Distal Venous Outlet	$-0.0021x^2$ + 0.042x + 2.6891	-0.0042x + 0.042	-0.0042
Proximal Venous Outlet	$-0.0042x^2$ + 0.057x + 2.883	-0.0084x + 0.057	-0.0084

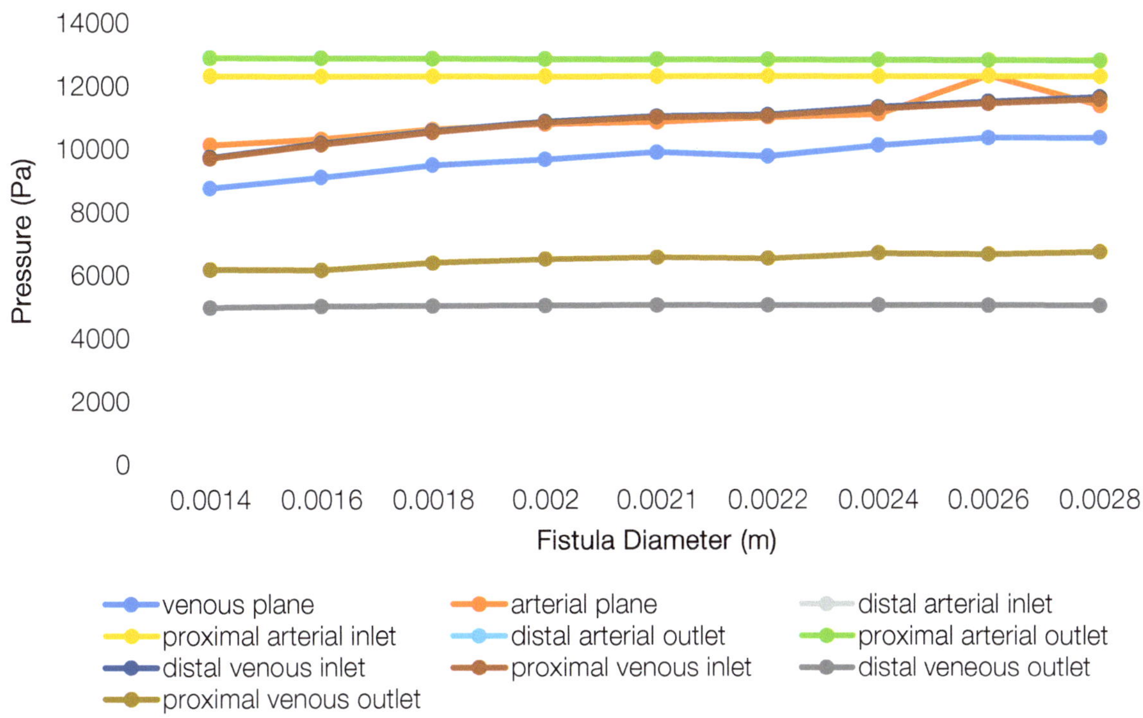

Figure 15.24 Pressure change with increasing Diameter.

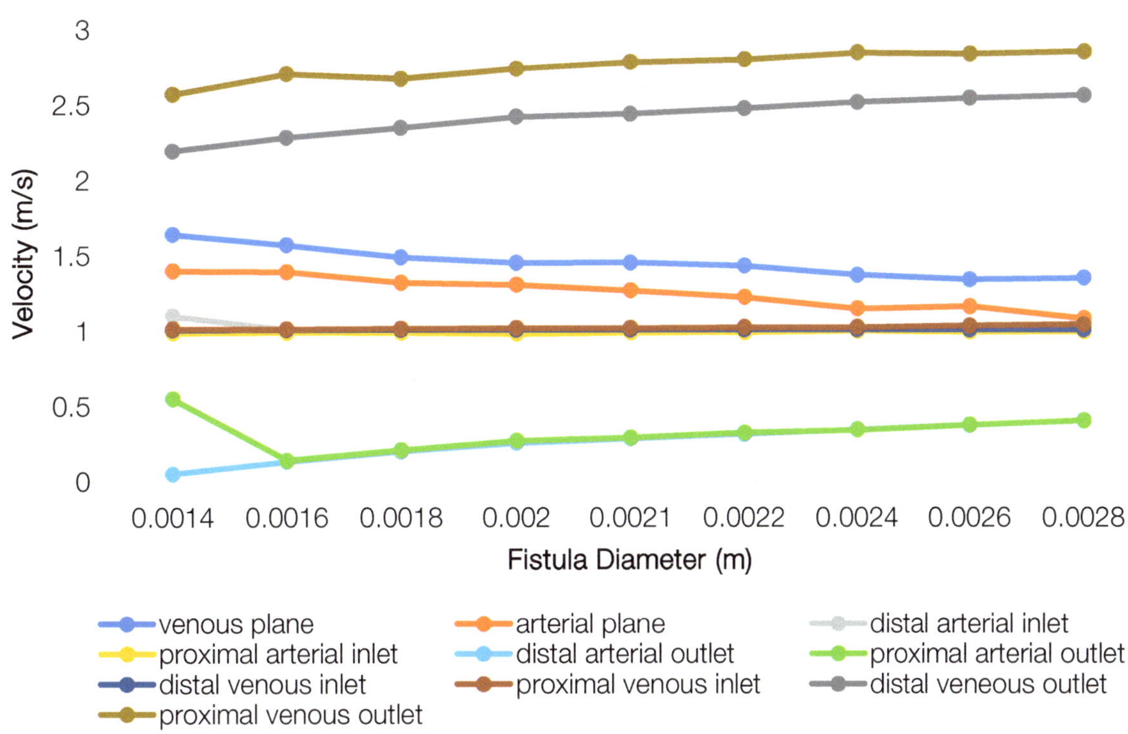

Figure 15.25 Test 2.4 Velocity Plot.

Table 15.9 First and Second Derivatives calculated of Outlet flow.

Section	Location	Equation ($y =$)	$\frac{dy}{dx}$	$\frac{d^2y}{dx^2}$
Fistula Diameter = 0.0014m to 0.002m	Artery Outlet	$-0.0002x^2 + 0.0013x - 0.0023$	$-0.0004x + 0.0013$	-0.0004
	Vein Outlet	$-6E\text{-}05x^2 + 0.0002x - 0.006$	$-0.00012x + 0.0002$	-0.00012
Fistula Diameter = 0.002m to 0.0028m	Artery Outlet	$3E\text{-}07x^2 + 6E\text{-}05x - 8E\text{-}05$	$0.0000006x + 0.0006$	0.0000006
	Vein Outlet	$-3E\text{-}07x^2 - 6E\text{-}05x - 0.0059$	$-0.0000006 - 0.00006$	-0.0000006

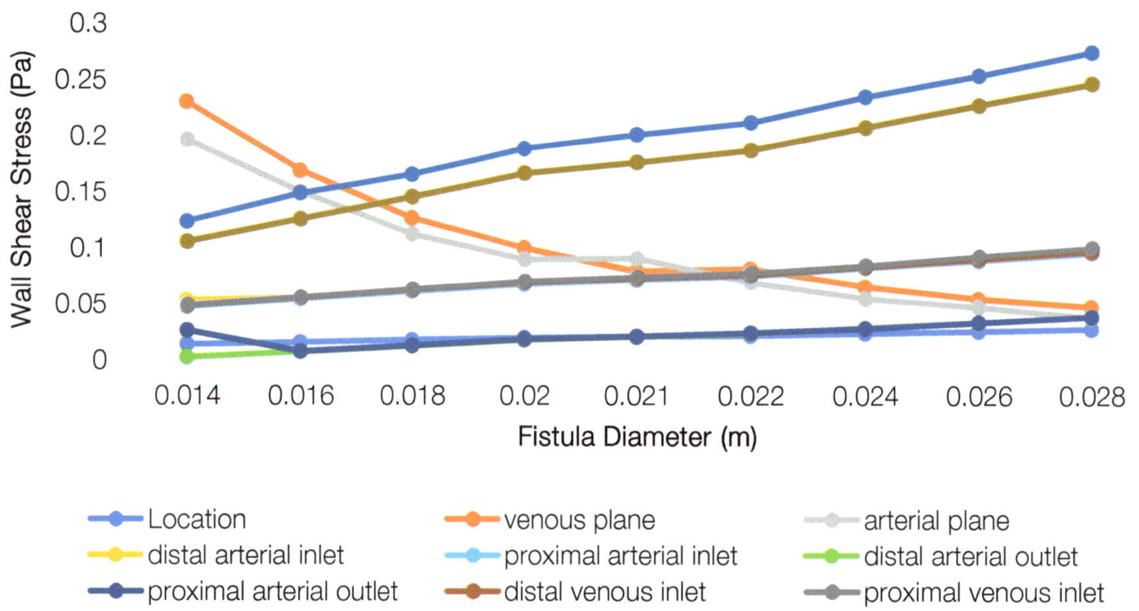

Figure 15.26 Test 2.4 WSS.

Wall shear stress was also measured at all model locations yielding the following Figure 15.26.

Test 3: Controlled flow

The further testing conducted to observe blood flow in the AVM yielded interesting results. Figure 15.27 indicates the change in maximum pressure which occurs across the points of examination.

The pressure across all points, excluding the venous outlet segment, appears relatively unchanged. The arterial segment of the AVM shows minimal change in arterial blood pressure, contradicting much of the research found regarding the effects of pressure (Young[355], Sorimachi[306] & Duong[72]).

Figure 15.28 depicts the velocity curves obtained from this trial. Table 15.10 and 15.11 illustrate the equations yielded prior to and after steal onset.

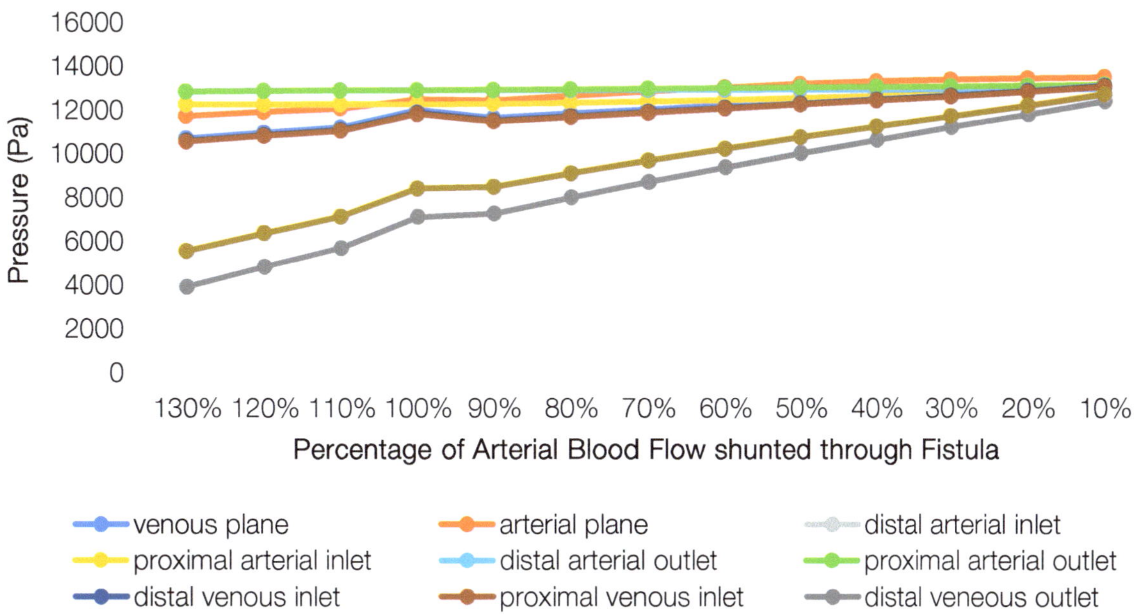

Figure 15.27 Test 3 Pressure Plot.

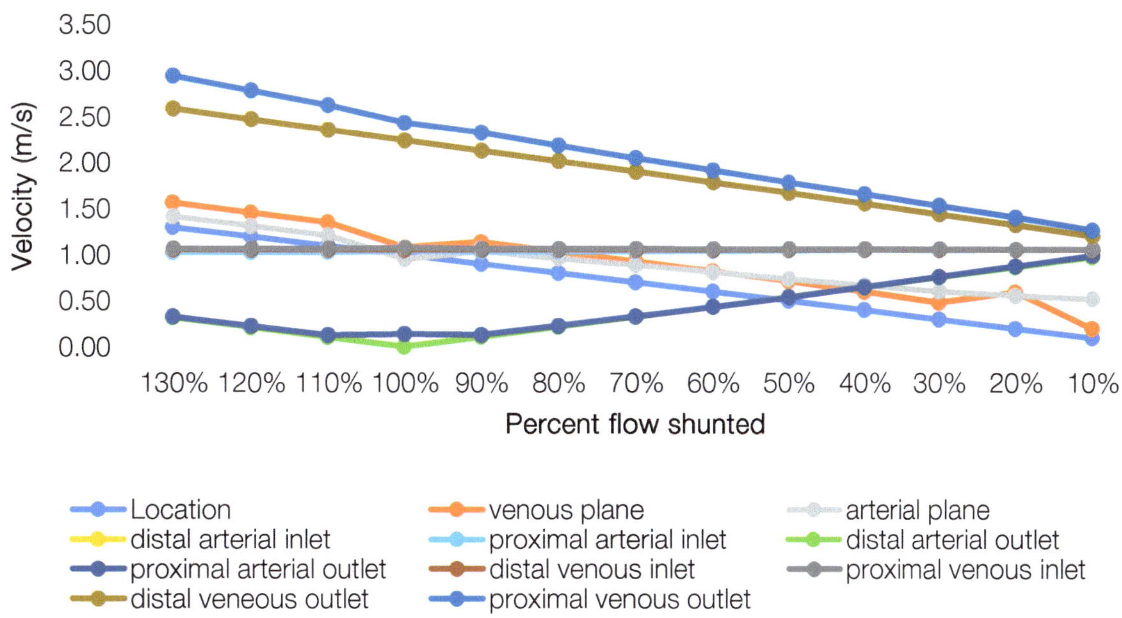

Figure 15.28 Test 3 Velocity profile.

Table 15.10 Velocity equations measured for Test 2.3 between D = 0.0014m and D = 0.002m.

Location	Equation ($y =$)	$\frac{dy}{dx}$	$\frac{d^2y}{dx^2}$
Arterial Plane	-0.0476x + 1.4116	-0.0476	
Venous Plane	-0.035x + 1.5242	-0.035	
Distal Arterial Inlet	-0.0591x + 1.3734	-0.0591	
Proximal Arterial Inlet	-0.0598x + 1.3523	-0.0598	
Distal Arterial Outlet	$0.0779x^2$ - 0.5381x + 0.9254	0.01558x – 0.5381	0.01558
Proximal Arterial Outlet	$0.0916x^2$ - 0.5855x + 0.9704	0.1832x – 0.5855	0.1832
Distal Venous Inlet	$0.049x^2$ - 0.3035x + 1.6157	0.098x – 0.3035	0.098
Proximal Venous Inlet	$0.0504x^2$ - 0.3097x + 1.6282	0.1008x – 0.3097	0.1008
Distal Venous Outlet	$0.0263x^2$ - 0.1007x + 2.4733	0.0526x – 0.1007	0.0526
Proximal Venous Outlet	$0.0043x^2$ + 0.0045x + 2.6509	0.0086x + 0.0045	0.0086

Table 15.11 Velocity equations measured for Test 2.3 between D = 0.002m and D = 0.0028m.

Location	Equation ($y =$)	$\frac{dy}{dx}$	$\frac{d^2y}{dx^2} =$
Arterial Plane	-0.0504x + 1.3167	-0.0504	
Venous Plane	-0.0227x + 1.4149	-0.0227	
Distal Arterial Inlet	-0.00002x + 1.1766	-0.00002	
Proximal Arterial Inlet	0.0027x + 1.1495	0.0027	
Distal Arterial Outlet	$0.0009x^2$ + 0.0188x - 0.0164	0.0018x + 0.0188	0.0018
Proximal Arterial Outlet	$0.0057x^2$ - 0.0125x + 0.0845	0.0114x – 0.0125	0.0114
Distal Venous Inlet	$0.000006x^2$ + 9E-05x + 1.1756	0.000012 + 9E-05x	0.000012
Proximal Venous Inlet	$0.001x^2$ - 0.003x + 1.189	0.002x – 0.003	0.002
Distal Venous Outlet	$-0.0006x^2$ + 0.031x + 2.4523	-0.0012x + 0.0313	-0.0012
Proximal Venous Outlet	$-0.0032x^2$ + 0.0441x + 2.7058	-0.0064x + 0.0441	-0.0064

Figure 15.29 indicates the wall shear stress measured across the AVM.

Test 4: Examination of Ratio of Artery and Fistula

Test 4 offered complementary results to Test 1 and 2, by maintaining a constant arterial diameter. Figure 15.30 indicates blood flow at the arterial outlet and venous outlet. This provides a clear representation of the way in which increased fistula diameter results in the occurrence of cerebrovascular steal in the arterial outlet region. Similarly, a larger amount of fluid leaves the AVM system via the arterial outlet with increased steal occurring.

Figure 15.31 shows the change in pressure across various data points of the AVM as the

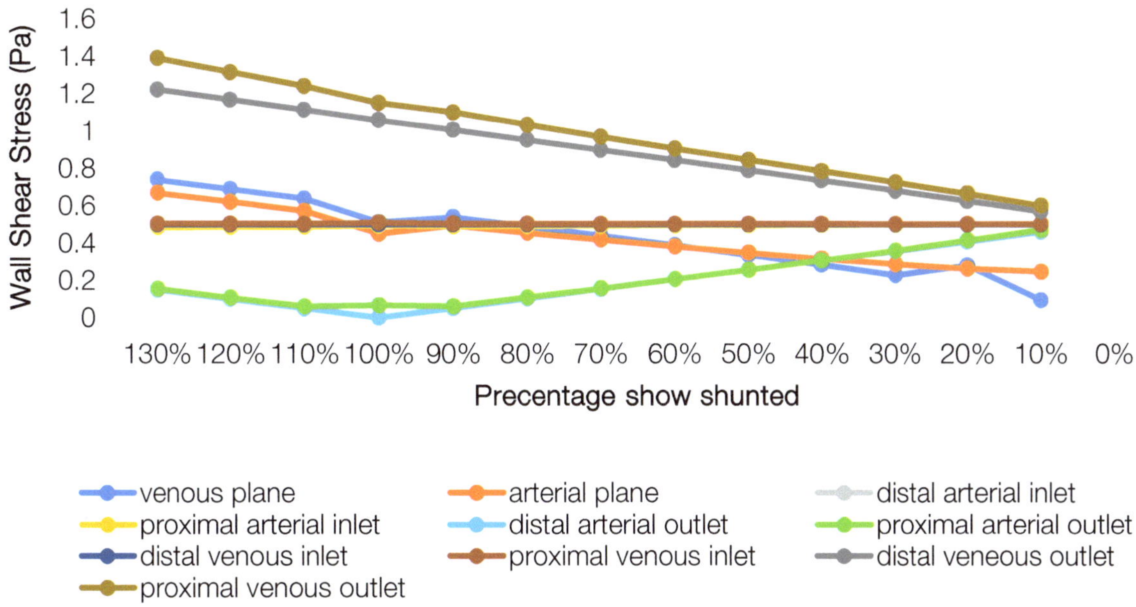

Figure 15.29 Test 3 Wall Shear Stress.

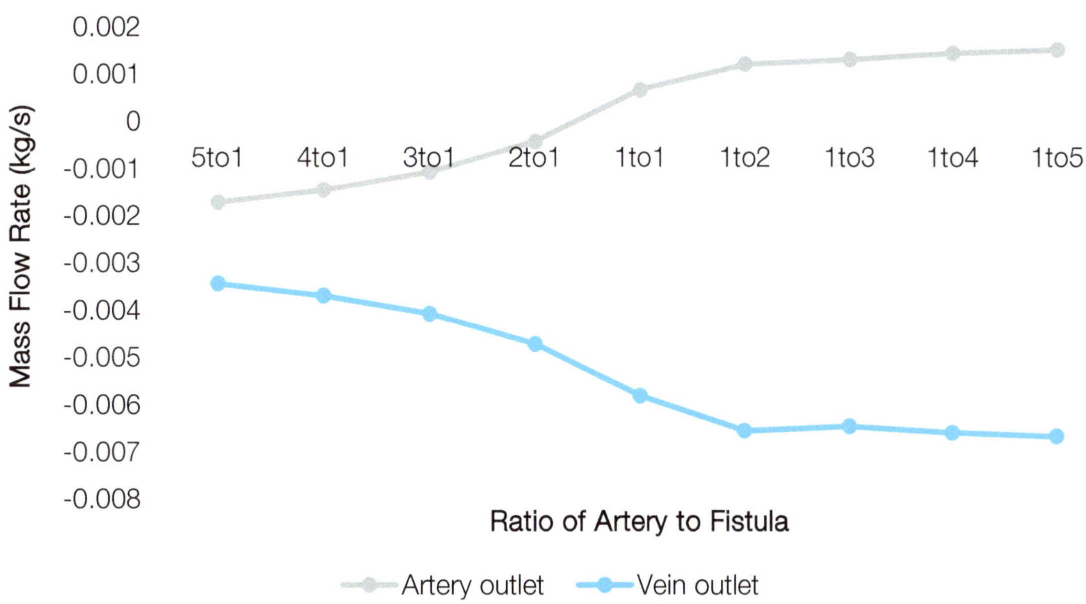

Figure 15.30 Flow at Outlets.

fistula size increases according to the artery to fistula ratio. With consideration that pressure conditions were applied at the artery outlet and venous outlet to direct blood flow, the other data points offer insights into the way in which flow changes. Similar to the results obtained above, there is a significant change in the curvature of the lines generated for values of the fistula, across the arterial and venous planes and the draining vein.

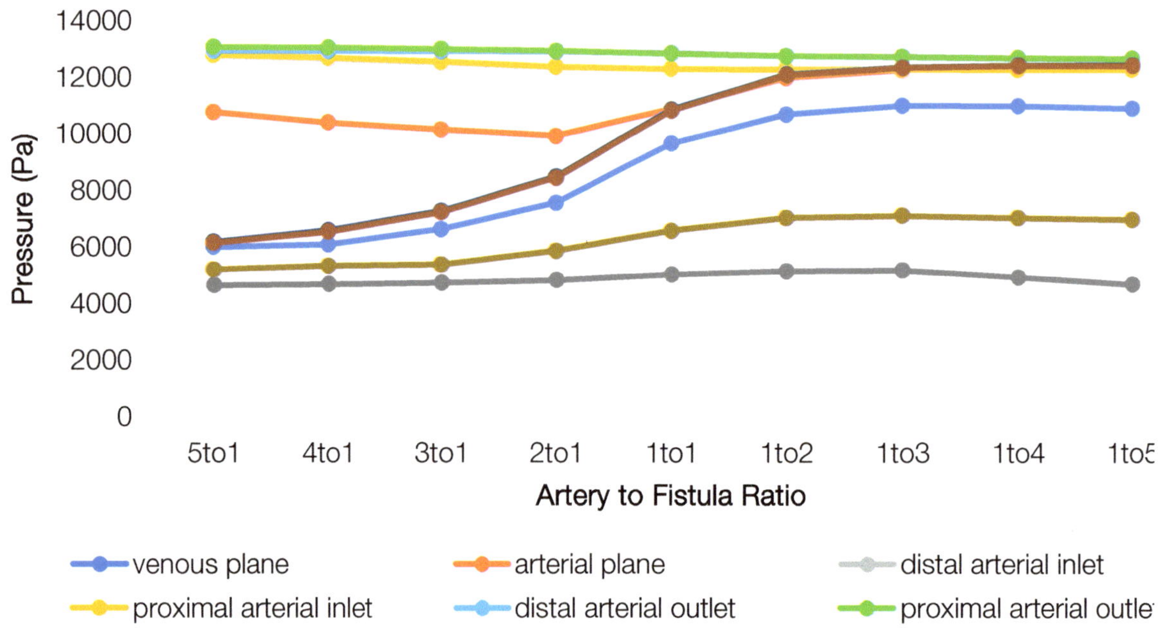

Figure 15.31 Test 4 Pressure Plot.

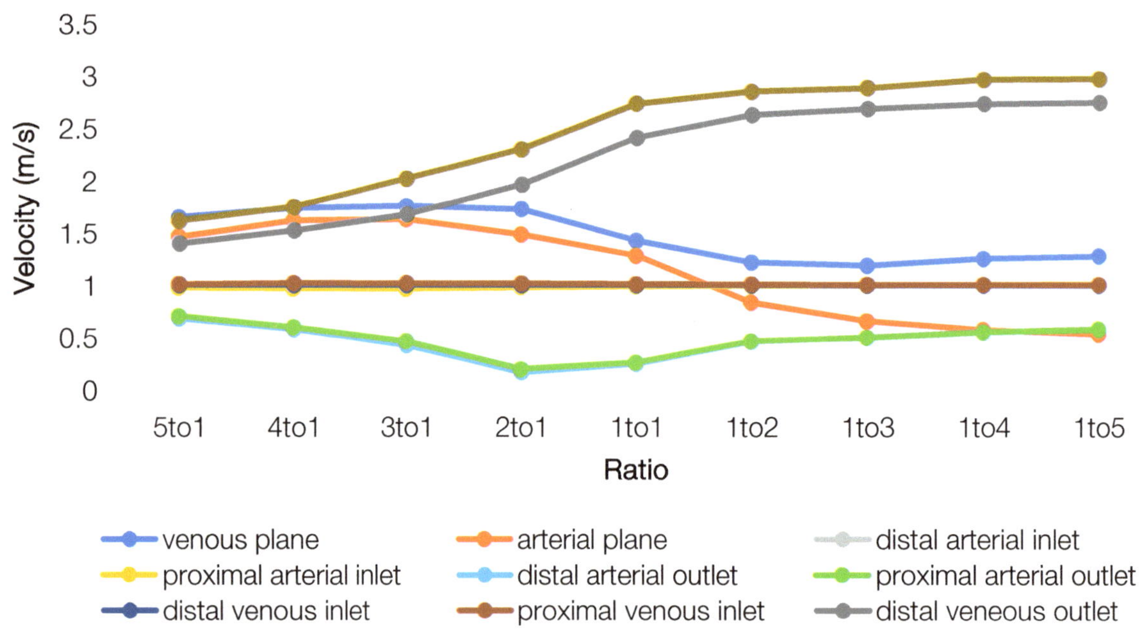

Figure 15.32 Test 4 Velocity Plot.

Test 4 Pressure Plot

Figure 15.32 depicts the velocity values obtained across all points. The graph explains that there is some significant change in the flow regime between ratios 1:1 and 2:1. Figure 15.30 shows that cerebrovascular steal occurs. Tables 5.12 and 5.13 highlight the equations found prior to and after steal onset.

Figure 15.33 shows the wall shear stresses across the locations.

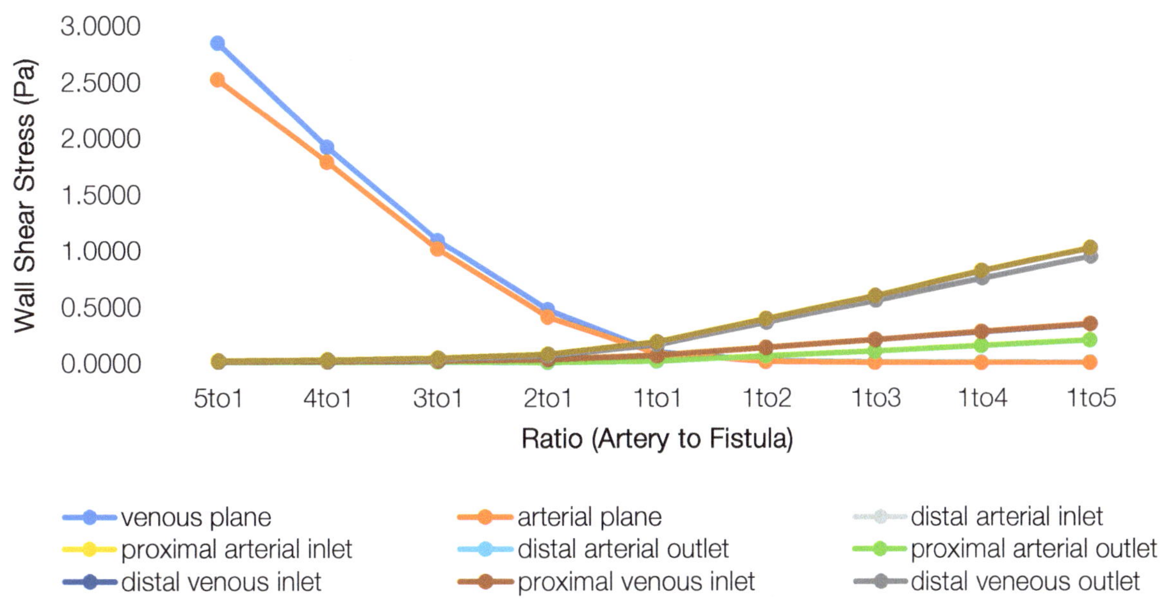

Figure 15.33 Test 4 Wall Shear Stress.

Analysis of the experimental findings

Various patterns have been found in this analysis, and provide a greater overall understanding of the effects of individual factors upon the progression of AVMs. As multiple tests were conducted, each test and the respective results are deconstructed in this discussion.

Blood swirling as described by Ha ,et.al[106] alters much of the flow regime within the AVM model, causing the velocity to decrease through the length of the fistula and causing pressure changes within the system (Drake[70])

Note that in all models, the swirling of fluid occurs in the same plane of the fistula length, thus not generating a vortex occurring in the cross-sectional plane of the model. As explained by Parida and Chand[239], vortexes occurring in the cross-sectional plane cause a rapid decrease in pressure in the area, thereby resulting in an increase in mass flow at that point.

Additionally, the expected drop in pressure in the system based on gravitational forces and directionality alone did not completely match the actual effect that was found. Examining the specific boundary conditions applied to the system, the expected pressure drop is more evident. The equations below utilise the specific values obtained by Casikar[41] at the inlet conditions. For purposes of examination in the *CFX module* in *ANSYS Workbench,* the outlet conditions were critical for measurement, and basic pipe flow principles were employed (Brady[29] & Pritchard[257])

As a result, the expected pressure changes within the feeding artery and draining vein are equivalent to the additional variables in the equations below ($\rho g \Delta h$), which equals a reduction by 3.3 mm Hg, and an increase by 3.3 mm Hg respectively.

$$P = P_{inlet} - \rho g \Delta h$$

$$P_{artery\ outlet} = 100 \text{ mm Hg} - 1280(9.81)(0.035)$$

$$P_{artery\ outlet} = 96.7 \text{ mm Hg}$$

$$P_{vein\ outlet} = 30 \text{ mm Hg} + 1280(9.81)(0.35)$$

$$P_{vein\ outlet} = 33.296 \text{ mm Hg}$$

Several errors have been identified within this examination, which may result from various factors. One critical factor could be that the analysis is conducted utilising computational methods. Such an analysis may lead to errors which are associated with the mesh generation, positioning of measurement points relative to geometry and the mesh, and the convergence of all data (Pritchard[257] & Oberkampf[222])

Essentially, if a measurement point lies close to an element boundary, or lies directly over a node, the result is skewed relating to the shape of the measurement point. Additionally, a point along a boundary line between elements pertains documented errors in calculation (Oberkampf[222]). Additional errors relate to the convergence data through the *CFX module*. To maintain validity of the study, a low convergence point of 0.0000001 was selected in the solving module, with 200 iterations to perform the analysis (Duong.et.al[72]). In some cases, 200 iterations were completed prior to all points converging and thus may have resulted in some overall errors in the final results obtained from specific trials of specific diameters. To maintain validity of the testing procedure, the convergence point and number of iterations were maintained as constant for all trials(Oberkampf[222]).

As auto-regulation of the blood pressure and blood vessel diameter is unaccounted for in this examination. It cannot be determined whether its occurrence is specific to the circulatory system is continually adjusting to the flow change which occurs during AVM progression (Young[355] &Duong[72]) The absence of auto-regulation of blood diminishes the overall validity of the model. However, it was essential in the simplification of the CFD analysis.

The analysis conducted justified the disproportionate change in pressure across the venous outlet and inlet (likely related to mass flow rate), and ignores the factor of auto-regulation of the vessels which exists in order to maintain suitable blood pressure in all regions of the body . Although mass flow through the region significantly increases, the lowering of blood pressure in the venous outlet is indicative that the vessels may constrict in order to return the blood pressure of this region to the acceptable range for the body (Young[355]). The constriction as a result of decreased blood flow, however coupled with a larger increase in blood flow through the venous outlet region provides a graphical and mathematical identification of the critical region for analysis for AVM progression and treatment. Future research should incorporate the findings in this examination that fistula blood flow, and venous outlet draining from an AVM, is independent of arterial outlet pressure. Additionally, future research could examine the specific forces and stresses experienced between the proximal and distal regions of the venous outlet, using pressure in the region, mass flow and autoregulation as analysis factors.

There are errors with the analysis because pulse rate was not included. The validity of this work is therefore lessened, although the exclusion was deemed necessary to prepare a cohesive, concise and simple experiment process. The assumption of negligible effects of pulse rate, though invalid, allow for the examination of the geometrical factors specifically in relation to mass flow and pressure. The incorporation of pulse rate, however, would also require modelling of vessel movement, and variance, in accordance to the wave forms generated by pulsatile flow.

Overall the tests conducted pertained a high level of reliability, owing to the repeated testing procedures within this examination. Each CFD analysis was tested thrice over, to identify errors and ensure reliable testing procedure and results obtained. Each test yielded the same, or highly similar, data sets, identifying conclusively the overall reliability of the data obtained. These results can be reproduced.

The examination of wall shear stress in blood vessels, explored by Papaioannou[238], offer some insight into the role of this factor in vascular endothelial functions. In particular, the paper explores additional mechanisms of vessel wall remodelling resulting from changes in wall shear stress experienced by the vessels. The article finds that increasing wall shear stress in the region results in an increase in wall thickness and vessel diameter in order to normalise the values.

Across all models, it was found that wall shear stress increased steadily, particularly in the venous region, as shunted flow increased. The velocity plots obtained, across all tests, indicate the rapid increases in velocity in the draining vein particularly in the outlet region, and as a result causing the overall increase in the wall shear stresses obtained. Test 2.3 and 2.4 specifically indicated increasing wall shear stresses in the arterial outlet segment upon the onset of steal modelling in the system. This is essentially related to the increase in velocity found in the region due to the reversed blood flow.

With increasing fistula diameter throughout Test 2, it can be expected through analysis of the Hagen-Poiseulle equation that wall shear stresses should decrease significantly through the fistula unless velocity increases proportionally (Alaraj[4] et al). Figure 15.15, 15.18, 15.22, 15.25, 15.28 and 15.32 however emphasise that velocity through the fistula decreases with fistula dilation, related to the occurrence of blood swirling occurring in the region. Test Two indicated that wall shear stresses decreased in the fistula, which may lead to blood stagnation and increase blood cell attachment in this region (Alaraj[4], Copley[50] & Bessonov[2]1). Increasing blood pressure in the fistula region, also, may be indicative of the high volatility of the environment in a progressing AVM, causing rapid changes in blood flow regime.

Test 3 explored controlled flow amounts through the fistula, which yielded that all testing points experience an increase in wall shear stress overall. The arterial outlet, also, showed decreasing wall shear stress until cerebrovascular steal modelling, after which a steady decrease followed. This relates to the influx of blood flow as a result of steal. Through the fistula, the velocity of the blood is shown to increase overall, with minimal blood swirling regions, resulting in increasing wall shear stresses across the vessel. The increase in wall shear stress, however, should result in fistula dilation owing to vascular remodelling that follows (Alaraj[4] & Rossitti[277]). Essentially, as identified in Tests 2 and 4, this should follow with a decrease in wall shear stress through the region Jo-Yu,W[145]. This may lead to the hindrance of further dilation of the fistula, therefore not allowing the normalisation of flow that was observed in Test 4.

With respect to the results calculated from Test 1, Reynold's number was not considered critical compared to pressure, velocity and wall shear stresses in the vessel. Though considered suitable for this study, Reynold's number and the flow regime are still pertinent for future work. There is onset of turbulent flow and high Reynold's number in the AVM system, probably at the junctions of the two-dimensional models (Lasheras[161], Knisely[149] & Pritchard[257]). The laminar flow assumption, hence, may not be completely valid for this examination. Laminar flow however was deemed suitable for purposes of performing a coherent CFD analysis (Knisely[149]).

Test 1: Buckingham Pi

Prior to addressing the results obtained from testing, the Buckingham Pi theorem presents interesting components related to all subsequent results. The dimensionless groups obtained comprise primarily of ratios between the dimensions of the AVM and the velocities of the inlet and outlets. This presents some theory to identify that proportionality of the AVM is more significant than the size of the AVM as a whole, in terms of the disease progression.

The Buckingham Pi analysis identifies dimensionless groups void of Reynold's number as a critical analysis point, due to the absence of dynamic viscosity of blood. This analysis thus postulates that blood viscosity has negligible effect upon the blood flow through the AVM. The importance of Reynold's number upon cerebral blood flow, particularly in the examination of strokes, is substantiated by Hademenos and Massoud[31] who reported that Reynold's Number is key to the pattern of flow within cerebral blood vessels.

Though the findings from this test provide important information regarding the disorder, the analysis is conducted with various assumptions thus rendering the final dimensionless groups not accurate. The assumptions were made relative to literature found. This included equating arterial inlet and venous inlet flow, owing to the lack of ability to measure venous blood flow at this stage. Additionally, pulsatile flow was ignored for this analysis, due to unknown method by which this flow could be incorporated into a computational model, as explored in methodology.

Test 2.1: Okell& Chappell[228] assumption

Examining the Okell& Chappell assumption trial provides insights into the overall flow through an AVM model, even though cerebrovascular steal was not modelled. The critical factors, as identified through the Buckingham Pi analysis, were explored and a better understanding of blood flow in the system can be achieved through the exploration of these individually. The point at which steal would be modelled can be estimated by identifying the governing equation of arterial outlet flow as follows:

$$y_{arterial\ outlet\ test\ 2.1} = 0.1475x - 0.00755441$$

Cerebrovascular steal would be modelled after

$$x = 0.0511m$$

Further examining the pressure plots obtained, the lack of deviation across the arterial and venous outlets is expected, from the set boundary condition applied to the system. In the computational model, this was to drive flow, and without the application of this condition the model would be considered under-defined and thereby not possible to solve.

The artery and venous inlet location show interesting results. It is evident in Figure 15.14 that the two artery inlet location plots follow very closely. Both are observably parallel, and increase together as fistula diameter increases. On the other hand, though evidently parallel, there is a more significant pressure gradient between the distal and proximal venous outlet points. The venous outlet pertains to a pressure boundary condition. This implies that in the small section between the proximal and distal venous outlet there is a significant pressure gradient. This can be considered a comparable model to the way in which the human body auto-regulates to maintain blood pressure and stresses in vessels. Essentially, the pressure across the length of the draining vein increases, thereby forcing fluid flow out of the outlet at a faster rate.

Deconstructing the results obtained for velocity, shown in Figure 15.15 at all measurement points also shows interesting factors. In this trial there appears, on average, no significant change in the flow velocity across the fistula. This may essentially be due to the high mass flow through the sections, and no considerable alteration to the flow regime. In addition, there is no change in the velocity across the venous and arterial inlet conditions. Though the inlets themselves have boundary velocity conditions, some change was expected. Secondary to the high volume of fluid, it is likely that this effect was more significant compared to the model and pressure gradient in the system. Figure 15.15 further shows slight decrease of arterial outlet flow, and a slight increase in the velocity outlet flows. This relates to the decreasing and increasing flows in the respective sections, the equations of which are shown in Table 15.7. This essentially emphasises that as fistula diameter increases, the flow through the arterial outlet diminishes, and is diverted through to the fistula.

All the equations for the measurement of velocity are linear, shown in Table 15.7. The equations emphasise the decreasing nature of the velocity across the fistula as the geometry increases, and as the flow progresses from the arterial to venous plane.

There is a decrease in the velocity at the distal arterial inlet, whereas the gradient at the proximal arterial inlet indicates that by this point the velocity increases. The initial decrease may be a result of the overall system not experiencing as significant a shunting of fluid flow, directly related to the high flow in the vessels and the lack of steal phenomenon.

A closer look at the fistula highlights the occurrence of swirling shown in Figure 15.7. Fluid swirling leads to an overall reduction in fluid velocity. The diminished velocity of the flow through the malformation is explained by the overall characteristics of the results obtained.

The test consisted of some errors, and noise in data, which are identified in further analysis. Re-testing of the entire set of conditions yielded no change in the results across a series of three repetitions. There is apparent noise at different measurement locations and different diameter trials, which may be largely indicative of the data point coinciding or in close proximity of an element boundary in the mesh (Oberkampf[222]).

Test 2.2: Stock et.al[316]

The Stock, Wetzel assumption did not model cerebrovascular steal, but rather provided information regarding critical factors and flow regime within an AVM. Examining outlet flow, it can be summarised that as fistula diameter dilates, the mass flow rate of the arterial outlet decreases. Similarly, the mass flow rate at the venous outlet steadily increases with fistula dilation. This is due to an increase in fluid flow through the fistula. It can further be expected that eventually steal will be found as the fistula diameter further dilates. This point has been estimated using the formula governing arterial outlet flow as follows:

$$y_{arterial\ outlet} = 0.2x - 0.0782$$

Now, the diameter at which mass flow through the outlet equals zero, after which steal is expected to occur is

$$x = 0.0391m$$

Examining the velocity plots further, Figure 15.18 indicates an overall decrease in velocity through the arterial outlet and fistula. This decrease can be expected in the outlet due to the decreased mass flow rate measured in the region and the increased flow in the fistula. Similarly, the venous outlet has consistently increasing velocity, expected owing to the increases flow in the region. As steal is not observed the critical changes in the velocity profile cannot be examined. This test however exemplifies the significance of inlet mass flow rate upon the AVM system, which is also shown in the Buckingham Pi analysis. Inlet flow rates, as shown in Figure 15.18 are critical to the onset of cerebrovascular steal in the body owing to the mass flow rate relative to pressure.

Table 15.8 describes the overall linear equations obtained for each velocity plot across all locations, to further explicate the pattern of velocity flow. Examining the fistula itself, the equation listed in Table 15.8 and the visual plot in Figure 15.18 highlight that the velocity across the plane is decreasing, as the blood flow enters into draining vein. This slowing of the fluid, though minor, is likely due to the occurrence of swirling through the fistula which is unhindered in that zone. Further study shows that velocity measured at the arterial inlets too decreases as the fistula dilates. Though the arterial inlet mass flow rate was pre-determined as a boundary condition in the CFX solver, there is minute decreasing occurring at the distal arterial inlet point. This may relate to the dilation of the fistula itself, potentially alleviating the pressure in the arterial region, thus causing a relaxation in the velocity (Drake[70], Hamel[114] & Constantiono[53]). The arterial outlet experiences increasing velocity, however, moving at a parabolic method. Similarly, the venous outlet indicates an overall increase in the velocity of the blood in the region.

The equations identified in Table 15.6 emphasise the critical differences occurring across small regions of the AVM model. Between the arterial and venous plane the gradient increases by roughly 2.3 times, indicating that through the fistula there is a larger decrease in the blood velocity, as the blood progresses closer to the draining vein when the fistula diameter dilates. This is a pattern identified in various articles exploring the results of vasodilation and vasoconstriction, and the relationship with blood flow rate (Drake[70]& Constantino[53]).

The distal and proximal arterial inlets also exhibit a similar alteration across a small region, with the proximal arterial inlet gradient, or rate of change, is 15 times the rate of change of the distal arterial inlet. As such between the arterial blood entry to the system, and the entrance of the fistula at the artery, there is a significant amount of acceleration occurring of the blood. This is largely a result of the pressure gradient within arterial section of the system, and the requirement of the system to maintain equilibrium which is altered with the introduction and dilation of the fistula (Brady[29] & Pritchard[257]). The differential factor between the distal and proximal arterial outlet regions is equivalent to 1.611, showing that the acceleration at the artery inlet region is significantly greater than the artery outlet region. This is likely causal to the influx of blood flow diverted through the fistula, with lesser blood flow in the arterial outlet. Figure 15.7.

Blood swirling, as explored is a critical component to analyse in this examination. Figure 15.8 depicts the swirling which occurs in the same plane as the length of the fistula.

Examination of pressure drop from the proximal arterial outlet and distal arterial outlet, to the outlet point itself, compared to that gradient developed in the inlet region, provides explanation for the rapid acceleration of the blood between the distal and proximal arterial inlets. This data is presented in Figure 15.17. Similarly, the venous region exhibits larger pressure gradient of the venous blood flow approaching the fistula, compared to the physically draining outlet venous region. This may be indicative of the significant of AVM geometry. However this pattern is not fully explained by its existence or the dilation of the vessel. Further examination of these regions and the effects of changing fluid variables upon the region may provide greater detail as to the causal factors for this pattern observed.

The pressure plots yielded, in Figure 15.17, indicate little deviation of the values across the location as fistula diameter increases in the models. This is largely due to the set pressure value upon the outlets to the AVM, and further the lack of substantial blood flow disturbance. Without the occurrence of steal, it cannot be expected that the pressure would alter significantly within the model. The venous outlet pressure however shows different pressure levels compared to all other locations. Though the venous outlet pressure condition is set in the model, the deviation between the proximal and distal venous outlets is disproportionate compared to the matching 2 venous inlet locations, and arterial locations. Thus, within the small section of 0.0035m between the distal and proximal venous outlet, there is a considerable pressure gradient, which further explains the increased velocity in the region.

The situation explains the attempts by the system to regulate pressure according to the boundary conditions applied to the model. Similarly, in the human body, this occurrence can be explained by the need to regulate pressure within blood vessels (Ornestein[231] & Kamiya[146]). In response to this mechanism, if blood flow in the venous region is identified by the body, there may be dilation of the inlet region in order to maximise the pressure gradient within the draining vein thereby forcing the fluid at a higher velocity out of the nidus (Gao[87&88]& Schwartz[296]].

Finally examining wall shear stress, it can be seen that all values continually decrease as diameter increases shown in Figure 15.19. To identify the differences in the wall shear stress progression across the locations of the AVM, the equations pertaining to the curves were measured. The steeper curves yielded for the 2 venous outlets, is indicative that within the venous outlet region the flow is subject to significant alteration of the regime causing this drastic difference in the wall shear stresses. Decreasing wall shear stress with the dilation of fistula diameter is an expected response from the body as it naturally attempts to normalise the system(Papaioannou[238]).

Errors are apparent in two specific diameter models, which when tested again, yielded the same results. These results however are pertinent to two particular measurement points which indicate that these points lie upon an element boundary or in very close proximity to this boundary (Oberkampf[222]). These two specific diameter trials, furthermore, did not converge at the set point after 200 iterations.

Test 2.3: 0.003 kg/s assumption

Examining results obtained from Test 2.3 utilising inlet mass flow rate of 0.003 kg/s identified interesting flow progression. Looking firstly at outlet flows alone, the occurrence of the steal phenomenon is clearly indicated by the change in directionality of the fluid. Clarified in Figure 15.20, the section between 0.002m and

0.0021m encourages steal onset. Finding the exact modelled diameter whereby steal occurs, yields the following equation

$$y = 0.662303x - 0.0013377441$$

the equation solves

$$x = 0.0020198m$$

Table 15.9 shows the first and second derivatives measured for outlet flow rate, explicating the changes occurring with steal onset. The second derivative values obtained emphasise that across the values, where steal is not modelled, between fistula diameter 0.0014m and 0.002m, there is a decreasing curve obtained. The section between fistula diameter 0.002m and 0.0028m, however, indicates a more substantial alteration. The increasing curve measurement at the arterial outlet as fistula diameter increases is expected due to the influx of modelled blood through the outlet – the occurrence of steal. The venous outlet shows a much less significant alteration in the rate at which the curve changes with increased diameter. This may relate to the slowing velocity of the blood, through the fistula, as the fistula dilates and thus the overall change in mass flow rates at the draining section are decreased (Drake[70] & Hamel[114]).

Looking at the velocity curves in this trial, three clusters are observable in Figure 15.22. The arterial plane and venous plane curves, alongside the distal inlets and proximal inlets are positioned together. This is an expected occurrence due to the fixed boundary condition applied to the inlet itself. The distal and proximal venous outlets have continually increasing fluid velocity leaving the AVM system. There is no observable change in velocity between diameters 0.002m and 0.0021m where the cerebrovascular steal is modelled. Finally, the arterial outlet locations show decreasing velocity between 0.0014m to 0.002m, expected due to fluid leaving the system. After approaching the critical position between 0.002m and 0.0021m, where cerebrovascular steal is modelled, the velocity of blood flow at the venous outlet locations continually increases. This rate of velocity increase, however, is at a lower rate compared to the velocity drop seen earlier.

Examining the way in which flow continues, through analysis of the equations of the velocity plots, shown in Figure 15.22 and Table 15.1. The equations indicate the significant changes occurring in the arterial outlet and entire draining vein. The degree to which the velocity changes in these regions is explicated by the second derivatives identified for the measurement points. The distal arterial region shows the level of change in velocity slowing, potentially reaching a plateau prior to steal phenomenon occurring in the system. This phenomenon is most likely a result of the opening of the fistula, causing a rapid change in the velocity in that immediate section, after which the flow normalises near the outlet. Similarly, the proximal venous inlet, the point of which approaches the draining point of the fistula, shows that the rate of change exceeds that measurement at the distal venous inlet. The results essentially emphasise the overall effect of the fistula , and how the geometrical change causes changes in the blood flow. (Hademenos[107&110], Nornes[217&218] & Krauss[152]).

Examining further the other diameter models, more information regarding the changes in overall fluid flow is obtained. Table 15.11 illustrates the velocity equations measured between the models of fistula diameter equal to 0.002m and 0.0028m. As shown in Figure 15.22 after the onset of steal, the velocity decreases only along the arterial and venous plane, and the distal arterial inlet. All other locations experience an increase in velocity as the fistula dilates more, and steal volume through the fistula increases. Similar to the results explored above, there is a more rapid change occurring at the proximal arterial outlet compared to the distal end. The proximal venous inlet similarly experiences more rapid change compared to the distal venous inlet. The distal venous outlet experiences a slowing of velocity faster than the proximal venous region. This may relate to the slowing of large amounts of fluid through the fistula, or may be indicative that after steal onset occurs, as fistula dilates further, the velocity in the region approaches a convergence point.

Represented in Figure 15.9, it can be observed that the level of blood swirling occurring at the entrance of the fistula is to a lesser degree than found in Test 2.1 and 2.2. This suggests that the level of decrease in velocity is less than that found in Test 2.1 and 2.2 also. Comparing the Figures 15.15, 15.18 and 15.22 alone, it can be seen that the velocity change in Test 2.3 across the fistula is significantly less. There is some swirling observable at the proximal arterial outlet region which, (with steal), feeds into the fistula. In doing so there is decrease in the flow velocity in this region also. Blood entering the low-pressure system of the draining vein however, results in a significant increase in velocity as observed in Figure 15.22. Interestingly, the flow rate in Test 2.3 is less than that of Tests 2.1 and 2.2, implying that the high flow results in a larger onset of swirling within the fistula.

In contrast Pressure values had little deviation, the most significant changes occurred across the fistula, and the inlets. Figure 15.21. This is however an expected situation as the outlet pressure condition was set. The increase in pressure at the venous inlet the may be causal for the increase in velocity of the fluid from the artery into the vein, by essentially generating a less gradual pressure drop across the system. Drawing information from the Buckingham Pi analysis, the change in pressure across the fistula is identified as a critical factor for analysis within the AVM, and a possible determinant for potential rupture of the nidus.

The results shown in Figure 15.21 highlights the changing pressure within the AVM system, and emphasises the need to further examine the venous region. There is evidence that the venous inlet region experiences a slowing down of the rate at which the pressure increases. This may suggest that as the fistula dilates further equilibrium point in terms of pressure may be achieved, essentially reaching a value at which the pressure converges. The convergence identified may relate to the system eventually fulfilling the pressure and flow requirements sufficiently (Pritchard[257]).

In this examination errors were observed in the first trial set with diameter equal to 0.0014m. Subsequent testing yielded the same results. This result, occurring at the arterial outlet locations only, may highlight a rapidly changing system at particular velocity thereby causing a drastic change between fistula diameter 0.0014m and 0.0018m. Alternatively this may indicate that the changes in the arterial outlet are relative to the mass flow rate and not the fistula diameter, with consideration of other results obtained. As steal is not modelled at fistula diameter equal to 0.0014m, the change in flow regime cannot account for the value measured.

There is also some skewed velocity value at fistula diameter equal to 0.0028m at the venous plane. This could be attributed to the dilation of the vessel itself. Whether this particular value is an error cannot be determined through the formulation of equations or through the visual graphs (Oberkampf[222]).

Test 2.4: 0.0025 kg/s assumption

Examining Test 2.4, utilising the assumption of mass flow rate through the cerebral arteries and veins to be equal to 0.0025 kg/s in order to further observe the effects of mass flow rate, and thus velocity of fluid, upon the progression of the AVM model. Table 15.12 illustrates that steal phenomenon. The smallest fistula diameter, of 0.0014m, produced a result close to the intercept across the graph. An equation was thus formulated to identify the diameter at which steal began in this trial set. The following equations was calculated

$$y = 1.0733x - 0.00137111$$

Steal is modelled after fistula diameter (x) is

$$x = 0.001277m$$

Examining the pressure plots obtained in Figure 15.24, shows results differing from prior tests. The proximal venous outlet, however, indicates a slight increase as diameter increases, while the distal venous outlet remains unchanged with a zero gradient. This linearity is due to the set pressure condition in the CFX module, while the gradient developed between the proximal and distal venous outlet is likely to be the reason for additional fluid flow passing through the area. The arterial inlet locations indicate linear progression with a zero gradient also. The venous inlet conditions along with the arterial plane and venous plane show increasing pressure as diameter increases. This behaviour identifies that the pressure increase and changing pressure gradient is likely to be the cause for the flow regime alteration, and it is the draining vein that encourages the onset of steal in the model. Prior studies have indicted that the arterial outlet drives the flow through the AVM, however this study shows otherwise (Mast[194&195], Nornes[217-219] & Ornstein[231]).

The above factors are more clearly observed in Table 15.13 through the examination and measurement of the governing equation of velocity, along with the first and second derivatives. There is a clear reduction in the rate of change of velocity between the proximal and distal arterial outlet, highlighting a reduction in velocity, though steal is occurring, as the fistula dilates further. This observation essentially identifies that after the appearance of cerebrovascular steal in the AVM network, the change in velocity gradually reduces potentially converging to essentially result in some constant velocity – the system normalises as the fistula further dilates (Pedley[242] & Pritchard[257]). The linearity of the distal venous inlet values highlight that with steal modelling, the velocity in the immediate venous region is largely unaffected, with velocity changes occurring closer to the opening of the fistula at the proximal venous inlet. Interestingly the venous outlet section shows that the rate at which the velocity

Table 15.12 Mass Flow Rate of Outlets.

Location	Diameter (m)								
	0.0014	0.0016	0.0018	0.002	0.0021	0.0022	0.0024	0.0026	0.0028
Artery outlet	0.000132	0.000346	0.000516	0.000662	0.000733	0.000807	0.000885	0.000960	0.001037
Vein outlet	-0.00529	-0.00550	-0.00567	-0.00582	-0.00589	-0.00597	-0.00605	-0.00612	-0.00620

decreases is higher at the proximal region, and the rate of change is less at the distal point. This further suggests that the system is approaching some point where the system is in equilibrium, and expands the notion that after cerebrovascular steal, as fistula diameter further dilates, the system begins to normalise.

The generation of a changing pressure gradient condition within the venous outlet region is the likely cause for the various velocity plots obtained in Figure 15.25. There is a clear increase in velocity of the fluid at the venous outlet locations as diameter increases, and a clear decrease in the velocity across the fistula. Decreasing velocity in the fistula itself is expected due to the dilation of the diameter, thus increasing the area through which the flow passes. There is additionally a significant increase in the velocity at the arterial outlet owing to the influx of fluid in order maintain balanced flow within the AVM. This is documented as the same situation occurring in cerebral vessels caused by the body and its auto-regulatory mechanisms aiming to satisfy pressure conditions in the body (Mast[194&195], Hademenos[107-110], Nornes[217-219] & Numaguchi[221]).

The pressure curves obtained explain the changes occurring in the curves, showing that the arterial inlets and outlets experience decreasing pressure at a consistently increasing rate. The pressure changes are likely a result of the velocity changes occurring, as explored by Nornes[217-219]. This relates to concepts of the auto-regulation mechanism which is employed in response to changes. The introduction of the fistula along with the velocity and flow regime changes that follow are highlighted in Figure 15.25. Similarly, the draining vein experiences an overall increase in pressure in the system however at a consistently decreasing rate. This again relates to the requirement of the system to adjust to the changes occurring (Spetzier[307-310]). The combination of decreasing pressure at the high pressure feeding artery and increasing pressure at the low-pressure vein indicates that the system as a whole is working to reach a level of equilibrium (Ornstein[231] & Spetzler[307-310]).

As with previous tests, blood swirling was found in this trial. The existence of steal throughout all diameter sets of this trial, thus shows interesting flow characteristics pertaining to the phenomenon itself. Figure 15.10

Table 15.13 Velocity equations measured for Test 2.4.

Location	Equation ($y =$)	$\frac{dy}{dx}$	$\frac{d^2y}{dx^2}$
Arterial Plane	-0.0397x + 1.4557	-0.0397	
Venous Plane	-0.0349x + 1.6309	-0.0349	
Distal Arterial Inlet	9E-06x + 1.012	0.000000006	
Proximal Arterial Inlet	0.0012x + 0.9856	0.0012	
Distal Arterial Outlet	-0.0027x^2 + 0.0609x + 0.0868	-0.0054x + 0.0609	-0.0054
Proximal Arterial Outlet	-0.0031x^2 + 0.0628x + 0.0935	-0.0062x + 0.0628	-0.0062
Distal Venous Inlet	0.0001x + 1.0109	0.0001	
Proximal Venous Inlet	0.0005x^2 - 0.0009x + 1.0167	0.001x – 0.0009	0.001
Distal Venous Outlet	-0.0034x^2 + 0.0694x + 2.2249	-0.0034x + 0.0694	-0.0012
Proximal Venous Outlet	-0.0016x^2 + 0.0403x + 2.6401	-0.0032x + 0.0403	-0.0032

indicates that there is a small region where swirling occurs, to a lesser degree than observed in previous trials. This provides further evidence that with lesser flow, the level of blood swirling respectively decreases and as a result the overall reduction in blood velocity, as shown in Figure 15.25, diminishes.

The trial using diameter equal 0.0026m found a small spike in pressure at the arterial plane. The existence of this error may pertain to the location of the plane relative to the elements present in the immediate region (Oberkampf[222]). There is likely a large boundary, or multiple boundaries coinciding with the arterial plane as defined in CFX. With consideration that all other locations appear to follow the same patterns as previous and subsequent trials, other potential error factors can be ignored. Another error is apparent at the velocity calculation at the proximal arterial outlet, which cannot be linked to steal modelling as the entire trial experiences the same error. Pressure additionally does not undergo drastic alteration after the first diameter model, where fistula diameter is equal to 0.0014, and thus the apparent error in velocity measurement cannot be attributed to this (Pritchard[257] & Oberkampf[222]). It is likely the distal arterial outlet probe exists upon or close to an element boundary, and was thus subject to noise in calculation through CFX [95]

Test 3: Controlled flow examination

The results obtained from the fixed flow test conducted, examining fluid flow in a controlled flow environment, indicated results which contradict much of the literature found (Young[355], Sorimachi[306] & Duong[72]). Essentially, research reports that the feeding artery is the largest factor affecting blood flow through the AVM and fistula, and in general is the biggest factor governing overall cerebral blood flow (Schwartz[294&295]). Thereby any pressure condition of flow rate which exists should govern the results obtained (Sorimachi[306]).

Casikar[41] hypothesised, during animal testing, that fistula blood flow may be independent of any pressure condition which exists at the arterial outlet, thereby not governing the amount or direction of fluid flow through this outlet, or the draining vein. Our results indicate minimal pressure change, and where 100% of arterial blood flow is shunted through the fistula, a pressure condition is still measured through the arterial outlet. Basic pipe flow theory should identify that this region, essentially void of blood at 100% blood flow shunting, would pertain a static pressure condition of considerable adjustment (Pritchard[257]).

With consideration that mass flow rate through the arterial outlet varies from 100% of arterial inlet flow, equal to 0.0027 g/s, to -30%, equal to 0.00081 g/s in the reverse direction, it is expected that pressure should adjust accordingly. Figure 15.27 better represents the arterial segment of the AVM model, and indicates the distal arterial outlet pressure changes little across the different flow regimes. This does not completely explain the reversal of flow, as the pressure drop from 100% to 130% is considerably smaller than that which occurs in the draining vein. The disproportionate change in pressure is indicates that the pressure condition of the feeding artery is negligible, or is proportionally less significant to the mass flow rate, and the venous pressure condition. Examining Figure 15.27 it is evident that the draining vein is likely to drive the fluid flow through the AVM. The analysis of the fluid flow, rather, indicates, a more significant importance of the venous outlet.

This test offers clear insight into the governing conditions in an AVM and the flow characteristics overall. The identification of independence between flow direction of the arterial outlet and arterial pressure condition indicates that this direction is dependent upon the draining vein, a factor which has been largely undocumented due to the difficulty in quantifying venous blood flow and the existing difficulties explored in computational examination of cerebral blood vessels. Graphically, it is evident that the pressure condition pertaining to the venous inlet and venous outlet have significant deviation shown in Figure 15.27. Based on pipe flow theory, and the effect of change in location upon pressure is governed by:

$$P_1 = P_0 + \rho g \Delta h$$

Based off this linear formula, the expectation of the deviation between venous inlet and venous outlet should be consistent essentially yielding two parallel lines. As a result, it can be extrapolated that the additional mass flow of blood entering the vein via the fistula affects the pressure measured at the venous outlet in a multiplicative manner, resulting in the generation of a parabolic curve. This data presents that mass flow rate significantly affects pressure in the draining vein, and does so in a non-linear manner.

The velocity in this trial follows a generally linear progression, across all locations (Figure 15.28). The arterial outlet, however, shows an increase in velocity occurring after steal is modelled in the system. In the arterial and venous planes there is a noticeable spike (Figure 15.28), occurring at 100% flow shunting, and zero modelling of cerebrovascular steal. Equations shown in Tables 15.14 and 15.15 are measured based of the curves obtained in Figure 15.28. These equations identify that overall the artery experiences increasing velocity as the amount of flow shunted decreases, excluding the arterial inlet which experiences very slight increases in fluid flow velocity. All other variables continually decrease in velocity as shunted volume decreases through the fistula. This is expected as increased shunt volume should translate to increase velocity through the vein (Pritchard[257]).

The velocity curves obtained after steal onset in modelled (table 15.15) explicates that as the fistula is approached, there is a rapid increase in the velocity as the shunted flow volume increases. This change is not proportional to all other changes in the system, and thus it can be postulated the existence of the fistula causes some additional acceleration of the flow, after steal phenomenon is modelled. This particular result may also provide some evidence as to the onset of symptoms when the overall velocity profile changes drastically after this point (Mast[194&195] & Constantino[49]).

Observing blood swirling in the fistula identifies that blood flow velocity decreases upon entry into the fistula shown in Figure 15.11.

Table 15.14 Velocity equations Test 3 prior to steal modelling.

Location	Equation $(y =)$	$\frac{dy}{dx} =$	$\frac{d^2y}{dx^2} =$
Arterial Plane	-0.1489x + 1.5954	-0.1489	
Venous Plane	-0.1559x + 1.7538	-0.1559	
Distal Arterial Inlet	5E-05x + 1.0584	5E-05	
Proximal Arterial Inlet	$0.0029x^2$ - 0.0092x + 1.0357	0.0058x – 0.0092	0.0058
Distal Arterial Outlet	-0.1057x + 0.4229	-0.1057	
Proximal Arterial Outlet	$0.0284x^2$ - 0.2083x + 0.5142	0.0568x – 0.2083	0.0568
Distal Venous Inlet	0.0001x + 1.0579	0.0001	
Proximal Venous Inlet	$0.0027x^2$ - 0.0106x + 1.0772	0.0054x 0.0106	0.0054
Distal Venous Outlet	-0.1153x + 2.7021	-0.1153	
Proximal Venous Outlet	-0.1685x + 3.1168	-0.1685	

Table 15.15 Velocity equations Test 3 prior to steal modelling.

Location	Equation ($y =$)	$\frac{dy}{dx} =$
Arterial Plane	-0.0595x + 1.101	-0.0595
Venous Plane	-0.0949x + 1.2804	-0.0949
Distal Arterial Inlet	-1E-05x + 1.0586	-1E-06
Proximal Arterial Inlet	0.0022x + 1.0355	0.0022
Distal Arterial Outlet	0.1082x - 0.1081	0.1082
Proximal Arterial Outlet	0.1009x - 0.0467	0.1009
Distal Venous Inlet	-3E-05x + 1.0583	-3E-05
Proximal Venous Inlet	-0.0011x + 1.0718	-0.0011
Distal Venous Outlet	-0.1147x + 2.3577	-0.1147
Proximal Venous Outlet	-0.1299x + 2.5702	-0.1299

Comparing data and the patterns observed to the Buckingham Pi analysis, the results obtained are consistent with the overall trends found in prior tests. Controlling the flow led to data with significantly different curves, compared to Tests 2.1-2.4, the importance of the inlet flow and outlet flow occurring across the system is evdent. Figure 15.27 and 15.28 however highlight that the venous outlet must pertain some additional factor to result in the vast change in the curve. This indicates that some constant factor must be present in the mathematical calculation for this variable. This was not found through the Buckingham Pi analysis. Further research, or a more extended Buckingham Pi measurement could identify the existence of such a factor.

The results infer that this highly volatile situation of increasing wall shear stress would result in significant remodelling responses in the vasculature leading to vessel dilation and even thinning. The reduction in vessel thickness in response may lead to a further diminished capacity to withstand the high wall shear stresses experienced in the vasculature, which in turn could accelerate the potential rupture of the vessel (Papaioannou[238], Fung[83] & Ornstein[231]). Future research could aim to identify this physiological response, and the degree to which this affects the progression of the disorder.

The values obtained in Figure 15.29 detailing wall shear stress calculations at each point, show significant effects from flow changes to the AVM. The turning point of the parabolic curves for the arterial outlet at 100% shunted flow through the AVM indicate the absolute value of flow passing through the outlet. On the other hand, wall shear stress appears to progress linearly through the outlet. Figure 15.29 largely indicates expected results from the wall shear stress calculation, showing the higher stresses encountered by the draining vein outlet as mass flow through the region increases, and indicates the effect of volume of blood , irrespective of direction, upon the arterial outlets. As expected the wall shear stress remains unchanged across the arterial inlet and venous inlet, as a result of the fixed flow condition set to the AVM model.

The linearity of the changes in wall shear stress, is expected with consideration that the blood volume through the system incrementally increases and diameter remains constant, as made evident by the Hagen-Poiseulle equation (Shojiama[301]). With respect to the results, this linearity indicates the validity of the two-dimensional model in representing blood flow in the AVM, which follows expected patterns according to the accepted mathematical model (Hademenos[107-110] Alaraj[4] & Papaioannou[238]). The findings from the controlled flow test highlights the predicative nature of the equation in its application to study blood flow in AVMs.

The spike occurring at the point where 100% flow is shunted through the fistula may be attributed to some computational or meshing error apparent in Figure 15.27 to 15.29 (Oberkampf[222]). The occurrence however is found at multiple points in the venous region, which may give indication to the existence of a turning point in the data, whereby the overall governing equation change drastically across these points. In order to identify the true nature of these points, and to specifically identify whether this point is a true point of significant change in flow regime, further models should be developed.

These models should follow smaller percentage flow(shunt) increments.

Test 4: Observing ratio between artery diameter and fistula diameter

Test 4, observing the ratio between artery diameter and fistula diameter, presented a number of interesting results. Firstly, this test largely expands on Test 2 and 3, offering a wide spectrum of change of the fistula diameter. Linking this to the Buckingham Pi analysis, this test offers strong evidence to exemplify the importance of the ratio between artery and fistula diameters, as opposed to exact value of measurement, to study AVM progression.

The critical ratio, upon examination of flow rates at the arterial and venous outlet, exists between 2:1 and 1:1, as clear by Figure 15.30. Measurement and calculations were thus conducted to find the linear equation which governs the graph. To do this, the section between ratios 2:1 and 2:1 was examined alone and yielded the following equation:

$$y = -0.00109113x + 0.00174786$$

Thus, the y-intercept, the ratio at which cerebrovascular steal begins is 1.60188: 1

Similar to the pressure pattern observed across the arterial outlet and venous outlet, the rapid change in curvature is observed between ratio 2:1 and 1:1 of artery diameter to fistula diameter, in Figure 15.31. Interestingly, these results further indicate some convergence of the data to a plot approaching a linear line, before decreasing in value. This is particularly evident in the distal venous outlet plot and proximal venous outlet.

Data from Figure 15.31 shows that between ratios 2:1 and 1:3 plots follow the left arm of a quadratic equation eventually reaching its turning point within the region of ratio 1:2 and 1:3. Within exception only to the arterial plane, all other points indicate the right arm of positive quadratic plots, with a smaller gradient however. Between ratio 5:1 and 2:1, the changes in pressure occur at a lesser rate though continually increasing. Essentially these plots indicate that with increasing fistula diameter, or reducing the artery diameter to fistula diameter ratio, pressure increases. Upon the occurrence of the steal phenomenon, the rate of pressure increase accelerates and approaches a linear line with zero gradient. After a certain level of dilation of the diameter of fistula , the pressure follows a decreasing linear plot. This highlights that dilation of the fistula will potentially cause blood flow to return to normal blood flow, if vessel rupture does not occur.

The results additionally are indicative that the draining vein has a more significant role in the progression of AVMs, as was indicated in Test 3 during controlled flow testing. The significant change in curvature for all venous testing points, and the venous end of the fistula, highlight this. The comparatively lesser change in curvature for arterial testing points shows that the artery has a lesser effect, and is less affected by, the AVM and flow regime. The results indicate how narrowing of the fistula causes a rapid reduction in the wall shear stress measured across the AVM.

Table 15.16 explores the equations yielded for the velocity curves obtained in Test 4 between ratios 5:1 to 1:1. The curves in Figure 15.32 show that the venous and arterial planes experience some rise in velocity, before the velocity decreases as the ratio of fistula to artery approaches parity. The equations shows that the changes in the velocity are occurring at an overall decreasing rate. The arterial outlet on the other hand exhibits decreasing velocity which rises as the ratio approaches equivalence. The changing of velocity in the outlet region occurs at a lesser rate, compared to that measured for the fistula. The arterial and venous inlet follow a linear progression, showing little change in velocity depicted in the Figure 15.32. Examining the venous outlet region, it can be seen that there is significant change occurring in the velocity profiles. The distal venous outlet, in particular, shows the most drastic change in Figure 15.32. Table 15.16 also emphasises the comparatively steep increasing rate of the curve.

Table 15.16 indicates the velocity equations obtained in Test 4 between ratios 1:1 to 1:5. Firstly examining the arterial and venous planes, as shown in Figure 15.32, the arterial plane experiences a more significant change in velocity. The overall decrease in velocity is emphasised by the decreasing equation obtained, and higher negative rate at which the changes occur, compared to the venous plane. The distal arterial and venous inlet show little deviation from the linear plot obtained in Figure 15.32, and is also indicative in the minute gradient of change measured in Table 15.17. The proximal arterial inlet experiences some positive change in velocity, resulting directly from the opening of the fistula, and the overall dilation the fistula experiences across the trial set. The arterial outlet region experienced an overall increase in velocity likely resulting from the onset of steal phenomenon through the system (Mast[194&195]). Similarly, the venous outlet experienced an overall increase velocity- to a larger degree than compared to all other locations. The overall rate of change occurring in the velocity in this region rapidly rises. There is evidence that the venous region undergoes more significant alteration due to fistula dilation, and steal influx, and is likely the cause for the onset of steal and the changes which follow (Pedley[242] & Papaioannou[238]).

The wall shear stresses found in Test 4, shown in Figure 15.33 indicate decreasing parabolic curves, showing that diameter change

Table 15.16 Velocity equations Test 4 ratios 5:1 to 1:1.

Location	Equation ($y =$)	$\frac{dy}{dx} =$	$\frac{d^2y}{dx^2} =$
Arterial Plane	$0.0643x^2 - 0.5619x + 1.7631$	$0.1286x - 0.5619$	0.1286
Venous Plane	$0.0397x^2 - 0.2633x + 1.6348$	$0.0794x - 0.2633$	0.0794
Distal Arterial Inlet	-3E-05x + 1.0121	-3E-05	
Proximal Arterial Inlet	$-0.0007x^2 + 0.0083x + 0.9894$	$-0.0014x + 0.0083$	-0.0014
Distal Arterial Outlet	$-0.0254x^2 + 0.2282x + 0.0724$	$-0.0508x + 0.2282$	-0.0508
Proximal Arterial Outlet	$0.0147x^2 - 0.2171x + 0.9415$	$0.0294x - 0.2171$	0.0294
Distal Venous Inlet	$-0.0002x + 1.0115$	-0.0002	
Proximal Venous Inlet	$0.0006x^2 - 0.005x + 1.0232$	$0.0012x - 0.005$	0.0012
Distal Venous Outlet	$-0.0297x^2 + 0.2569x + 2.2062$	$-0.0594x + 0.2569$	-0.0594
Proximal Venous Outlet	$-0.0125x^2 + 0.1337x + 2.6252$	$-0.025x + 0.1337$	-0.025

Table 15.17 Velocity equations Test 4 ratios 1:1 to 1:5.

Location	Equation ($y =$)	$\frac{dy}{dx} =$	$\frac{d^2y}{dx^2} =$
Arterial Plane	$-0.063x^2 + 0.3291x + 1.208$	$-0.126x + 0.3291$	-0.126
Venous Plane	$-0.0595x^2 + 0.3108x + 1.3887$	$-0.119x + 0.3108$	-0.119
Distal Arterial Inlet	8E-05x + 1.0116	8E-05	
Proximal Arterial Inlet	$0.0035x^2 - 0.0167x + 0.9947$	$0.007x - 0.0167$	0.007
Distal Arterial Outlet	$0.0192x^2 - 0.2431x + 0.9473$	$0.0384x - 0.2431$	0.0384
Proximal Arterial Outlet	$0.0147x^2 - 0.2171x + 0.9415$	$0.0294x - 0.2171$	0.0294
Distal Venous Inlet	-3E-05x + 1.0114	-3E-05x	
Proximal Venous Inlet	$-0.0025x^2 + 0.0151x + 1.0054$	$-0.005x + 0.0151$	-0.005
Distal Venous Outlet	$0.0554x^2 - 0.0858x + 1.4501$	$0.1108x - 0.0858$	0.1108
Proximal Venous Outlet	$0.0436x^2 + 0.0176x + 1.5579$	$0.0872x + 0.0176$	0.0872

affects the wall shear stress within vessels to negative power of 2. This is also an expected result - Hagen-Poiseulle equation. As the fistula dilates, the wall shear stress in the system drastically decreases, at an increasing rate, across all points. The values found were, however, within suitable bounds for cerebral vessels (Shojiama[301]). Overall the venous region shows the most rapid changes shown in Figure 15.33.

Blood Swirling was found in all the models for this trial. With fistula dilation the velocity through the fistula clearly decreases, as shown in Figures 15.12 and 15.13, and the blood swirling occurs in a larger region. At smaller diameters, the velocity through the fistula is clearly high, compared to the feeding artery, and the blood swirling region appears small. This region is however, unclear at the small diameters. Further research to isolate these small fistula diameters may yield better results and improve the understanding of the potential vasoconstriction that may ensure. This may increase the understanding relating to the opening of a small fistula which dilates over a period of time. This may also explain the reasons for a silent fistula (in the embryo) manifests it's presence during the second or third decade in life.

No clear errors were observed in the data obtained, as no spikes or outliers were identified. There are however chances of errors pertaining to computational error, particularly in the meshing tools. This error pertains to all the models explored, and in this data set there is no appearance that any measurement location lies in close proximity of, or directly over, an element boundary (Oberkampf[222]).

The figures obtained show that AVM fistula diameter increase, with all other variables constant, the pressure and velocity across the entire system shows significant changes. The computational evidence suggests that the critical change for both pressure and velocity are directly related steal phenomenon in the system. This further solidifies the various hypotheses relating to the critical nature of both diameter and the effect of the onset of steal phenomenon. The sudden alteration in pressure and velocity of blood in the AVM after during and after the onset of vascular steal may present further explanation for the dormant nature of the symptoms of the disorder where the symptoms are found to largely present only after steal occurs (Mast[194&195] & Constantiono[49]].

It was found that the AVM system normalises with extensive fistula dilation, though this occurrence is hindered in the body as a result of low wall shear stresses existing in the fistula as the vessel diameter increases. High wall shear stresses, however, resulting from increased volume through the fistula, should encourage remodelling to dilate the fistula.

Blood swirling was another important factor identified, causing the rapid decrease in blood velocity through the fistula. This combined with low wall shear stress would likely lead to blood stagnation and increase cell adhesion in the vessel, causing additional stress on the AVM (Ha[106]).

The results obtained in this study highlight relationship between mass flow rate, fistula diameter, and amount of flow shunting upon the overall progression of an AVM. The increasing blood volume entering and exiting the fistula through the outlet of the draining vein results in a significant alteration in the pressure in this region. The venous outlet was found to be of most significant alteration as a result of the influx of fluid flow in the area. This is contrary to traditional research conducted on the arterial outlet, as the critical region of examination (Desai[63] & Pietila[4247&248]].

This study postulates that the combination of vessel dilation, and diminished capacity of auto-regulation of the vessels may render the AVM incapable of approaching a point of equilibrium. This study has found evidence to explain the onset of symptomology of AVMs as a result of steal phenomenon and create highly volatile clinical conditions.

Endovascular treatment of AVMs is the current approach. This method of treatment relies on the flow dynamics of the fistula. Occlusion of the arterial feeding vessels or the occlusion of the fistula by venous route are popular modes of present day management. In appropriate occlusion of the feeders or the venous outflow create steal phenomenon with disastrous damage to the brain. The understanding of the flow dynamics is essential for this method of treatment. The present study highlights some of the flow features. However there are still many unresolved issues that need further study.

This study offers many potential avenues for future research. Much of the future work should focus on incorporating biological processes, such as autoregulation and cell renewal, into the computational model. This would allow realistic modelling of blood flow, reflecting real-time or time-step based progression of the disease. The time variable could be introduced into the study of arteriovenous malfunctions, which offers many potential benefits to both engineers and physicians. Methods of classification of the arteriovenous malfunction and determination of treatment options would improve. The ability to produce a time map of the progression of an AVM provides significant potential for patient specific mapping offering diagnostic value to the clinicians. This would enable the generation of a time model detailing the potential progression allowing a physician to qualify the risk of the disorder with and without treatment.

The introduction of autoregulation in addition to the time factor, furthermore, would enable a detailed analysis of largely hypothesised phenomena occurring in the AVM (Kim[148] & Alaraj[4]]. Through computational analysis it may be possible to identify specific responses to the changes which occur in the AVM such as the auto-regulatory response to dilatation of blood vessels in response to increases wall shear stress in a vessel. In terms of diagnostics this would allow the visualisation of the patient specific responses owing to the various biological factors in an individual such as acquired medical conditions, congenital and genetic factors. A better analysis of the methods by which auto-regulation or cell renewal follow in the body in response to AVM progression would additionally offer scientific value to the computational studies. This information has the potential to validate many theories and hypothesis proposed by clinicians and engineers.

Additional research should be conducted to quantify pressure and wall shear stress thresholds which exist in cerebral blood vessels in order to identify points of critical flow for rupture. Much research has been conducted aiming to quantify these values. However significant contention exists as to the values obtained and the clinical applicability of these values (Shojiama[301]& Fung[83]]. Wall shear stress and other thresholds within the body are largely dependent on various genetic and physiological factors. A better representation of these values may arise from the development of governing equations relating these together (Komiama[150]).

As discussed before the quantification of arterial and venous blood flow is difficult to measure and calculate (Casikar[41], Mast[194&195], Shakur[298], Stock[316] & Duong[71&72]). The field of neuroscience and research into brain vasculature requires significant work to accurately quantify and produce some mathematical relationship to quantify, a value for both arterial and venous blood mass flow rate. Currently several estimates, arbitrary values and single research values are utilised thereby generating unreliable results and the production of large discrepancies in findings. The identification of mass flow rate through cerebral arteries and veins would provide value in research enabling clinicians and engineers to accurately model fluid flow and thus develop coherent, valid and reliable results. This would further solidify much of the hypotheses, or current theorems utilised in AVM and cerebral vasculature theory.

The number of feeding arteries and draining veins have been restricted in this experimentation, in order to simplify the model utilised and the study itself. This situation does not occur naturally and presents a large flaw in the assumptions used and the testing. As a result of the exclusion of this factor, this study cannot qualify whether the number of feeding arteries and draining veins plays a role in the progression of an AVM.

Using basic fluid mechanics properties it can be postulated that the number of feeding and draining vessels should have varied effect on the various factors pertaining to AVMs. Future avenues of research could aim to include this factor and attempt to understand the effects of additional vessels in the system. The generation of a complete understanding of the effects of additional vessels could potentially provide additional diagnostic value to the current methods of AVM assessment, and assist in the correct selection of vessels during treatment. For engineers and scientists, this research would further expand the potential of research to be conducted in the field, moving further toward a near-human representation of the disorder.

One of the most significant hindrances to generating a cohesive model that replicates natural AVM progression in the brain is the inability to apply a pulsatile flow rate to the vessel network. The pulse rate, caused by the heart, essentially serves as the driving force to circulate blood in the blood vessels of the body. The representation of this action is thus essential to the creation of a model that appropriately provides the physiological processes under which the disorder is governed and changes. The pulsatile flow and its effects upon the AVM is largely an elusive factor, one which many academics have noted would provide not only provide greater validity to the results. Some have hypothesised the adverse effects of certain changes of pulse upon disorder progression (Hademenos[107-110]). Future models which could encompass the pulsatile effects, over time, could greatly enhance the value of diagnostic modelling conducted and offer a better understanding of the progression of an AVM.

The possibility of generating a model based of MRI data would provide significant value in terms of patient specific diagnostics and modelling, beneficial to clinical and research purposes. The segmentation of the AVM though simplistic when utilising *ScanIP* and the various modules within the program, the addition of boundary conditions, increases the difficulty with which the disorder is modelled. Future research and development in the field of cerebral computational fluid dynamics using ScanIP data would be interesting. This particular model development would account for the various vessel geometries found in the human body, not conforming to regular shapes as utilised thus far in this thesis. Additionally, there are many variable factors that were assumed constant or negligible for simplicity which cannot be made in such a scenario. This includes vessel thickness, number of feeding arteries or draining veins, positioning of the nidus, and location of the AVM.

This study explicates the need to explore the effects of pulse rate upon the progression of the AVM, and the relationship between pulse rate with pressure and blood volume through the nidus. This study identifies the critical region of the draining vein, and the considerable pressure drop, which if controlled, may hinder the blood volume through the system. As discussed by Marmarou[178], the significant changes may have a direct relationship with pulse rate, causing it to change in response to the system variables.

Additional factors largely ignored in this examination could also form the crux of future research in the field. In particular the role of various nutrients upon the body and the way in which flow is affected. This concept is exemplified by the finding of Schaller[285] and the identification that oxygenation and water levels within blood have significance upon the velocity and blood flow rate through vessels in the body (Fritz[82]). Potential research could thus examine blood flow in a further simplified pipe flow model in order to accurately visualise and quantify the effects of factors such as temperature, water, oxygen, plasma, sodium and hormones have upon the mass flow rate with which blood is transported in the body. Though not specific to AVMs, such research will provide greater value to all computational fluid models generated for body fluid modelling and may also prove instrumental in solving many of unanswered questions pertaining to the ambiguity of AVM and cerebral blood flow (Sojiama[301] & Fritz[82]).

16

Summary

As in other parts of the body, arteriovenous malformations of the brain occur when there is a direct pathological communication between arteries and veins, without the intervention of a capillary system. Although trauma is responsible for most of the arteriovenous fistulae, cerebral arteriovenous malformations manifest in the intrauterine period because of defective development of the vessel walls in certain critical regions of the brain.

Since in the brain the pathological process occurs in an immature system (primitive brain), the severity of the lesions are more extensive when compared with those in other regions of the body. The manner in which the primitive cerebral vascular system adjusts to the abnormal circulatory condition is governed by certain general principles of embryology. The complex variations seen in the post-natal period follow a definite predictable pattern.

The primitive brain (notochord) is segmental in origin. Each segment has a pair of arteries and veins. The segmental veins drain laterally into longitudinal channels. This pattern is repeated in every segment. Around the 40-mm stage, these arteries and veins (pia-arachnoidal vessels) cross each other at right angles. If, at their points of intersection, the development of their vessel walls is defective, creating potential weakness, arteriovenous fistulae result.

The development of the arteries progress at a faster pace, compared with that of the veins. At the 40-mm stage, the arterial system is nearly complete. The effects of an arteriovenous fistula on the arterial system, therefore, tend to be localised.

On the contrary, the venous system lags behind in its development. The influx of abnormal quantities of blood creates severe circulatory problems in the immature veins. The effects often extend to the regions distant from the primary lesion. The extent of these changes is related to the size of the shunt and the capacity of the venous channels that receive the excess flow. If there is a small shunt in a large vein, the latter accommodates the overflow easily. If, on the other hand, there is a large shunt in a relatively small vein, the adjacent venous channels are also used to accommodate the influx.

During the development, the cerebral venous system constantly adjusts its anatomy to suit the changing needs of the developing brain. Inefficient and roundabout routes are replaced by efficient and direct channels. When there is an arteriovenous fistula, the vascular channels that normally undergo atritic process are retained to assist in the drainage. The embryo does not produce any new vessels exclusively to deal with the fistula. Existing channels are used to the best advantage. In cerebral arteriovenous malformations, the abnormal venous channels seen represent these persistent embryonic veins.

The spinal cord retains the segmental pattern to a large extent. When there is an arteriovenous fistula in any of these segments, the corresponding venous channels drain the blood laterally into the longitudinal spinal veins. If the fistula is large, the venous channels in the adjacent segments are also used. In the adult, these channels will be seen as distended and tortuous veins extending along the length of the spinal cord.

The myelencephalon and metencephalon retain the segmental pattern to some extent. The inferior and superior cerebellar arteries represent the segmental arteries, respectively. The myelencephalic and the metencephalic veins (segmental veins) drain laterally into the transverse sinus which corresponds to the longitudinal spinal veins. These segmental veins are retained in their embryonic form when there is an arteriovenous fistula.

Although in the mesencephalon the segmental pattern can be seen, the secondary changes in the vascular system obscure the basic plan. The arterial component (mesencephalic artery) and the venous drainage are both annexed by the adjacent diencephalon. Therefore, the anatomical features of the arteriovenous malformations in this segment resemble those of the diencephalon (see below).

The anterior choroidal, posterior choroidal, and posterior cerebral arteries represent the segmental arteries of the diencephalon. The ventral and dorsal diencephalic veins drain laterally into the transverse sinus via the tentorial sinus. The backward swing of the brain stretches the tentorial sinus. A decrease in the size of the lumen creates problems in drainage. A second longitudinal channel (basal vein) develops as a substitute and drains medially into the great cerebral vein. If there is an arteriovenous fistula, these problems are magnified.

The diencephalic veins will be seen in the adult draining medially into the great cerebral vein through the components of the primitive basal vein. As an exception, the primary lateral drainage may persist, and then segments of tentorial sinus will be represented in the adult.

Similar changes occur in the telencephalic arteriovenous malformations also. The arterial components consist of the anterior and middle cerebral arteries. The venous drainage occurs laterally through the telencephalic veins into the tentorial sinus. When the tentorial sinus is unable to function efficiently, the basal vein takes over. The persistent telencephalic vein in the adult courses backwards and medially into the great cerebral vein, incorporating segments of the basal vein.

In addition to this, there are two other regions in the telencephalon where arteriovenous malformations occur frequently, namely, in the regions of the basal ganglia and the surface of the cerebral hemisphere. The persistent embryonic veins drain into the anterior end of the internal cerebral vein and the superior sagittal sinus, respectively.

The dural malformations also follow the same basic pattern seen in the brain. The persistent embryonic veins drain either into the transverse sinus or into the superior sagittal sinus. These dural lesions are often classified with the scalp malformations, on the assumption that the meningeal vessel (middle meningeal artery) is a branch of the external carotid artery. The middle meningeal artery is primarily a branch of the internal carotid artery and, therefore, has features similar to those of the latter. The scalp arteries alone are purely external carotid in origin and cannot be compared with the rest of the cerebral vessels.

In short, if the course and termination of the embryonic pia-arachnoidal veins are known, the anatomical and radiological features of arteriovenous malformations can be easily predicted.

Application to Treatment

Obliteration of the fistula is the ideal method of treatment (Gibson[93]). The problems and complication of ligating the feeding artery alone in the presence of collateral circulation are well documented in the field of vascular surgery (extracranial) (Svien[319&320]). Excision of the plexus of vascular tissue in the region of the fistula in the limbs or in the chest is never attempted! It stands to reason to apply the same principles when dealing with the vascular fistulae in the brain, with appropriate modification.

Obliteration of the Shunt

Good and permanent results have been claimed by both irradiation (DXR) and surgery. The occurrence of fibrosis in irradiated tissues is, perhaps, responsible for the 'good cases'. If there is fibrosis around the fistula, it might effectively either obliterate it completely or sufficiently reduce the shunt. Of course, complete obliteration would produce a permanent cure.

But where it is partial, it will reduce the size of the shunt. By so doing, it might create a situation where the feeding artery is able to deal with the problem without the help of the collaterals, or a feeder which is directing all its flow into the shunt will now be able to have some flow distally.

Both these changes will naturally improve the radiological appearances and perhaps reduce the severity of clinical symptoms (Von Der Max[345], Weir[346], Wickbom[347], Willis[348].

Surgical treatment claims similar results when the malformation has been completely excised. This is accomplished in two situations (Vinken[342], Wyburn[353], Zulch[357]:

1. When the entire lesion (artery, shunt, and the dilated veins) is small and is situated in an area where the removal with the sacrifice of surrounding normal brain tissue is feasible
2. When a 'radical excision' (removal of all the vascular elements) is undertaken in an accessible situation

In both these instances, the actual removal of the shunt in the process is responsible for the good results.

'Exsanguination'

The fibrosis initiated by DXR, if it restraints the feeding artery partially or completely, will reduce the degree of shunting. This is likely to be temporary as collateral channels will re-form to satisfy the needs of the fistula.

The surgical approach is probably more effective here, as the treatment is more specific.

Contrary to the earlier statement, ligation of the feeding artery alone may be most effective in some situations.

When an arterial feeder is just about able to maintain the fistula by diverting all its blood (without collaterals), the above-mentioned method is justified. This apparent exception can be explained based on the concepts of development.

In the beginning, the fistula, as per classical description, will contain the proximal and distal arterial and venous segments connected by the shunt. If the relative sizes of the feeder and the fistula are such that all the flow is diverted into the shunt, the distal arterial limb, having been rendered functionless, will disappear, a process common in the developmental stages. Since the patency of the distal limb is essential to produce a reversed flow, recurrence is unlikely in these cases.

But radiological appearances of an artery feeding into the vein do not necessarily mean that the distal arterial segment is absent. The contrast might have just opacified the blood flow, thus excluding the distal segment. This fallacy probably accounts for some of the recurrences with new feeders following the procedure (see 'Dural Arteriovenous Malformations').

When more than one arterial feeder is seen, clipping of either all or the principal vessels will only produce a temporary improvement. Development of fresh collaterals will occur soon. The very existence of collateral channels indicates the need to obliterate the actual fistula to produce permanent results.

The size of the feeding vessels is no guide to identify the primary feeder. If the primary feeder is small, but the fistula is large, the collateral vessel may be diverting more blood than will the principal fistula in maintaining the shunt.

The Angioma

The collection of amorphous, dilated arteries and capillaries in the vicinity of many arteriovenous malformations corresponds to the entire area of collateral vessels, arterialised veins, and hypertrophied capillaries in extracranial situation (Boucquey[27], Brock[31] Caram[38] Crawford[55] Fincher[80] Gerlach[91] Hamby[111-113] Krayenbuhl[153&155] Mackenzie[185] Manuelidis[186] Margolis[187] Northfield[220] Odom[225], Paterson[241] Potter[254] Prensky[256] Raynor[266] Schneider[291] Sutherland[318] Worster-Drought[352], McGuire[182], Norlen[216]). Attempts to excise the latter are never made. A similar principle may be applicable in dealing with these angiomata.

These remarks on the treatment are only meant to demonstrate how the general principles of surgery of arteriovenous fistula are applicable to those of the nervous system also. The consideration of the feasibility of application of these principles in individual cases is outside the scope of the present book (Alexander[5], Bassett[15] Beck[17] Carton[40] Edgar[73] Eisenbrey[74] Gannon[85] Hamby[111&112] Hook[136&137] Jaeger[123&124] Johnson[142&143] Locke[168] Penfield[243], Parkinson[240], Pool[250-252], Robles[275], McKissock[184]).

The results obtained in the study of CFD highlight relationship between mass flow rate, fistula diameter, and amount of flow shunting upon the overall progression of an AVM. The increasing blood volume entering and exiting the fistula through the outlet of the draining vein results in a significant alteration in the pressure in this region. The venous outlet was found to be of most significant alteration as a result of the influx of fluid flow in the area. This is contrary to traditional research conducted on the arterial outlet, as the critical region of examination (Desai[63] & Pietila[248]].

This study postulates that the combination of vessel dilation, and diminished capacity of auto-regulation of the vessels may render the AVM incapable of approaching a point of equilibrium. This study has found evidence to explain the onset of symptomology of AVMs as a result of steal phenomenon and create highly volatile clinical conditions.

Using basic fluid mechanics properties it can be postulated that the number of feeding and draining vessels should have varied effect on the various factors pertaining to AVMs. Future avenues of research could aim to include this factor and attempt to understand the effects of additional vessels in the system. The generation of a complete understanding of the effects of additional vessels could potentially provide additional diagnostic value to the current methods of AVM assessment, and assist in the correct selection of vessels during treatment. For engineers and scientists, this research would further expand the potential of research to be conducted in the field, moving further toward a near-human representation of the disorder.

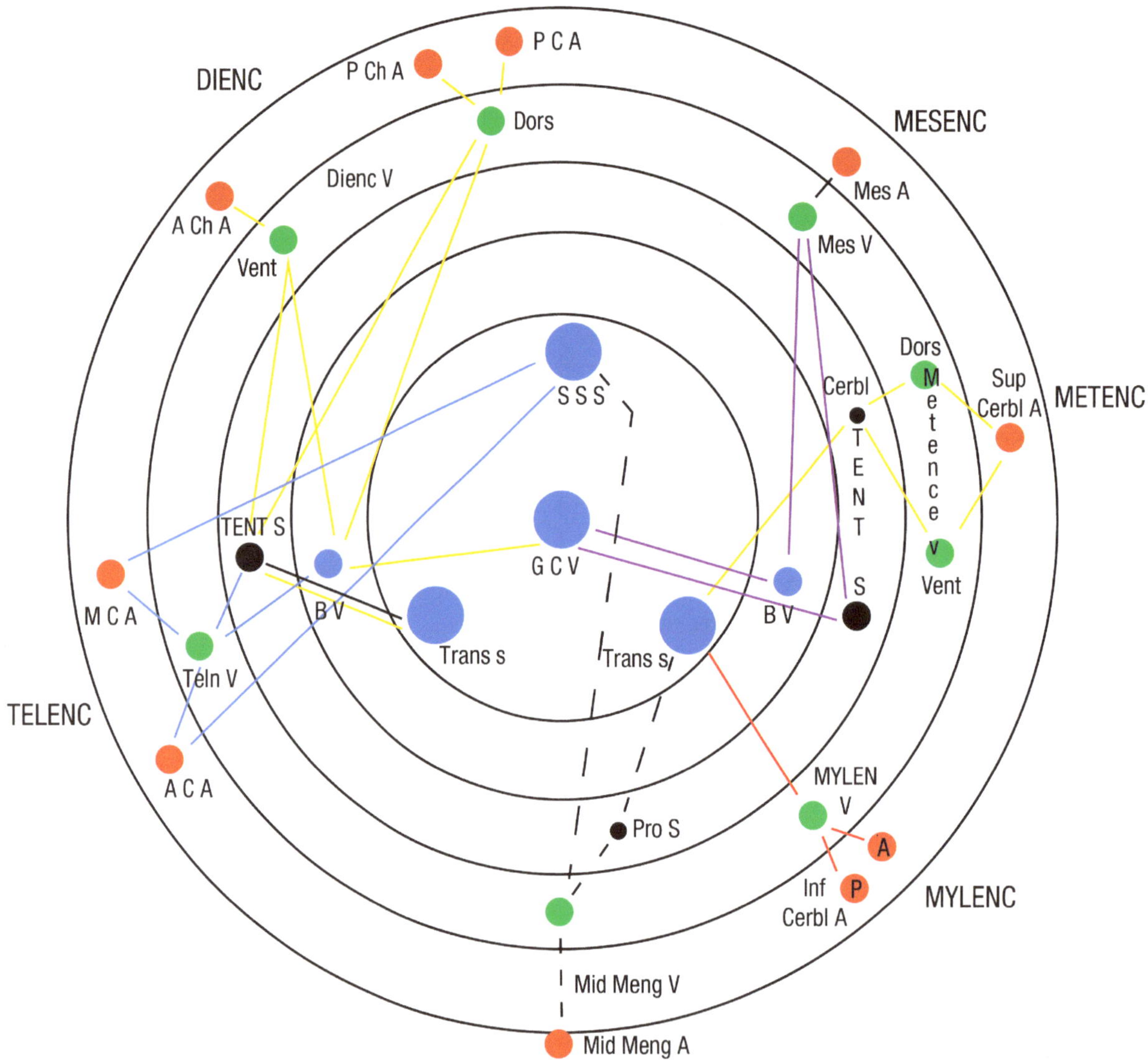

Figure 14.15 Diagrammatic representation of the persistent venous channels in cerebral AVMs.

References

1. Adams, W. E. — 'The Possible Homologies of the Occipital Artery in Mammals, with Some Remarks on the Phylogeny and Certain Anomalies of the Subclavian and Carotid Arteries'. Acta. Anat. 1957, 29: 90–113.
2. Agee, O. F., & Green, M. — 'Anomalous Cephalic Venous Drainage in Association with Aneurysm of the Great Vein of Galen'. Radiology 1967, 88: 725–729.
3. Agee, O. F., Musella, R., & Tweed, C. G. — 'Aneurysm of the Great Vein of Galen – Report of 2 Cases'. J. Neurosurg. 1969, 31: 346–351.
4. Alaraj, A., et al. — *Changes in Wall Shear Stress of Cerebral Arteriovenous Malformation Feeder Arteries After Embolization and Surgery.* Stroke, 2015. 46(5): p. 1216-1220.
5. Alexander, W. S. — 'Cerebral Calcification Epilepsy: Report of a Case of Epilepsy Caused by a Calcified Haematoma of the Brain'. J. Neurosurg. 1953, 10: 69–74.
6. Alpers, B. J., & Forster, F. M. — 'Arterio-venous Aneurysm of the Great Cerebral Vein and Arteries of the Circle of Willis'. Arch. Neurol. Psychiat. 1945, 54: 181–185.
7. Amacher, A. L., & Shillito, J. — 'The Syndromes and Surgical Treatment of Aneurysm of the Great Vein of Galen'. J. Neurosurg. 1973, 39: 89–96.
8. Amico, G., Macchi, L., & Parmeggiani,A. — 'Malformazioni Vascolari Epicraniche Drenantisi nei Seni Durali Posteriori'. Minerva Neurochir. 1970, 14: 324–329.
9. Antoni, N. — 'Spinal Vascular Malformation (Angioma) and Myelo melecia'.correct Neurology 1962, 12: 795–804.
10. Arey, L. B. — *Developmental Anatomy (W. B. Saunders, Philadelphia and London, 1965).*
11. Arieti, S., & Gray, E. W. — 'Progressive Multiform Angiosis'. Arch. Neurol. Psychiat.1944, 51: 182–189.
12. Askenasy, H. M., Herzberger, E. E., & Wijsenbeek, H. S. — 'Hydrocephalus with Vascular Malformation of the Brain: A Preliminary Report'. Neurology 1953, 3: 213–220.
13. Bailey, O. T. — 'The Vascular Component of Congenital Malformations in the Central Nervous System'. J. Neuropath. Exp. Neurol. 1961, 20: 170–184.
14. Balo, J. — 'The Dural Venous Sinuses', in Symposium of Intracranial Abnormalities, Anatomical Records, 1950, 106: 319–325.
15. Bassett, R. C. — 'Surgical Experience with A.V. Anomalies of the Brain'. J. Neurosurg. 1951, 8: 59–74.
16. Batjer HH, Devous MD, Seiber GB, Purdy P, Ajmani AK, Delarosa M and Bont F. — Intracranial arteriovenous malformation. Relationships between clinical and radiographic factors and ipsilateral steal severity. Neurosurgery 23(3): 322- 327, 1988.
17. Beck, D. J. K. — 'Operable Intra-cranial Haemorrhage'. Proc. R. Soc. Med. 1954, 47: 700–701.
18. Bedford, T. H. B. — 'Great Vein of Galen and Syndrome of Increased Intra-cranial Pressure'. Brain 1934, 57: 1–24.

19. Benda, C., Henke, F., & Lubarsch, O. — Handbuch Der Speziellen Pathologischen Anatomie, Vol. 2 (Berlin: Julius Springer, 1924).

20. Bergstrand, H. Olivecrona, J. Ladenheim — Congenital Arterio-venous Aneurysms of the Carotid and Vertebral Arterial Systems (Berlin, Gottingen, Heidelberg: Springer-Verlag, 1957).

21. Bessonov, N., et al. — *Methods of Blood Flow Modelling.* Mathematical Modelling of Natural Phenomena, 2016. **11**(1): p. 1-25. Page | 75

22. Blair, G.S. — *An equation for the flow of blood, plasma and serum through glass capillaries.* 1959. Methods in Angiology. Martinus Nijhoff Publishers,The Hague/Burton/London.

23. Bloom, W., Fawcett, D. W. — *A Textbook of Histology, 10th edn. Philadelphia-London-Toronto: W.B. Saunders Company; Tokyo: Igaku Shoin Ltd., 1975.*

24. Boldrey, E., & Miller, E. R. — 'A.V. Fistula of the Great Cerebral Vein of Galen and Aneurysm of the Circle of Willis. Report on 2 Patients Treated by Ligation'. Arch. Neurol. Psychiat. 1949, 62: 778–784.

25. Bort, J.D. — Beitrag zur Kenntnis des Angioma Racemosum des Gehirns, Inaug. Dissert. Leipzig, Arb. a.d. Geb. d. Path. Anat. Inst. zu Tubingen, 1920.

26. Bosher, Jnr., L. H., Harper, F., & Bigger, I. A. — 'A Study of the Collateral Circulation after Excision of Arterio-venous Fistula'. Surgery 1949, 26: 918.

27. Boucquey, J. P. — 'Angiomes Arterioveineux et Aneurysmes de la fosse Posterieure'. Acta. Neurol. Belg.1965, 65: 335–348.

28. Boyd, W. — *Pathology for the Physician, 7th edn. (London: Henry Kimpton, 1965).*

29. Brady, A., — *Simulating cerebral arteriovenous fistula blood flow as both pipe and duct flow*, in *School of Engineering and IT*. 2005, University of Sydney.

30. Brion, S., Netsky, M. G., & Zimmerman, H. M. — 'Vascular Malformations of the Spinal Cord'. Arch. Neurol. Psychiat. (Chicago) 1952, 68: 339–361.

31. Brock, S., & Dyke, C. — 'Venous and Arterio-venous Angiomas of the Brain'. Bull. Neurol. Inst. New York 1932, 2: 247.

32. Brown, RD, Wiebers, DO, Torner, JC & O'fallon, MW — 'Incidence and prevalence of intracranial vascular malformations in Olmsted County, Minnesota, 1965 to 1992', *Neurology,* vol. 46, no. 4, pp. 949-952, 1996.

33. Browne, Sir T. — Religio Medici, 1642, 14. That is an old ref correct

34. Buis DR, van den Gerg R, Lycklama G, van derWorp HB, Driven CM, vandertop WP. — Spontaneous regression of brain arteriovenous malformations – a clinical study and a sytematic review of the literature. J. Neurol 251(11):1375-82, 2004.

35. Bushby D. and Burton A. — The effect of age on the elasticity of the major brain arteries.Can J Physiol Pharmacol. 43:185- 190, 2002.

36. Callander, C. L. — 'Study of Arterio-venous Fistula with an Analysis of 447 Cases'. Ann. Surg. 1920, 71: 428.

37. Campbell, A. C. P. — 'The Vascular Architecture of the Cat's Brain. A Study of Vital Injection in the Circulation of the Brain and Spinal Cord'. Res. Publ. Assoc. Res. Nerv. Ment. Dis. Pub. Chap. 3. 18: 69–93.1946

38. Caram, P. C., Sharkey, P. C., & Alvord, Jnr., E. — 'Thalamic Angioma and Aneurysm of the Anterior Choroidal Artery with Intra-ventricular Haematoma'. J. Neurosurg. 1960, 17: 347–352.

39. Carroll, C. P., & Jakoby, R. K. 'Neo-natal Congestive Heart Failure as the Presenting Symptom and Cerebral Arterio-Venous Malformations'. J. Neurosurg. 1966, 25: 159–163.

40. Carton, C. A., & Hickey, W. C. 'Arterio-venous Malformation of Head of Caudate Nucleus. Report of Case with Total Removal'. J. Neurosurg. 1955, 12: 414.

41. Casikar, V., G.S. Ramaswamy, and V. Vidyasagar *Observations on the flow characteristics of blood flow in arteriovenous fistulae (experimental).* Cardiovasc Eng, 2010. 10(2): p. 66-77.

42. Castellano, F., Troisi, F., & Vitale, A. 'Intracranial Arterio-venous Aneurysm of Vertebro-Basilar System. Preliminary Note (in Italian)'. Minerva Neurochir. 1962, 6: 103.

43. Chapman, W. B. 'The Effect of the Heart-beat on the Vascular System in the Chick'. Am. J. Anat. 1928, 23(1): 175.

44. Cipolla, M.J. *Control of Cerebral Blood Flow*, in *The Cerebral Circulation*. 2009, Morgan & Claypool Life Sciences: San Rafael: CA.

45. Ciminello, V. J., & Sachs, Jnr., E. 'Arterio-venous Malformations of the Posterior Fossa'. J. Neurosurg. 1962, 19: 602–604.

46. Claireaux, A. E., & Newman, C. G. 'Arterio-venous Aneurysm of the Great Vein of Galen with Heart Failure in Neo-natal Period'. Arch. Dis. Child. 1960, 35: 605–612.

47. Clark, E. R. 'Studies on the Growth of Blood Vessels in the Tail of the Frog Larva – By Observation and Experiment on the Living Animal'. Am. J. Anat. 1928, 23(1): 37.

48. Cohen, M. M., Kristiansen, K., & Hival, E. 'Arteriovenous Malformations of the Great Vein of Galen'. Neurology 1954, 4: 124–127.

49. Constantiono A, Vintners HV. A pathogenic correlate of the "Steal" phenomenon in a patient with cerebral arteriovenous malformation, Stroke 17: 103-106, 1986.

50. Copley, A. *Apparent viscosity and wall adherence of blood systems*. 1960: Pergamon Press, Oxford, UK.

51. Corliss, C. E. *Patten's Human Embryology. New York: McGraw-Hill Book Co., 1976.*

52. Corrin, B. 'Three Cases of Intracranial Vascular Malformations in Infants'. American Journal Of Clinical Pathology.1959, 12: 412–418.

53. Costantino, A. and H. Vinters *A pathologic correlate of the'steal'phenomenon in a patient with cerebral arteriovenous malformation.* Stroke, 1986. **17**(1): p. 103-106.

54. Courville, C. B., & Abbott, K. H. 'Angioblastic Group of Meningiomas. Study of 13 Verified Cases'. Bull. Los Angeles Neurol. Soc. 1940, 5: 47.

55. Crawford, J. V., & Russell, D. S. 'Cryptic Arterio-venous and Venous Haematomas of the Brain'. J. Neurol. Neurosurg. Psychiat. 1956, N.S. omit19: 1–11.

56. Cronqvist, J., Granholm, L., & Lundstrom, N. R. 'Hydrocephalus and Congestive Heart Failure Caused by Intra-cranial Arterio-venous Malformations in Infants'. J. Neurosurg. 1972, 36: 249–254.

57. Cushing, H., & Bailey, P. Tumours Arising from the Blood Vessels of the Brain: Angiomatous Malformations and Haemangioblastomas (Springfield, IL: Charles C. Thomas, 1928, p. 219).

58. Cushing, H., & Eisenhardt, L. Meningioma (Springfield, IL:Charles C.Thomas,1938, ch1, p.506

59. Dandy, W. E. 'Arterio-venous Aneurysms of the Brain'. Arch. Surg. 1928, 17: 190–243.

60. Davidoff, L. M. 'Intra-cerebral Haemorrhage Associated with Hypertension and Arterio-sclerosis'. J. Neurosurg. 1958, 15: 322–328.

61. Delman, M. 'Posterior Fossa Arterio-venous Malformations'. Am. J. Ophthalmol. 1963, 56: 409–413.

62. De Haan, R. L. yes 'The Heart', in J. W. Hurst and R. B. Logue (Eds.), Embryology of the Heart (McGraw-Hill Book Co., The Blakiston Division, New York, St. Louis, San Francisco, London, Sydney, Toronto, Mexico, Panama, 1970).

63. Desai, D.P.K. *Cerebral arteriovenous malformation*, in *Radiopaedic*, L.i.c.a.L. projection, Editor. n.d., Radiopaedic. p. DSA angriogram confirms AVM on right side with PCA and MCA feeding branches on ipsilateral side. Venous drainage apparent into superior sagittal sinus. PCA feeder artery has a aneurysm.

64. Deshpande DH, Vidyasagar C. Histology of persistent embryonic veins in arteriovenous malformations of brain; Acta Neurochirurgica 52:,227-236, 1980.

65. Deutsch G. Blood flow changes in arteriovenous malformation during behavioural activities, Ann Neurol 13: 38-43, 1983.

66. Di Chiro, G., & Wener, L. 'Angiography of the Spinal Cord. A Review of Temporary Techniques and Applications'. J. Neurosurg. 1973, 39(1): 1–25.

67. Djurberg HG, Tjan GT. Anaesthesia for Superselective Embolisation of Cerebral Arterio-Venous Malformations. Pan Arab – Journals 12; 1-17, Oct 1996.

68. Doane, J. C., & Kravitz, C. H. 'Pathological and Physiological Consideration in Arterio-venous Fistulas'. Am. J. Surg. 1947, 73: 713–716.

69. Dott, N. M., & MacCabe, J. *Arterio-venous Malformations of the Brain, Ann. Mtg. Harvey Cushing Soc., Philadelphia, April 1963.*

70. Drake, C.T. and C. Iadecola *The role of neuronal signalling in controlling cerebral blood flow.* Brain Lang, 2007. **102**(2): p. 141-52. Parida, A. and P. Chand, *Turbulent swirl with gas—solid flow in cyclone.* Chemical Engineering Science, 1980. **35**(4): p. 949-954.

71. Duong DH, Vang MC, Sciacca RR, Mast H, Koennecke H, Hartman A, Joshi S, Mohr JP, Pile-Spellman J. Feeding Artery Pressure and Venous Drainage Pattern Are Primary Determinants of Hemorrage From Cerebral Arteriovenous Malformations. Stroke 29:1167-1176, 1998.

72. Duong, D.H., et al. *Feeding artery pressure and venous drainage pattern are primary determinants of haemorrhage from cerebral arteriovenous malformations.* Stroke, 1998. **29**(6): p. 1167-76. Page 76- 81.

73. Edgar, R., & Baldwin, M. 'Vascular Malformation Associated with Temporal Lobe Epilepsy'. J. Neurosurg. 1960, 17: 638.

74. Eisenbrey, A. B., & Hegarty, W. M. 'Trigeminal Neuralgia and Arterio-venous Aneurysm of Cerebello-pontine Angle'. J. Neurosurg. 1956, 13: 647.

75. Elkin, D. C. 'Cirsoid Aneurysm of the Scalp'. Ann. Surg. 1924, 80: 332.

76. Elkin, D. C., & Warren, J. V. 'Arterio-venous Fistulas. Their Effects on Circulation'. J. Am. Med. Assoc. 1947, 134: 1524–1528.

77. Evans, N. G., & Courville, C. B. 'Notes on the Pathogenesis and Morphology of New Growths, Malformations and Deformities of the Intra-cranial Blood Vessels'. Bull. Los Angeles Neurol. Soc. 1939, 4: 145–167.

78. Fadhli, H. A. — 'Congenital Arterio-venous Fistula Involving the Occipital Artery and Lateral Venous Sinus – Case Report'. J. Neurosurg. 1969, 30: 299–300.

79. Fincher, E. F. — 'Arterio-venous Fistula Between the Middle Meningeal Artery and Greater Petrosal Sinus. Case Report'. Ann. Surg. 1951, 133: 886–888.

80. Fincher, C. M. — 'The Pathology and Pathogenesis of Intra-cerebral Haemorrhage', in W. S. Fields (Ed.), Pathogenesis and Treatment of Cerebro-vascular Disease (Springfield, IL: Charles C. Thomas, 1961, xii, pp. 562.

81. French, L. A., & Peyton, W. T. — 'Vascular Malformations in the Region of the Great Vein of Galen'. J. Neurosurg. 1954, 11: 488–498.

82. Fritz, S., L. Chaitow, and G.M. Hymel — *CHAPTER 6 - Review of Pertinent Anatomy and Physiology*, in *Clinical Massage in the Healthcare Setting*. 2008, Mosby: Saint Louis. p. 140-195.

83. Fung, Y.C. and S.Q. Liu — *Determination of the mechanical properties of the different layers of blood vessels in vivo.* Proceedings of the National Academy of Sciences of the United States of America, 1995. **92**(6): p. 2169-2173.

84. Gagnon, J., & Boileau, G. — 'Anatomical Study of an Arterio-venous Malformation Drained by the System of Galen'. J. Neurosurg. 1960, 17: 75–80.

85. Gannon, W. E. — 'Malformations of the Brain. Persistent Trigeminal Artery and Arterio-venous Malformations'. Arch. Neurol. (Chicago) 1962, 6: 496–498.

86. Garner yes, D. L., Dodds, T. C. — *Human Histology, 3rd edn. Edinburgh-London-New York: Churchill Livingstone, 1976.*

87. Gao E,Young WL,Ornstein E, Pile-Spellman J, Qiyuan MA. — Theoretical Model of Cerebral Haemodynamics. Application to the Study of Arteriovenous Malformations,Journal of CerebralBlood Flow & Metabolism 17:905-918, 1997.

88. Gao, E.Z., et al. — *Theoretical modelling of arteriovenous malformation rupture risk: a feasibility and validation study.* Medical Engineering & Physics, 1998. **20**(7): p. 489-501.

89. Geibpraser,S MD ,Pongpech, S MD • Jiarakongmun, P MD • Shroff, M MD Armstrong, D MD , Krings,T MD, PhD — Radiographics

90. Gerbode, F., Holman, E., Dickenson, E., & Spencer, R. — 'Arterio-venous Fistula and Artery Aneurysm'. Surgery 1952, 32: 259.

91. Gerlach, J., & Jensen, H. P. — a) 'Mikroangiome des Gehirns'. Arch. Klin. Chir. 1960, 293: 481–493.

b) 'Die Intracerebralen Hamatome Bei Mikroangiomen'. Acta. Neurochir. 1961, 7 (Suppl.) 367–373.

92. Gibbs, E. L., & Gibbs, F. A. — 'The Cross Section Area of the Vessels That Form the Torcula and the Manner in Which Flow Is Distributed to the Right and to the Left Lateral Sinus'. Anat. Rec. 1934, 59: 419–425.

93. Gibson, J. B., Taylor, A. R., & Richardson, A. E. — 'Congenital Arterio-venous Fistula with an Aneurysm of the Great Cerebellar Vein and Hydrocephalus Treated Surgically'. J. Neurol. Neurosurg. Psychiat. 1959, 22: 224–228.

94. Gillingham, J. — 'Arterio-venous Malformations of the Head'. Edin. Med. J. 1953, 60: 305–315.

95. Glatt, B. S., & Rowe, R. D. 'Cerebral Arterio-venous Fistula Associated with Congestive Heart Failure in the Newborn: Report of 2 Cases'. Paediatrics 1960, 26: 596–603

96. Globus, J. H ' Classification of Vascular Meningeal Tumors with Meningioma'. Arch. Neurol. Psychiat. 1937, 38: 677..

97. Gold, A., Ransohoff, J., & Carter, S. 'Vein of Galen Malformation'. Acta. Neurol. Scand. 1964, 11(40, Suppl.): 1–31.

98. Goldberger AL, West BJ. Fractals in Physiology and Medicine. Yale Journal of Biology and Medicine 60:421-435, 1987.

99. Goldberger AL,West BJ. Chaos and Fractals in human physiology. Scientific American :36-41, Feb 1990.

100. Golkar A Personal collection

101. Gomez, M. R., Whitten, C. F., Nolke, A., Bernstein, J., & Meyer, J. G. 'Aneurysmal Malformation of the Great Vein of Galen Causing Heart Failure'. Paediatrics 1963, 31: 400–411.

102. Grant, J. C. B. *An Atlas of Anatomy (London: Bailliere, Tindall & Cox, 1947).*

103. Grinker, R. R., & Sahs, A. L. *Neurology, 6th edn. (Springfield, IL: Charles C. Thomas, 1966, pp. 947–961).*

104. Gross, S. W., & Ralston, B. L. 'Vascular Malformations of the Spinal Cord'. Surg. Gynaecol. Obstet. 1959, 108: 673–678.

105. Gurdjian, E. S., Thomas, L. M., Scrath, G. P., & Darmody, W. R. 'Intra-cranial Aneurysms, Arterio-venous Malformations and Subarachnoid Haemorrhage', W. S. Fields and A. L. Sahs (Eds.). Springfield, IL: Charles. C. Thomas, 1965, pp. 143–183.

106. Ha, H., et al. *Effect of swirling blood flow on vortex formation at post-stenosis.* Proc Inst Mech Eng H, 2015. **229**(2): p. 175-83.

107. Hademenos GJ, Massoud TF, Vinuela F: A Biomathematical Model of IntracranialArteriovenous Malformations Based on Eletrical Network Analysis: Theory and Hemodynamics. Neurosurgery 38(5):1005-1015, May 1996.

108. Hademenos GJ, Massoud TF. Risk of Intracranial Arteriovenous Malformation Rupture Due to Venous Drainage Impairment. Stroke 27: 1072-1083, 1996.

109. Hademenos, GJ, Massoud, TF 'Biophysical mechanisms of stroke', *Stroke,* vol. 28, no. 10, pp. 2067-77, 1997.

110. Hademenos, G.J., T.F. Massoud, and F. Vinuela *A biomathematical model of intracranial arteriovenous malformations based on electrical network analysis: theory and hemodynamics.* Neurosurgery, 1996. **38**(5): p. 1005-14; discussion 1014-5.

111. Hamby, W. B. 'Pathology of Supra-tentorial Angioma'. J. Neurosurg. 1958, 15: 65.

112. Hamby, R. I., & Desposito, F. 'Congenital Intradural Arterio-venous Fistula and Congestive Heart Failure in Infancy'. J. Paediat. 1962, 61: 590–594.

113. Hamby, W. B., & Gardner, W. J. 'Treatment of Pulsating Exophthalmos'. Arch. Surg. 1933, 27: 676–685.

114. Hamel, E. *Perivascular nerves and the regulation of cerebrovascular tone.* J Appl Physiol (1985), 2006. **100**(3): p. 1059-64.

115. Hamilton, W. J., Boyd, J. D., & Mossman, H. W. *Human Embryology (Cambridge: W. Heffer & Sons, Ltd., 1962).*

116. Hanford, J. M., & Wheeler, J. M. 'Pulsating Exophthalmos'. Arch. Surg. 1930, 92: 8–22.

117. Hassler, O. 'Medical Defects in the Meningeal Arteries'. J. Neurosurg. 1962, 19: 337–340.

118. Hayashi K, Handa H, Nagasawa S, Okumura A, Moritaki K. Stiffness and elastic behahvior of human intracranial and extra cranial arteries. J Biochem 13:175-179, 1980.

119. Hedon, C. E. Etude Anatomique sur la Circulation Veineuse de l'Encephale. Doctoral Thesis, Bordeaux, 1888, p. 96.

120. Heine, L. Ztschr F. Augena 51: 1, 1923.

121. Hernandez, Jnr., A., Schwartz, H. G., & Goldring, D. 'Cerebral Arterio-venous Fistula and Congenital Heart Disease'. J. Pediat. 1962, 61: 590–594.

122. Herren, R. Y., & Alexander, L. 'Sulcal and Intrinsic Blood Vessels of the Human Spinal Cord'. Arch. Neurol. Psychiat. 1939, 416: 678–687.

123. Hirano, A., & Solomon, S. 'Arterio-venous Aneurysm of the Vein of Galen'. Am. Arch. Neurol. 1960, 3: 589–593.

124. Hochstetter, F. Ueber eine Varietat der Vena Cerebralis basialis des Menschen nebst Bemerkungen uber die Entwicklung bestimmter. Hirnvenen. Ztschr. f. Anat. v. Entwicklungesch 1938, 108: 311–336.

125. Holden, A. M., Fyler, D. C., Shillito, Jnr., J., et al. 'Congestive Heart Failure from Intracranial Arterio-venous Fistula in Infancy – Clinical and Physiological Considerations in 8 Patients'. Paediatrics 1972, 49: 30–39.

126. Holman, E. 'The Physiology of an Arterio-venous Fistula'. Arch. Surg. 1923, 7: 64.

127. Holman, E. 'Arterio-venous Fistula. Dilatation of the Artery Distal to the Abnormal Communication'. Arch. Surg. 1929, 18: 1672.

128. Holman, E. *Arterio-venous Aneurysm (New York: McMillan Co., 1937).*

129. Holman, E. 'The Anatomic and Physiologic Effects of an Arterio-venous Fistula'. Surgery 1940, 8: 362.

130. Holman, E. 'Problems Encountered in the Dynamics of Blood Flow. I. Conditions controlling collateral Circulation in the Presence of an Arterio-venous Fistula Following Ligation of an Artery'. Surgery 1949, 26: 889.

131. Holman E. Arteriovenous fistula, dilatation of the artery distal to abnormal Communication Arch. Surg 18: 1672-1680, 1929.

132. Holman E. The anatomic and physiological effects of an arteriovenous fistula, Surg 8: 362-368, 1940.

133. Holman E. Problems encountered in the dynamics of blood flow me. Conditionscontrolling collateral circulation in the presence of an arteriovenous fistula following the ligation of an artery. Surg. 26: 889 – 894, 1949

134. Holman, E., & Taylor, G. 'Problems in the Dynamics of Blood Flow. II. Pressure Relations at Site of an Arterio-venous Fistula'. Angiology 1952, 3: 415–430.

135. Homan RW, Devous MD, Strokely EM, Bonte FJ. Quantification of intracerebral steal in patients with arteriovenous malformations Arch Neurol 13 (8): 779 – 85, Aug 1986.

136. Hook, O., & Johanson, C. 'Intracranial Arterio-venous Aneurysms: A Follow-up Study with Particular Attention to Their Growth'. Arch. Neurol. Psychiat. 1958, 80: 39–54.

137. Hook, O., Werko, L., & Ohrberg, G. 'Intracranial Arterio-venous Aneurysms. A Study of Their Effects on the Cardio-vascular System'. Arch. Neurol. Psychiat. (Chicago) 1958, 79: 622–632.

138. Houdart, R., Djindjian, R., & Hurth, M. 'Vascular Malformations of the Spinal Cord. The anatomic and Therapeutic Significance of Arteriography'. J. Neurosurg. 1966, 24: 583–594.

139. Huang, Y. P., Wolf, B. S., & Antin, S. P. 'The Veins of Posterior Fossa, Anterior or Petrosal Draining Group'. Am. J. Roentgenol. 1968, 104: 36–56.

140. Hyman, L. H. *Comparative Vertebrate Anatomy (Chicago and London: The University of Chicago Press, 1968).*

141. Jacas, R., Ley, A., & Campillo, D. 'Congenital Intra-orbital Arterio-venous Aneurysm'. J. Neurol. Neurosurg. Psychiat. 1959, 22: 330.

142. Jaeger, R. 'Arterio-venous Aneurysm of the Brain: Report of Case Cured by Clipping Middle Cerebral Artery'. J. Neurosurg. 1951, 8: 335.

143. Jaeger, J. R., Forbes, A. P., & Dandy, W. E. 'Bilateral Congenital Cerebral Arterio-venous Communication Aneurysm'. Trans. Am. Neurol. Ann. 1937, 63: 173–176.

144. Johnson, M. C., & Salmon, J. H. 'Arterio-venous Malformation Presenting as a Trigeminal Neuralgia'. J. Neurosurg. 1968, 29: 287–289.

145. Jo-Yu, W. and R. Lee *The advantages of triangular and tetrahedral edge elements for electromagnetic modelling with the finite-element method.* IEEE Transactions on Antennas and Propagation, 1997. **45**(9): p. 1431-1437.

146. Kamiya, A. and T. Togawa *Adaptive regulation of wall shear stress to flow change in the canine carotid artery.* Am J Physiol, 1980. **239**(1): p. H14-21.

147. Kaplan, H. A., Aronson, S. M., & Browder, E. J. 'Vascular Malformations of the Brain. Anatomical Study'. J. Neurosurg. 1961, 18: 630–635.

148. Kim, H., et al. *Brain arteriovenous malformation pathogenesis: a response-to-injury paradigm.* Acta Neurochir Suppl, 2011. **111**: p. 83-92.

149. Knisely, C.W., K. Nishihara, and M. Iguchi *Critical Reynolds Number in Constant-Acceleration Pipe Flow From an Initial Steady Laminar State.* Journal of Fluids Engineering, 2010. **132**(9): p. 091202-091202.

150. Komiyama, M. *Pathogenesis of Brain Arteriovenous Malformations.* Neurologica medico-chirurgica, 2016. **56**(6): p. 317-325.

151. Kosnik, E. J., Hunt, W. E., & Miller, C. A. 'Dural Arterio-venous Malformations'. J. Neurosurg. 1974, 40: 322.

152. Krauss, J.K., G.D. Kiriyanthan, and J.J. Borremans *Cerebral arteriovenous malformations and movement disorders.* Clin Neurol Neurosurg, 1999. **101**(2): p. 92-9.

153. Krayenbuhl, H. 'Discussion Des Angiomes Supratentoriels'. Brussels Acta. Med. Belgica 1957, vol 7 263–267. Int. Congr. Neurol. Surg. (Brussels, 1957).

154. Krayenbuhl, H., & Siebenman, R. 'Small Vascular Malformations as a Cause of Primary Intra-cerebral Haemorrhage'. J. Neurosurg. 1965, 22: 7–20.

155. Krayenbuhl, H., & Yasargil, M. G.
156. Krueger EG, Sobel GL. Schobinger RA

The function of the vertebral veins and their role in the spread of metastases. Ann Surg 1940 ...Cerebral Angiography (London: Butterworth & Co., 1968).

157. Krumhar D, Schulz U. Quantitative evaluation of retrograde arterial flow in chronic experimental AVFs Basic Res. Cardiol 70: 29-45, 1970.

158. Kushner, J., & Alexander, Jnr., E. 'Partial Spontaneous Regressive Arterio-venous Malformation: Case Report with Angiographic Evidence'. J. Neurosurg. 1970, 32: 360–366.

159. Laplace, L. B. 'Observations on the Effect of an Arterio-venous Fistula on the Human Circulation'. Am. J. Med. Sci. 1935, 189: 497–507.

160. Laplace, L. B. Cardio-vascular System'. Arch. Neurol. Psychiat. (Chicago) 1958.

161. Lasheras, J.C. *The biomechanics of arterial aneurysms.* Annu. Rev. Fluid Mech., 2007. **39**: p. 293-319.

162. Lazorthes, G., Gouuze, A., Zadeh, J. O., et al. 'Arterial Vascularization of the Spinal Cord: Recent Studies of the Anastomotic Substitution Pathways'. J. Neurosurg. 1971, 35: 253–262.

163. Lehman, Jnr., J. S., Chynn, K. Y., Hagstrona, J. W. C., et al. 'Heart Failure in Infancy due to Arterio-venous Malformations of the Vein of Galen. Report of a Case'. Am. J. Roentgenol. 1966, 98: 653–659.

164. Levine, O. R., Jameson, A. G., Hellhaus, G., & Gold, A. P. 'Cardiac Complications of Cerebral Arterio-venous Fistula in Infancy'. Paediatrics 1972, 30: 563–575.

165. Lewis, T. 'The Adjustment of Blood Flow to the Affected Limb in Arterio-venous Fistula'. Clin. Sci. 1940, 4: 277.

166. Lindegaard KF,Grolimund P, Aaslid R, Nornes H. Evaluation of cerebral AVM's using trancranial Doppler ultrasound., J. Neurosurgery 65(3):335-344, Sep 1986.

167. Litvak, J., Yahr, M. D., & Ransohoff, J. 'Aneurysms of the Great Vein of Galen and Midline Cerebral Arterio-venous Malformations'. J. Neurosurg. 1960, 17: 945–954.

168. Locke, C. E. 'Intracranial Arterio-venous Aneurysms or Pulsating Exophthalmos'. Ann. Surg. 1924, 80: 1–24.

169. Logue, V., & Monckton, G. 'Posterior Fossa Angiomas – Clinical Presentation of 9 Cases'. Brain 1954, 77: 252.

170. Lombardi, G., & Migliavacca, F. 'Angioma of the Spinal Cord'. Brit. J. Radiol. 1959, 32: 810–814.

171. Lombardi, G., & Passain, A. *Spinal Cord Diseases (Baltimore: William and Wilkins, 1964).*

172. Louge FC, Giobano JM, Hobson RW. Regional haemodynamics of large and small femoral arteriovenous fistulae in dogs, Surg. 79(3): 346-349, 1975.

173. Luessenhop AJ. Natural history of cerebral arteriovenous malformation. In Wilson CV, Stein BM (Ed) Intracranial arteriovenous malformation, Baltimore, Williams and Wilkins, 1984 pp 12-23.

174. Luessenhop, A. J., Kachmann, Jnr., R., Shevlin, W., & Ferrero, A. A. 'Clinical Evaluation of Artificial Embolization in the Management of Large Cerebral Arterio-venous Malformation'. J. Neurosurg. 1965, 23: 400–417.

175. Luessenhop AJ, Genrallie TA. Anatomical grading of supratentorial arteriovenous malformations through internal carotid and vertebral arteries, Long term results, J. Neurosurg 42: 443-451, 1997.

176. Lumsden, C. E. 'A Case of Aneurysm of the Vein of Galen'. J. Pathol. Bacteriol. 1947, 59: 328–331.

177. Manchola I F, De Sallesa AA, Kok FT, Ackerman RH, Candia GT, Kjellberg RN. Arteriovenous malformation haemodynamics:a transcranial Doppler study.1:Neurosurgery 33 (4): 556-562, Oct 1993.

178. Marmarou, A., K. Shulman, and J. La Morgese *Compartmental analysis of compliance and outflow resistance of the cerebrospinal fluid system.* J Neurosurg, 1975. **43**(5): p. 523-34.

179. Mast, H., et al. *'Steal' is an unestablished mechanism for the clinical presentation of cerebral arteriovenous malformations.* Stroke, 1995. **26**(7): p. 1215-20.

180. McCormick, W. F. 'Pathology of Vascular Malformations'. J. Neurosurg. 1966, 24: 806.

181. McCormick, W. F., & Boulter, T. R. 'Vascular Malformation "Angiomas" of the Dura Mater. Report of 2 Cases'. J. Neurosurg. 1966, 25: 309–311.

182. McGuire, J. 'Circulatory Studies on a Case of Arterio-venous Aneurysm'. Ann. Heart J. 1935, 10: 360–366.

183. McGuire, T. H., Greenwood, J., & Newton, B. L. 'Bilateral Angioma of Choroid Plexus. Case Report'. J. Neurosurg. 1954, 11: 428.

184. McKissock, W., & Walsh, L. 'Subarachnoid Haemorrhage Due to Intra-cranial Aneurysm'. Results of Treatment of 249 Verified Cases'. Brit. Med. J. 1956, 2: 559–565.

185. Mackenzie, I. 'Clinical Presentation of the Cerebral Angioma. Review of 50 Cases'. Brain 1953, 76: 184–214.

186. Manuelidis, E. E. 'Uber Hamangiome Des Gehirns'. Arch. Psychiat. 1950, 184: 601–645.

187. Margolis, G., Odom, G. L., Woodhall, B., & Bloor, B. M. 'The Role of Small Angiomatous Malformations in the Production of Intra-cerebral Hematoma'. J. Neurosurg. 1951, 8: 564–575.

188. Marks, MP, Odonahue, J, Fabricant, JI, Frankel, KA, Phillips, MH, Delapaz, RL & Enzmann, DR 'Cerebral blood-flow evaluation of arteriovenous-malformations with stable xenon ct', *American Journal of Neuroradiology,* vol. 9, no. 6, pp. 1169-1175, 1988.

189. Marks, MP, Odonahue, J, Fabricant, JI, Frankel, KA, Phillips arteriovenous-malformations with stable xenon ct', American

190. Markham, J. W. 'Arterio-venous Fistula of Middle Meningeal Artery and Greater Petrosal Sinus'. J. Neurosurg. 1951, 18: 847.

191. Maroun, F. B., Jacob, J. C., Markesteyn, P. H., & Mercer, D. R. 'Congenital Venous Malformation of the Scalp Associated with Plexiform Neurofibroma and Cranial Defects'. J. Neurosurg. 1969, 31: 465–467.

192. Martin, Jnr., J. D., & Mabon, R. F. 'Pulsating Exophthalmos. Review of All Reported Cases'. JAMA 1943, 121: 330.

193. Masherpa, F., & Valentino, V. Intra-cranial Calcification (Springfield, IL: Charles C. Thomas, 1959, pp. 58–63).

194. Mast, H, Mohr, JP, Osipov, A, Pile-Spellman, J, Marshall, RS, Lazar, RM, Stein, BM & Young, WL 'Steal' is an unestablished mechanism for the clinical presentation of cerebral arteriovenous malformations', *Stroke,* vol. 26, no. 7, pp. 1215-20, 1995.

195. Mast, H, Young, WL, Koennecke, HC, Sciacca, RR, Osipov, A, Pilespellman, J, Haceinbey, L, Duong, H, Stein, BM & Mohr, JP 'Risk of spontaneous haemorrhage after diagnosis of cerebral arteriovenous malformation', *Lancet,* vol. 350, no. 9084, pp. 1065-1068, 1997.

196. Mayer R. L 'Intra-cranial and Intra-spinal Vascular Anomalies in Children'. J. Neurosurg. 1969, 31:149-156

197. Mayer R L — Intra-cranial and intra spinal vascular Anomalies in children. J Neurosurg.1969,31:149-156.

198. Meleney, F. L. — 'Pathological Study of a Case of Cirsoid Aneurism'. Surg. Gynaecol. Obstet. 1923, 36: 547–553.

199. Miller, JD, Stanek, AE & Langfitt, TW — 'Cerebral blood flow regulation during experimental brain compression', *J Neurosurg,* vol. 39, no. 2, pp. 186-96, 1973.

200. Monson KL, Barbaro NM, Manley GT. — Biaxial response to passive human cerebral arteries. Ann Biomed Eng 36(12); 2028-2041, Dec 2008.

201. Moody, R. A., & Poppen, J. L. — 'Arterio-venous Malformations'. J. Neurosurg. 1970, 32: 503–511.

202. Mount, L. A. — 'Arterio-venous Angioma Derived from the Anterior Inferior Cerebellar Artery. Case Report'. J. Neurosurg. 1965, 22: 612–615.

203. Mourmouras D E, Tsagaadopoulas DG. — On the elastic properties of arteries . J Biomech Nov; 36(1);1727-31,2003.

204. Mulvihill, D. A., & Harvey, S. C. — 'The Mechanism of the Development of Collateral Circulation'. New England J. Med. 1931, 204: 1032.

205. Murayama Y, Usami S, Hata Y, Ganaha F, Hasegawa Y, Terao T, Abe S, Furuhata H, Abe T. — Transvenous Hemodynamic Asssement of Arterivenous Malformations and Fistulas. Stroke 29; 1167-1176, 1988.

206. Nagasawa S, Handa H, Okumura A, Naruo Y, Moritake K, Hayashi K. — Surg Neurol 12(4):297-304, Oct 1979.

207. Nakamura, K., Tsugane, R., Ito, H., Obata, H., & Narita, H. — 'Traumatic Arterio-venous Fistula of the Middle Meningeal Vessels'. J. Neurosurg. 1966, 25: 424–429.

208. Newman, M. J. D. — 'Racemose Angioma of the Spinal Cord'. Quart. J. Med. 1959, 28: 97–108.

209. Newton, T. H., & Cronqvist, S. — 'Involvement of Dural Arteries in Intra-cranial Arterio-venous Malformation.' Radiology 1969, 93: 1071–1078.

210. Newton, T. H., & Greitz, T. — 'Arterio-venous Communication Between the Occipital Artery and the Transverse Sinus'. Radiology 1966, 87: 824–828.

211. Newton, T. H., & Hoyt, W. F. — 'Dural Arterio-venous Shunts in the Region of the Cavernous Sinus'. Neuroradiology 1970, 1: 71–81.

212. Newton, T. H., Weidner, W., & Greitz, T. — 'Dural Arterio-venous Malformations of the Posterior Fossa'. Radiology 1968, 90: 27–35.

213. Nizzoli, N. — 'Dural Arterio-venous Malformations of the Posterior Fossa'. J. Neurosurg. Psychiat. 1968, 31: 514–519.

214. Nomura, T. — *Atlas of Cerebral Angiography (Tokyo: Igaku Shoin, 1970).*

215. Noran, H. H. — 'Intra-cranial Vascular Tumors and Malformations'. Arch. Path. 1945, 39: 393–416.

216. Norlen, G. — 'Arterio-venous Aneurysms of the Brain. Report of 10 cases of Total Removal of the Lesion'. J. Neurosurg. 1949, 6: 475–494.

217. Nornes H, Grip A. — Haemodynamic aspects of cerebral arteriovenous malformations, J. Neurosurgery 53:456-465, 1980.

218. Nornes H . Quantification of altered haemodynamics, in Wilson CB, Stein BM, (ed) Intracranial Arteriovenous Malformations, Baltimore, Williams and Wilkins, pp 32-43, 1984.

219. Nornes, H. and A. Grip *Hemodynamic aspects of cerebral arteriovenous malformations.* J Neurosurg, 1980. **53**(4): p. 456-64.

220. Northfield, D.W.C. 'Angiomatous Malformations of the Brain'. Guys Hosp. Rep. 1940, 90: 149.

221. Numaguchi, Y., et al. *The Arteriovenous Malformation Associated with Major Arterial Occlusion and Moyamoya Vessels: a Cerebral Blood Flow Study.* Interventional Neuroradiology, 2000. **6**(3): p. 185-193.

222. Oberkampf, W.L. and T.G. Trucano *Verification and validation in computational fluid dynamics.* Progress in Aerospace Sciences, 2002. **38**(3): p. 209-272.

223. O'Brien, M. S., & Schechter, M. M. 'Arterio-venous Malformations of the Galenic System'. Radiology 1971, 99: 218; Am. J. Roentgenol. 1970, 110: 50–55.

224. O'Brien, M. S., & Schechter, M. M.. Oberkampf, W.L. and T.G. Trucano Verification and validation in computational fluid dynamics. Progress in Aerospace Sciences, 2002. 38(3): p. 209-272.

225. Odom, G. L., Tindall, G. T., & Dukes, H. T. 'Cerebellar Haematoma Caused by Angiomatous Malformations. Report of 4 Cases'. J. Neurosurg. 1961, 18: 777.

226. Ogilvy C S., M.D. Brain Aneurysm & AVM Center. Combined Modality Treatment in the Management of Brain Arteriovenous Malformations

227. Ogilvy C S. Web Page

228. Okell, T.W., M.A. Chappell, and P. Jezzard *A theoretical framework for quantifying blood volume flow rate from dynamic angiographic data and application to vessel-encoded arterial spin labeling MRI().* Medical Image Analysis, 2013. **17**(8): p. 1025-1036.

229. Olivecrona, H., & Ladenheim, J. *Congenital Arterio-venous Aneurysms of the Carotid and Vertebral Artery (Berlin: Springer-Verlag, 1957, IV. p. 91.*

230. Olivecrona, H., & Riives, J. 'Arterio-venous Aneurysms of the Brain'. Arch. Neurol. Psychiat. 1948, 59: 567–602.

231. Ornstein, E., et al. *A computer simulation of the haemodynamic effects of intracranial arteriovenous malformation occlusion.* Neurol Res, 1994. **16**(5): p. 345-52.

232. Osherwitz, D., & Davidoff, L. M. 'Midline Calcified Intra-cranial Aneurysm Between Occipital Lobes. Report of a Case'. J. Neurosurg. 1947, 4: 539–541.

233. Padget, D. H. 'The Development of the Cranial Venous System in Man from the Viewpoint of Comparative Anatomy'. Contributions to Embryology, Vol. 36 (Washington DC: Carnegie Institute of Washington, Publ. No. 611, 1957, p. 79–140).

234. Padget, D. H. 'The Development of Cranial Arteries in Human Embryology'. Contributions to Embryology, Vol. 32 (Washington DC: Carnegie Institute of Washington, Publ. No. 575, 1948, p.205–261).

235. Padget, D. H. 'Cranial Venous System in Man with Reference to the Development of Adult Configuration in Relation to the Arteries'. Am. J. Anat. 1956, 98: 307–356.

236. Pakarinen, S. 'Arterio-venous Fistula Between the Middle Meningeal Artery and the Sphenoparietal Sinus. Case Report'. J. Neurosurg. 1965, 23: 438–439.

237. Pang Q, Lu X,Gregerson H, von Oettinger G, Astrup J. Biomechanical properties of porcine cerebral bridging veins with reference to the zero- stress state. J Vas Res 38(1);83-90, Jan-Feb 2001.

238. Papaioannou, T.G. and C. Stefanadis *Vascular wall shear stress: basic principles and methods.* Hellenic J Cardiol, 2005. **46**(1): p. 9-15.

239. Parida, A. and P. Chand *Turbulent swirl with gas—solid flow in cyclone.* Chemical Engineering Science, 1980. **35**(4): p. 949-954.

240. Parkinson, D. 'Cerebral Arterio-venous Aneurysm. Surgical Management'. Can. J. Surg. 1958, 1: 313.

241. Paterson, J. H., & McKissock, W. 'Clinical Survey of Intra-cranial Angioma with Special Reference to Their Mode of Prognosis and Surgical Treatment Report of 110 Cases'. Brain 1956, 79: 233.

242. Pedley, T.J., *The Fluid Mechanics of Large Blood Vessels*. 1980: Cambridge University Press.

243. Penfield, W., & Ward, A. 'Calcifying Epileptogenic Lesion'. Arch. Neurol. Psychiat. 1948, 60: 20–36.

244. Perret, G., & Nishioka, H. *Intra-cranial Aneurysms and Subarachnoid Haemorrhage. A Co-operative Study (Philadelphia and Toronto: J.B. Lippincott Co., 1969).*

245. Perret, G., & Nishioka, H. 'Report on the Co-operative Study of Intra-cranial Aneurysms and Subarachnoid Haemorrhage. Section VI. Arterio-venous Malformations'. J. Neurosurg. 1966, 25: 467–490.

246. Pfeifer, R. A. A) Die Angioarchitektonik der Grosshirnrinde (Berlin, 1928, 157 pp.).

B) Grundlegende Untersuchungen Fur Die Angioarchitetonik des Menschlichen Gehirns (Berlin, 1939, 220 p).

247. Pietila TA, Zabramski JM, Thellier-Janko A, Duveneck K, Bichard WD, Brock M, Spetzler RF. Animal model for cerebral arteriovenous malformation, Acta Neurochir (Wien) 142 (11); 1231-40, 2000.

248. Pietila, T.A., et al. *Animal model for cerebral arteriovenous malformation.* Acta Neurochir (Wien), 2000. **142**(11): p. 1231-40.

249. Pollock, A. R., & Lasleth, P. A. 'Cerebral Arterio-venous Fistula Producing Cardiac Failure in the Newborn Infant. Case Report and Review'. J. Neurosurg. 1960, 17: 347–352.

250. Pool, J. L. 'Treatment of Arterio-venous Malformations of Cerebral Hemispheres'. J. Neurosurg. 1962, 19: 136.

251. Pool, J. L. 'Excision of Cerebral Arterio-venous Malformations'. J. Neurosurg. 1968, 29: 312–321.

252. Pool, J. L., & Potts, D. G. *Aneurysms and Arterio-venous Anomalies of the Brain. Diagnosis and Treatment (Harper-Row, Hoeber Med. Division, New York, Evanston, and London).*

253. Poppen, J. L., & Avman, N. 'Aneurysms of the Great Vein of Galen'. J. Neurosurg.1960, 17: 238–244.

254. Potter, J. M. 'Angiomatous Malformations of the Brain, Their Nature and Prognosis'. Ann. R. Coll. Surg. Engl. 1955, 16: 227.

255. Prattipati, N.C. — Study of flow characteristics of blood in an arteriovenous malfunction, in School of Engineering and IT. 2004, University of Sydney 'Angiomatous Malformations of the Brain, Their Nature and Prognosis'. Ann. R. Coll. Surg. Engl. 1955, 16: 227.

256. Prensky, A. L., & Gado, M. — 'Angiographic Resolution of a Neonatal Intracranial Cavernous Haemangioma Coincident with Steroid Therapy'. J. Neurosurg. 1973, 39: 99–103.

257. Pritchard, P.J. — *Fox and McDonald's Introduction to Fluid Mechanics*. 8th ed. 2011, New Jersey, USA: John Wiley & Sons, Inc.

258. Qian Z, Climent MM, Uson-Garallo J, Lima-Rodrigues MA, Calles C, Robertson H,Castaneda-Zuniga WR. — A Simplified Arteriovenous Malformation Model in Sheep: Feasibility Study. American Journal of Neuroradiology 20: 765- 770, 1999.

259. Quick CM,Young WL, Leonard EF, Joshi S, Gao E, Hashmoto T. — Model of structural and functional adaptation of small conductance vessels to arterial hypotension. Am J Physiol Heart Circ Physiol. 279: H 1645- H 1653, 2000.

260. Quick CM, Leonard EF, Young WL. — Adaptation of ccerebral circulation to brain arteriovenous malformations increases feeding artery pressure and decreases regional hypotension. Neurosurgery 50 : 167- 175, 2002.

261. Raimondi, A. J. — *Paediatric Neuroradiology (Philadelphia, London, and Toronto: W.B. Saunders & Co., 1972).*

262. Ramamurthi, B., & Balasubramanian, V. — 'Arterio-venous Malformations with a Purely External Carotid Contribution'. J. Neurosurg. 1966, 25: 643–647.

263. Raskin, N. — 'Angiomatous Malformations of the Brain'. J. Neuropathol. Exp. Neurol. 1949, 8: 326–337.

264. Ratliff J, MD and Connolly E, MD Department of Neurosurgery; Louisiana State University Medical Center and Ochsner Clinic New Orleans, Louisiana — Department of Neurosurgery; Louisiana State University Medical Center and Ochsner Clinic New Orleans, Louisiana

265. Ray, B. S. — 'Cerebral Arterio-venous Aneurysm'. Surg. Gynaecol. Obstet. 1941, 73: 615–648.

266. Raynor, R. B., & Kingman, Jnr., A. F. — 'Haemangioblastoma and Vascular Malformation as One Lesion'. Arch. Neurol. 1965, 12: 39–48.

267. Reid, M. R. — 'Abnormal Arterio-venous Communications, Acquired and Congenital. III. The Effects of Abnormal Arterio-venous Communications on the Heart, Blood Vessels and Other Structures'. Arch. Surg. (Chicago) 1925, 2: 25–42.

268. Reid, M. R. — 'Studies of Abnormal Arteriovenous Communication, Acquired and Congenital. I. A Report of a Series of Cases'. Arch. Surg. 1925, 10: 601; 11: 25–237.

269. Reid, M. R. — 'Abnormal Arterio-venous Communication, Acquired and Congenital. II. The Origin and Nature of Arterio-venous Aneurysm, Circoid Aneurysm and Single Angioma'. Arch. Surg. 1925, 10: 996.

270. Reid, M. R., & McGuire, J. — 'Arterio-venous Aneurysm'. Ann. Surg. 1938, 108: 643–691;

271. Ribbert, H. — *Virchows Arch. F. of Pathol. Anat. 1898, 151: 381.*

272. Richter, D. 'The Stability of the Nervous System During Development', in (G. E. W. Wolstenhome, M. O'Connor. (Eds.), Ciba Foundation Symposium on Somatic Stability in the Newly Born (Boston: Little Brown & Co., 1961, p. 393; see pp. 296–316).

273. Rienhoff, Jnr, W. F. 'Congenital Arterio-venous Fistula. An Embryological Study with the Report of a Case'. Bull. Johns Hopkins Hosp. 1924, 35: 271–284.

274. Robinson, J. L., & Sedzimir, C. B. 'External Carotid-Transverse Sinus Fistula. Case Report'. J. Neurosurg. 1970, 33: 718–721.

275. Robles, C., & Carrasco-Zanini, J. 'Treatment of Cerebral Arterio-venous Malformations by Muscle Embolization'. J. Neurosurg. 1968, 29: 603–608.

276. Rosenberg, A. W. 'A Vascular Malformation Drained by the Great Vein of Galen. Report of a Case'. Bull. Los Angeles Neurol. Soc. 1955, 20: 196–199.

277. Rossitti, S. and P. Svendsen *Shear stress in cerebral arteries supplying arteriovenous malformations.* Acta Neurochir (Wien), 1995. **137**(3-4): p. 138-45, discussion 145.

278. Roux, W. 'Uber Die Verzweigungen der Blutgefasse des Menschen', Jenaische Zeitscher F. Naturw. 1878, 12: 205–206.

279. Russel, D. 'Discussions on Vascular Tumours of the Brain and Spinal Cord'. Proc. R. Soc. Med. 1931, 24: 383.

280. Russell, D. S. 'Spontaneous Intracerebral Haemorrhage'. Proc. R. Soc. Med. 1954, 47: 689–693.

281. Russell, D. S., & Nevin, S. 'Aneurysm of the Great Vein of Galen Causing Internal Hydrocephalus. Report of Two Cases'. J. Pathol. Bacteriol. 1940, 51: 375–383.

282. Russell, D. S., & Rubinstein, L. J. *Pathology of Tumours of the Nervous System (London: Edward Arnold, 1959, p. 72–92).*

283. Russell, W., & Newton, T. H. 'Aneurysm of the Vein of Galen'. Am. J. Roentgenol. 1964, 92: 756–760.

284. Sabin, F. R. 'Origin and Development of the Primitive Vessels of the Chick and of the Pig'. Cont. Embryol 1917, 6: 61–124. Carnegie Inst. of Washington, Publ. NO. 226.

285. Schaller, B. *Physiology of cerebral venous blood flow: from experimental data in animals to normal function in humans.* Brain Res Brain Res Rev, 2004. **46**(3): p. 243-60.

286. Scharrer, E. 'Arteries and Veins in the Mammalian Brain'. Anat. Rec. 1940, 78: 173–196.

287. Schenk, W. G., Martin, J. W., & Portin, B. A. 'The Regional Hemodynamics of Chronic Experimental Arterio-venous Fistulas'. Surg. Gynaecol. Obstet. 1960, 110: 44–50.

288. Schenk, W. G., Bahn, R. A., Cordell, A. R., & Stephens, J. G. 'The Regional Hemodynamics of Acute Experimental Arterio-venous Fistula'. Surg. Gynaecol. Obstet. 1957, 105: 733.

289. Schlesinger, B. 'Venous Drainage of the Brain with Special Reference to the Galenic System'. Brain 1939, 62: 274–291.

290. Schmid-Schonbein, H, Wells, R & Goldstone, J 'Influence of deformability of human red cells upon blood viscosity', *Circ Res,* vol. 25, no. 2, pp. 131-43, 1969.

291. Schneider, R. C., & Liss, L. 'Cavernous Haemangiomas of the Cerebral Hemisphere'. J. Neurosurg. 1958, 15: 392–399.

292. Schnurer, L. B., & Stattin, S. 'Vascular Supply of Intra-cranial Dura from Internal Carotid Artery with Special Reference to its Angiographic Significance'. Acta. Radiol. (Chicago) 1963, 1: 441–450.

293. Schultz, E. C., & Hvston, W. A. 'Arterio-venous Aneurysm of the Posterior Fossa in an Infant. Report of a Case'. J. Neurosurg. 1956, 13: 211.

294. Schwartz, AE, Sandhu, AA, Kaplon, RJ, Young, WL, Jonassen, AE, Adams, DC, Edwards, NM, Sistino, JJ, Kwiatkowski, P & Michler, RE 'Cerebral blood flow is determined by arterial pressure and not cardiopulmonary bypass flow rate', *Ann Thorac Surg,* vol. 60, no. 1, pp. 165-9; discussion 169-70, 1995.

295. Schwartz, A.E., et al. *Cerebral blood flow is determined by arterial pressure and not cardiopulmonary bypass flow rate.* Ann Thorac Surg, 1995. **60**(1): p. 165-9; discussion 169-70.

296. Seljeskog, E. L., Rogers, H. M., & French, L. A. 'Arterio-venous Malformations of the Inferior Sagittal Sinus in an Infant'. J. Neurosurg. 1968, 29: 623–628.

297. Shakur, SF, Amin-Hanjani, S, Mostafa, H, Charbel, FT & Alaraj, A 'Hemodynamic Characteristics of Cerebral Arteriovenous Malformation Feeder Vessels With and Without Aneurysms', *Stroke,* vol. 46, no. 7, pp. 1997-1999, 2015.

298. Shakur, S.F., et al. *Hemodynamic Characteristics of Cerebral Arteriovenous Malformation Feeder Vessels With and Without Aneurysms.* Stroke, 2015. **46**(7): p. 1997-1999.

299. Shenkin, H. A., Spitz, E. B., Grant, F. C., & Kety, S. S. 'Physiologic Studies of Arterio-venous Anomalies of the Brain'. J. Neurosurg. 1948, 5: 165–172.

300. Shi YQ, Chen XC. A proposed scheme for grading intracranial arteriovenous malformations. J Neurosurgery. 65 (4): 484-9,Oct 1986.

301. Shojima, M., et al. *Magnitude and role of wall shear stress on cerebral aneurysm: computational fluid dynamic study of 20 middle cerebral artery aneurysms.* Stroke, 2004. **35**(11): p. 2500-5.

302. Shumacker, H. B., & Stahl, N. M. 'A Study Upon the Cardiac Frontal Area in Those Patients Found to have Arterio-venous Fistulae'. Surgery 1959, 26: 928.

303. Silverman, B. K., Breck, T., Craig, J., et al. 'Congestive Failure in the Newborn Caused by Cerebral Arterio-venous Fistula'. Am. J. Dis. Child. 1955, 89: 539–543;

304. Simmonds, M. Virchow's Arch. F. Pathol. Anat. 1903, 180: 280.

305. Smith FT, Purvis R, Dennis SCR, Jones MA, Ovenden NC, TADJFAR M. Fluid flow through various branching tubes. Journal of Engineering Mathematics. 47: 277-298, 2003.

306. Sorimachi, T., et al. *Blood Pressure Monitoring in Feeding Arteries of Cerebral Arteriovenous Malformations during Embolization: A Preventive Role in Hemodynamic Complications.* Neurosurgery, 1995. **37**(6): p. 1041-1048. Fluid flow through various branching tubes. Journal of Engineering Mathematics. 47: 277-298, 2003.

307. Spetzler RW, Martin N. A proposed grading system for arteriovenous malformation. J.Neurosurgery; 65:476-483, 1986.

308. Spetzler RW, Hargraves RW, McCormick PW, Zabramski JM, Flom RA, Zimmerman RS. Relationship of perfusion pressure and size to risk of hemorrhage from arteriovenous malformations. J. Neurosurgery 76 : 918-923, 1992.

309. Spetzler, RF & Hamilton, MG 'Pressure autoregulation is intact after arteriovenous malformation resection', *Neurosurgery,* vol. 33, no. 4, pp. 772-4, 1993.

310. Spetzler, R.F. and M.G. Hamilton, *Pressure autoregulation is intact after arteriovenous malformation resection.* Neurosurgery, 1993. **33**(4): p. 772-4.

311. Stattin, S. 'Meningeal Vessels of the Internal Carotid Artery and Their Angiographic Significance'. Acta. Radiol. (Chicago) 1961, 55: 329–336.

312. Steinhein, S. O. 'Ueber Einer Fall Von Vaix Aneurysmatica im Bereich der Gehirugefassie'. Inaug. Din Surzburg. Quoted by Dandy, W. E. (1928).

313. Stephanis CG, Mourmouras DE,Tsagaadopoulas DG. On the elastic properties of arteries . J Biomech Nov; 36(1);1727-31,2003.

314. Streeter, G. L. 'The Developmental Alteration in the Vascular System of the Human Embryo'. Cont. Embryol. 1918, 8: 5–38. Carnegie Inst., Washington, Publ. No. 271.

315. Streeter, G. L. 'The Development of the Venous Sinuses of the Dura Mater in the Human Embryo'. Am. J. Anat. Philadelphia, 1915, 18: 145–178. yes

316. Stock, K.W., et al. *Quantification of blood flow in the middle cerebral artery with phase-contrast MR imaging.* Eur Radiol, 2000. **10**(11): p. 1795-800.

317. Sugar, O. 'Anatomy and Angiography of Vascular Anomalies'. *J. Neurosurg.* 1951, 8: 3.

318. Sutherland, D. A., & Clark, H. 'Haemangioma Associated with Thrombocytopenia'. *Am. J. Med.* 1962, 33: 150–157.

319. Svien, H. J., & McRae, J. A. 'Arterio-venous Anomalies of the Brain. Fate of Patients Not Having Definitive Surgery'. *J. Neurosurg.* 1965, 23: 23–28.

320. Svien, H. J., & Peserico, L. 'Regression in Size of Arterio-venous Anomaly'. *J. Neurosurg.* 1960, 17: 493–496.

321. Takahashi, O. 'External Carotid Contribution to Intracranial Arterio-venous Malformations'. *Radiology* 1970, 95: 587.

322. Takekawa, S. D., & Holman, C. B. 'Roentgenologic Diagnosis of Anomalous Communication Between External Carotid and Intracranial Veins'. *Am. J. Roentgenol.*1965, 95: 822–825.

323. Thoma, R. 'Untersuchungen Uber Die Histogenese Und Die Pathogenese der Angiosklerose'. *Virchows Arch.* 1893, 204: 1.

324. Thoma, R. Textbook of General Pathology and Pathological Anatomy, translated by Bruce (London, 1896).

325. Thomson, J. L. G. 'Aneurysm of the Vein of Galen'. *Brit. J. Radiol.* 1959, 32: 680–684.

326. Tonnis, W., Schiefer, W., & Walter, W. 'Signs and Symptoms of Supratentorial Arterio-venous Aneurysm'. *J. Neurosurg.* 1958, 15: 471–480.

327. Torr, J. B. D. *The Blood Supply of the Human Spinal Cord*, Doctoral Thesis, Victoria University, Manchester, England.

328. Turner, O. A., & Kernohan, J. W. 'Vascular Malformations and Vascular Tumours Including the Spinal Cord'. *Arch. Neurol. Psychiat.* 1941, 46: 444.

329. Urdanibia, F., Silvela, J., & Soto, M. 'Occipital Dural Arterio-venous Malformations'. *Neuroradiology* 1974, 7: 57–64.

330. Van Der Eecken, H. M., & Adams, R. D. 'Anatomy and Functional Significance of Meningeal Arterial Anastomosis of the Human Brain'. *J. Neuropathol. Exp. Neurol.* 1953, 12: 132.

331. Venkatesan, J., et al. *Mathematical Analysis of Casson Fluid Model for Blood Rheology in Stenosed Narrow Arteries.* Journal of Applied Mathematics, 2013. **2013**: p. 11.

332. Verbiest, H. 'Arterio-venous Aneurysm of the Posterior Fossa. Analysis of 6 Cases'. *Acta. Neurochir. (Wien)* 1961, 9: 171–195.

333. Verbiest, H. 'Arterial and Arterio-venous Aneurysm of the Posterior Fossa'. *Psychiat. Neurol. Neurochir.* (Amsterdam) 1962, 65: 329–369.

334. Vidyasagar, C. Persistent embryonic veins in arteriovenous malformations of the brain, *Acta Neurochir. (Wien)* 40 (1978), 103–16.

335. Vidyasagar, C. Persistent embryonic veins in the deep midline arteriovenous malformation of the brain, Abstract 421, International Congress Series No. 418, Amsterdam, Oxford: Excerpta Medica, 1977.

336. Vidyasagar.Casikar, G.S. Ramaswamy, Vyshnavi Vidyasagar. Observations on the flow characteristics of blood flow in Arterio-venous fistula . Journal of cardio vascular engineering. 2010; 10:66-77.

337. Vidyasagar C. Persistent embryonic veins in the arteriovenous malformations of the Diencephalon. Acta Neurochirurgica 47: 63-82, 1979.

338. Vidyasagar C. Persistent embryonic veins in the arteriovenous malformations of the Telencephalon, Acta Neurochirurgica 47: 261-283,1979.

339. Vidyasagar C. Persistent embryonic veins in the arteriovenous malformations of posterior fossa, Acta Neurochirurgica 48: 199-214, 1979.

340. Vidyasagar C. Persistent embryonic veins in the arteriovenous malformations of the dura, Act Neurochirurgica 48: 199-214, 1979.

341. Vignon-Clementel, I.E., et al. *Outflow boundary conditions for three-dimensional finite element modeling of blood flow and pressure in arteries.* Computer Methods in Applied Mechanics and Engineering, 2006. **195**(29–32): p. 3776-3796.

342. Vinken, P. J., & Bruyn, G. W. *Handbook of Clinical Neurology. Part II* (Amsterdam: North Holland Publ. Co.; New York: The American Elsevier Publ. Co., 1972).

343. Virchow, R. 'Die Krankhaften Gescwulste'. A. Hirschwald, Berlin, 1863, Vol. 3, Lect. 25; 460.

344. Vita RP, Dixon SA. Annual review of biomedical engineering. 5: 413-439, 2003.

345. Von Der Max, H. 'Zur Vergleichenden Anatomie der Gehirnund Ruckenmarksvenen der Vertebraten'. Zeitschrift Fur Morphologie Und Anthropologie. Band III. 1901, 239–299.

346. Weir, B. K. A., Atkin, P. B. R., & Miller, J. D. R. 'Excision of Thrombosed Vein of Galen'. *J. Neurosurg*. 1968, 29: 619–622.

347. Wickbom, I. 'Angiographic Examination of Intracranial Arterio-venous Malformations'. *Acta. Radiol.* 1950, 34: 385–398.

348. Willis, R. A. — *The Borderland of Embryology and Pathology* (London: Butterworth & Co., 1958).

349. Wilson, C. B., & Cronic, F. — 'Traumatic Arterio-venous Fistula Involving the Middle Meningeal Vessels'. *JAMA* 1964, 188: 953–957.

350. Wolf, A., & Brock, S. — 'The Pathology of Cerebral Angiomas'. *Bull. Neurol. Inst. NY* 1935, 4: 144–176.

351. Wolfe, H. R. I., & France, N. E. — 'Arterio-venous Aneurysm of the Great Vein of Galen'. *Brit. J. Surg.* 1949, 37: 76–78.

352. Worster-Drought, C., & Ballance, C. A. — 'Venous Angioma of Cerebral Cortex with Report of a Case'. *Lancet* 1922, 2: 125.

353. Wyburn-Mason, R. — 'Arterio-venous Aneurysm of the Midbrain and Retina, Facial Nevi and Mental Changes', *Brain* 1943, 66: 163.

354. Yasargil, M. G. — 'Diagnosis and Treatment of Spinal Cord Arterio-venous Malformations'. *Proc. Neurol. Surg.* 1971, 4: 355–428.

355. Young, W.L., et al., — *Pressure autoregulation is intact after arteriovenous malformation resection.* Neurosurgery, 1993. **32**(4): p. 491-6; discussion 496-7.

356. Zingesser, L. H., Schechter, H. M., Kier, E. L.,& O'Brien, M. S. — 'Vascular Malformations of the Posterior Fossa, including the Tentorial Hiatus'. *Am. J. Roentgenol.* 1969, 105: 341–397.

357. Zulch, K. J. — *Brain Tumours: Their Biology and Pathology*. (New York: Springer, 1957, pp. 231–234).

358. 'Zur Vergleichenden Anatomie der Gehirnund Ruckenmarksvenen der Vertebraten'. — Zeitschrift Fur Morphologie Und Anthropologie. Band III. 1901, 239–299.

www.ingramcontent.com/pod-product-compliance
Lightning Source LLC
LaVergne TN
LVHW070950210926
848482LV00002B/164
* 9 7 9 8 9 0 0 9 4 0 0 3 8 *